www.whitbread.org/book
The 1997-98 Whitbread Round The World Race for the Volvo Trophy
produced by quokka sports

www.whitbread.org/book was extracted from the digital assets generated by the 1997-98 Whitbread Round The World Race for the Volvo Trophy, as presented on www.whitbread.org.

Each leg is divided into two-page graphic spreads that correspond with the days the boats were at sea. The spreads can be overlaid, using the numerical gridlines on each page, to form a complete map of The Whitbread.

We have retained the original formatting and spelling of the racers' emails in this book.

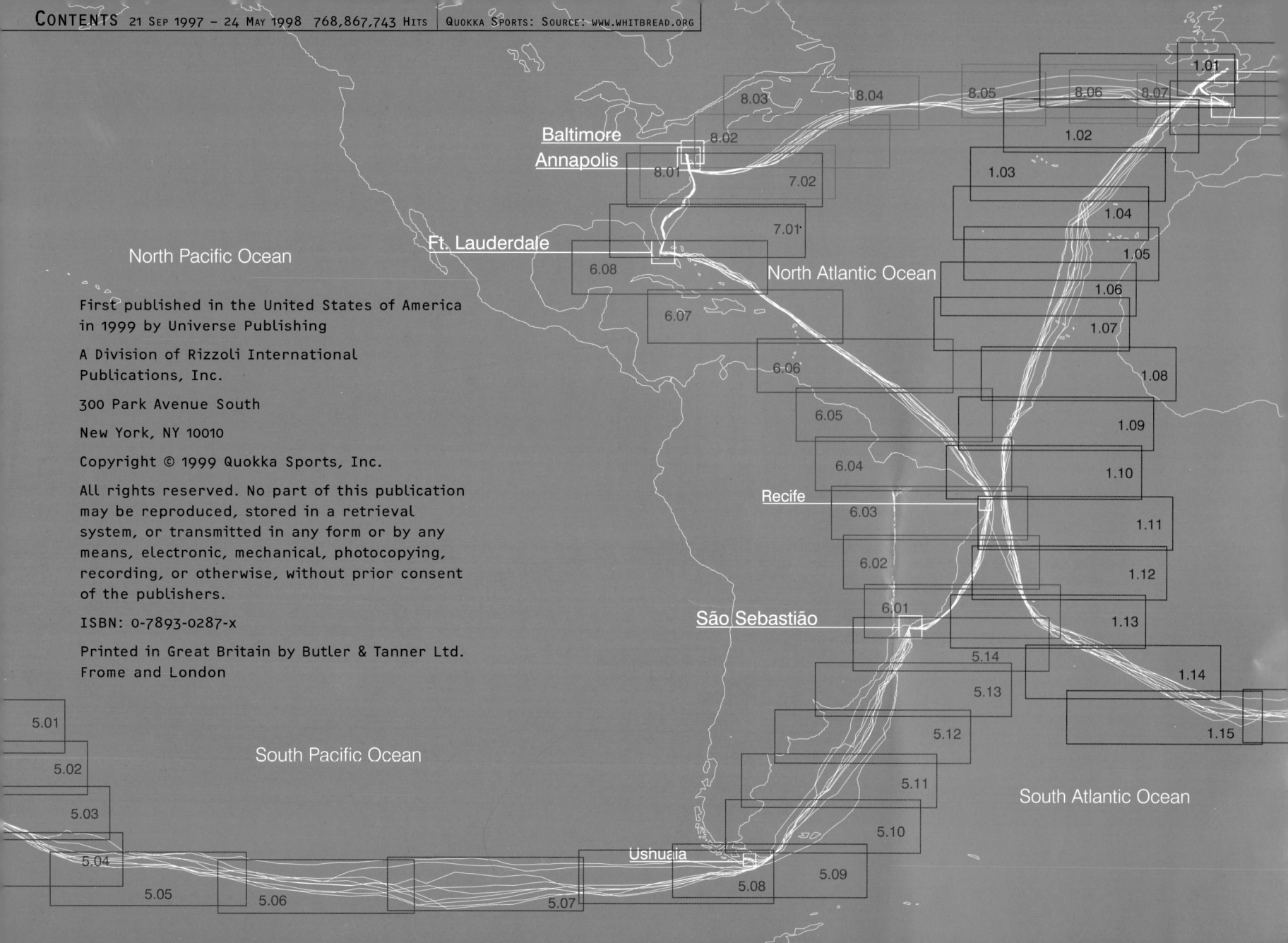

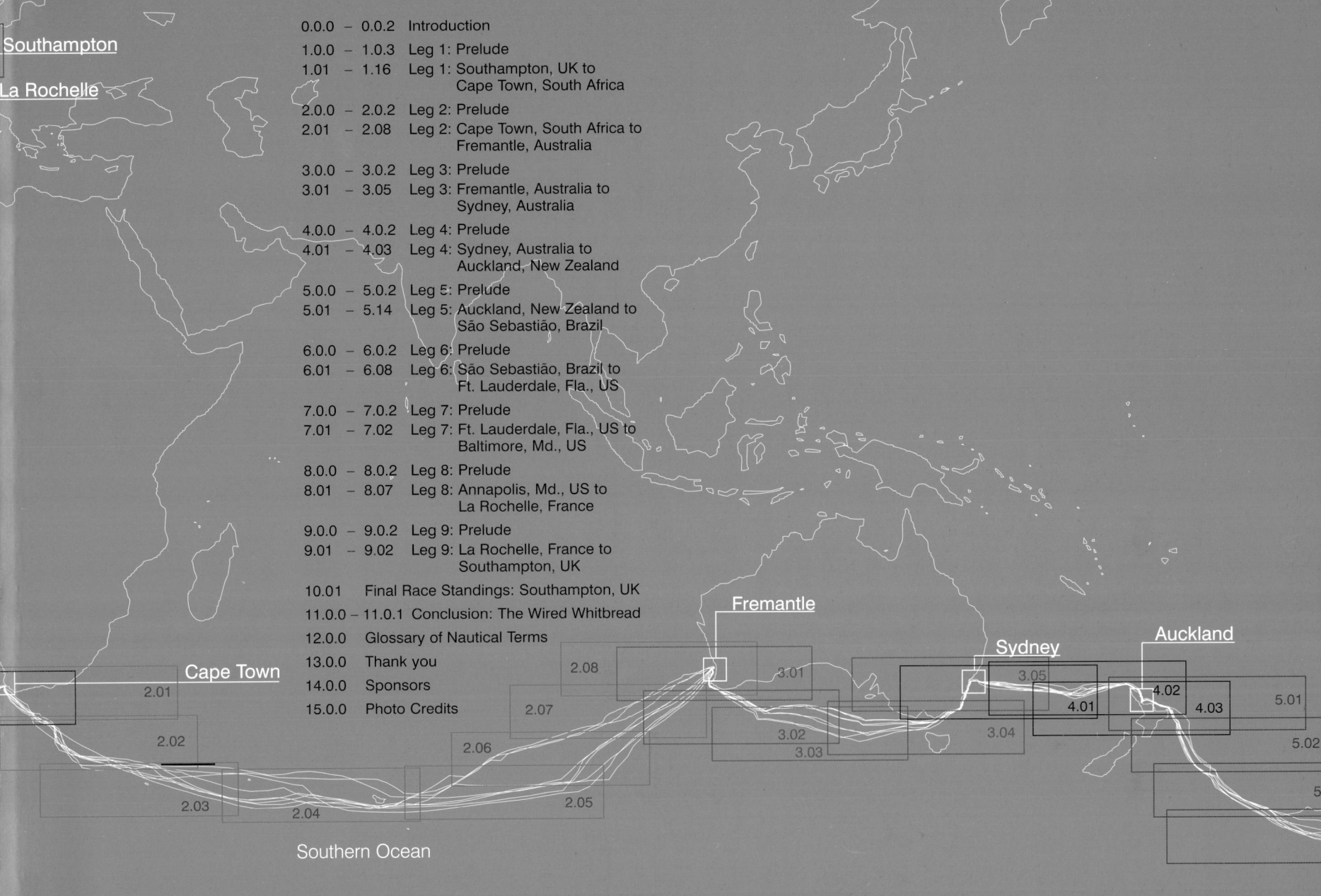

0.0.0 21 Sep 1997 – 24 May 1998   768,867,743 Hits | Quokka Sports: Source: www.whitbread.org

Distance:

Introduction

The 1997-98 Whitbread
Round The World Race for the Volvo Trophy | 31,600 nautical miles

> "It's blowing hard. With black snow squalls coming in from behind. And the yacht is on the verge of being out of control. The spray coming over the windward deck is turning to ice particles. The decks are covered in ice. The coils of ropes in the bottoms of the cockpits are full of snow. And it's so bitterly cold."
>
> Sir Peter Blake, Ocean Conquest

Sit long enough in any yacht club lounge or dockside bar, and eventually the conversation will drift to 'The Whitbread.' For the seasoned sailor, no further explanation is needed. It will take longer for the uninitiated to grasp that The Whitbread is one of the world's most challenging competitions: a nine-month circumnavigation through the toughest conditions Poseidon can dish out.

Saying that a sailor who just strolled through the door is someone who sailed the last Whitbread elevates that person into the company of those few hearty men and women who have scaled Mt. Everest. Both accomplishments extend the rights of membership to a small and exclusive club. No other sporting events today expose the competitors to such extremes as The Whitbread or Mt. Everest. In a time when 'extreme sports' are being embraced by thousands, these two events define the authentic edge of sport.

To understand why this is so, imagine what it is like for the teams of 12 crewmembers who sail in this remarkable race. The Whitbread demands all the teamwork and intensity of an America's Cup competition, but requires it be maintained 24 hours a day, for weeks on end. The Whitbread is not staged within the comfortable confines of a buoyed bay course, either, but runs crews through the most dangerous and feared oceans on Earth, thousands of miles from support staff or rescue.

And, unlike those well-organised around-the-cans races, a day of competition in The Whitbread is never called off due to bad weather. Whitbread crews sail as fast as they can, whether they are struggling through the fickle Doldrums or surfing at over 20 knots down the face of 40-foot waves in full-gale conditions. No Everest climber who ever dangled from an ice cliff in a storm has risked more than a Whitbread sailor who makes the two Southern Ocean crossings this race demands. The racers face days on end of bone-chilling cold, working and sleeping in wet clothing, fighting gale-force winds, and watching, always watching, for the iceberg that could doom boat and crew to an icy grave. Still, despite conditions, they rarely ease up on the accelerator. No matter how miserable or dangerous the conditions, or how battered the boat, Whitbread crews understand that the only hope of winning this race is to push harder than the others.

In this book, we recount the tale of one of these epic races, the 1997-98 Whitbread Round The World Race for the Volvo Trophy. It was the last race to bear the name of the venerable British company that first stepped forward in the spirit of adventuring to sponsor the race: Whitbread PLC. In the years 2001-2002, the Swedish auto maker, Volvo, will sponsor the entire race for the first time, changing the name to The Volvo Ocean Race. That's the future. Let's take a moment to recall how The Whitbread began.

A Short History

As the 1970s dawned, the notion of 'adventuring' was viewed as a quaint throwback to an earlier time. Nevertheless, many open-ocean sailors still felt an itch for one last great race. Whenever sailors gathered to down a few pints the conversation would often turn to the same subject: an around-the-world yacht race. If only someone could organise it, what an adventure it would be — boat and crew on a drag-race circumnavigation of the globe. Beginning from England, it would take boats around the Cape of Good Hope at the tip of Africa, through the icebergs and raging weather of the Southern Ocean, around South America's Cape

Horn and back to England. It would be a race that pushed sailors and boats to the brink, exposing them to every conceivable condition.

Around-the-world racing has its origins with the great clipper ships of the mid-19th century. These ships, built to cross oceans with speed, would compete to be the first into port and thus secure the best price for their cargoes. Some of the records they set for fast, long-distance sailing still stand today.

The first suggestions for a round-the-world yacht race came in 1924 following Conor O'Brien's successful circumnavigation, south of the Cape of Good Hope and Cape Horn, in Saoirse. Nothing came of the idea, although it was rekindled in 1967 when Sir Francis Chichester set a record for a single-stop circumnavigation of 226 days.

Who would finance such a race? Besides its inherent dangers, such an event would require a massive worldwide support network. Ports of call would have to be established, and rules and boat specifications would have to be established. Individual sponsors would have to be convinced to finance each team in a race that would be expensive and dangerous. On top of those difficulties, many in the sailing establishment believed that to try such a race was folly. At that time, fewer than ten private yachts had rounded Cape Horn — in one piece. In fact, critics were quick to note, just such a race already had been tried once, and had ended badly. In 1967, "The Sunday Times" of London had put up money to sponsor what it called the Golden Globe Race. Eight boats entered, but only one finished: Suhaili, navigated by Robin Knox-Johnston. The others gave up after near-catastrophic equipment failures, capsized or sank. One crewman became so despondent he committed suicide. These were not the sorts of events sponsors were eager to have associated with their names.

For a company to step forward to underwrite this new race, it would have to have a name and reputation so well respected it alone would reassure the most nervous of doubters.

In 1972, Whitbread & Company Ltd. (as it was called) stepped up to that challenge. The agreement was sealed with a handshake between Colonel Bill Whitbread and Rear Admiral Otto Steiner of the Royal Naval Sailing Association. It was a perfect fit for both sponsor and race. Whitbread's name stretched back to its founding in 1742, when Britain truly ruled the waves.

By September 1973, the first Whitbread Round The World Race was ready to begin. The course was established. The race would cover four legs totalling 27,000 miles, beginning and ending in Portsmouth, UK.

Six Whitbreads, Six Legends

On 8 September 1973, 17 boats hoisted their sails and raced out of Portsmouth harbour into the Solent to begin the first Whitbread Round The World Race. With the firing of a gun, this most dangerous and exciting of sailboat races was under way.

Those who warned that this race was too dangerous had plenty of reason to say "We told you so" before the first race was even half over. On Leg 2, just twelve days out of Cape Town, winds topping 50 knots lashed the fleet. The Italian yacht Tauranga, a Swan 55, sailing fast with her twin headsails boomed out, suffered a serious broach. A spar snapped off and began furiously beating at the hull. Crewman Paul Waterhouse climbed on deck and rushed forward to secure the boom before it pounded a hole in the deck or hull. He was tossed overboard by a sheet that was pulled taut when a sail abruptly filled with wind. His crewmates searched for hours, but it was no use. Waterhouse was lost.

Six days later, disaster struck again. The crew of a 60-foot French ketch, 33 Export, was changing sails in a full gale. Without warning, the boat was swept by a wave. Crewman Dominique Guillet's harness separated and he was washed overboard. A marker buoy was thrown into the water to mark his approximate position, but it was too late. The gale had built to the point where the boat was forced to run off downwind, so the crew was unable to conduct a search for their lost colleague. It was unavoidable, yet it was agonising for the crew.

If Leg 2 had proven deadly, Leg 3 proved no less so. Aboard the British entry Great Britain II, disaster struck. In the blink of an eye, crewman Bernie Hosking was washed overboard in a storm. Though his crewmates searched the area for hours, he was the third and final fatality of the race.

Nine months after it began, 14 of the 17 boats that started the race finished. The crews and their boats were the worse for wear, but sailed proudly back up the Solent to the finish line. As it has been through the ages, death at sea, though regrettable, was a risk all sailors understood and accepted when they signed on. The race's sponsor, Whitbread & Co., stood unshaken. It immediately announced that the race organisers were accepting applications for entry in the next race — 1977-78.

Back for More

The three fatalities during the first race focussed race organisers' minds on the issue of safety. The second Whitbread saw the first imposition of rules on boat size. In an effort to inject minimum boat standards into this event, the race committee mandated that no boat of less than 15.2 metres could enter. It would be the first of a series of boat rules that would eventually lead to the creation of a boat built solely for this race.

The 1977-78 Whitbread proved no less gruelling than the first. Though no one was lost at sea, injuries abounded. For example, aboard Great Britain II, an errant spinnaker guy whipped up off the deck as the sail filled, catching Nick Dunlop around the waist. With the pulling force of a team of horses, the full spinnaker began to squeeze the life out of Dunlop. By the time the line was cut all the blood vessels in his eyes had burst and he couldn't be moved without screaming in pain. Outside of injuries to crew, there were plenty of broaches and knockdowns.

However, at the end of the second race, all 15 boats that started the race finished. The high success rate of the second Whitbread encouraged a record 29 entries for the third running of the race in 1981-82. If the newcomers had any illusions this was an easy race, they disappeared on Leg 1. Of the 29 boats that left Southampton, UK, 21 arrived in Cape Town damaged. As if bad weather and high seas were not enough, the last boat to finish was Vivanapoli, arriving eight days behind the others. The boat had been stopped by an Angolan gunboat and boarded. When the Angolans discovered South Africans among the crew, they hauled the bunch in as spies. It was a week before the Italian embassy could arrange their release.

The competitors would learn during this race that they were not only sailing around the physical world, but the political world as well. The Vivanapoli incident would not be the only political hurdle the fleet would clear this time around. As the fleet rounded the Horn at the tip of South America and raced up the coast, they had no idea that they were sailing in troubled waters. Even as the boats worked their way past the Falkland Islands they couldn't know that Argentine and British naval ships were nervously manoeuvering in the area. The racers were sailing through waters that in just weeks would become an air and sea battle over the Falkland Islands. Only when the racers finished back in England did they learn that just days after they had departed on the last leg, Argentina had launched its invasion of the British-controlled Falklands.

Twenty of the 29 boats that started the 1981-82 race finished. It had been a rough trip around, and the beating taken by the Whitbread fleet, coupled with a worldwide recession, contributed to a smaller, 15-boat field for the fourth Whitbread in 1985-86. It proved to be another successful race, with all entrants finishing.

The Race Gets Tougher

The 1989-90 event marked a major change, as the race committee redrew the round-the-world course. The result was an addition of two legs, adding 5,000 miles to the overall length. The change bumped the race course from an already long 27,000 nautical miles to nearly 32,000 miles. Political rather than competitive considerations played a big role in this change. At the time, pressure had built in international sporting communities to boycott South Africa due to that country's apartheid policies. Dropping Cape Town from the ports-of-call list created major routing headaches for race organisers. A leg that stretched from Southampton all the way around the Cape of Good Hope to Australia was considered far too long and dangerous. So, to patch the hole left by the exclusion of Cape Town, Punta del Este, Uruguay, was added — twice. The boats would race to Punta del Este from Southampton; then from Punta del Este to Fremantle, Australia; from Fremantle to Auckland, New Zealand; from Auckland back to Punta del Este, then return to Southampton.

The fifth Whitbread also saw the first all-woman crew, skippered by Tracy Edwards, aboard the sloop Maiden. In all, 23 boats were at the starting line. Again, the second leg was rough on the fleet. Whitbread veterans said it was the roughest they had ever seen. A half-dozen boats saw crew-members washed overboard in gale conditions. Fortunately, most were tethered and were recovered unharmed. On the third leg, a crewman aboard the yacht Creighton's Naturally was not so lucky. Tony Phillips was washed into the raging seas and it took his fellow crewmen an hour to find and recover him. All efforts to revive Phillips failed. It was a reminder for everyone that this race was not for the faint of heart.

As if to keep the sailors on notice, after rounding Cape Horn on the fourth leg, a Finnish entry, Martela OF, lost her keel and capsized. The crew was rescued.

Sir Peter Blake made Whitbread history by winning all six legs of the race. However, some of the limelight was stolen by Tracy Edwards and her all-woman crew, who took second in their class. They proved that, as physically demanding as The Whitbread was, women could compete head to head with the men.

Not Blind to Safety

Race organisers remained anxious to find ways to mitigate the race's inherent danger where they could, without gutting the event of the very elements that distinguished it from tamer competitions. By the end of the fourth race it was becoming clear that allowing various kinds of boat designs, as had been the custom, made it hard to score the race. It also made it difficult to ensure uniform boat safety throughout the fleet. It was decided to come up with a design for a unique Whitbread boat.

Immediately the argument centred on whether to adopt a one-design rule, in which every boat in the race must be identical, or a development class, which allowed some variation and innovation between boats. Those who argued for the adoption of a one-design rule claimed it would keep the race affordable. It would mean no one team could develop an advantageous design using exotic and expensive materials. Those who wanted a development class argued that a one-design rule would stifle innovation and freeze boat technology developments. That, in a very few years, would make Whitbread boats non-competitive and the race boring.

When the dust cleared, both sides got a bit of what they wanted. Over the next few years a group of boat designers, sailors and race organisers developed a rule for a new class of boat, the Whitbread 60 — a development class. The group established basic parameters for overall boat design, while allowing for latitude in hull and keel designs. This would keep the 60-footers fairly similar, yet competitive within the confines of the new rule.

The W60 Makes Its First Appearance

The 1993-94 Whitbread was marked by the appearance of the new W60-class boats. These thoroughbreds of the sea had to prove themselves against Maxi yachts, which also competed in this race. In all, 15 boats raced; a handful of them skippered by the best in the business: Dennis Conner, Chris Dickson, Lawrie Smith and Ross Field. This race also saw the second all-woman team, this time headed by Dawn Riley.

Unfortunately, Lawrie Smith was forced to retire from the race when his Maxi, Fortuna, lost her mast just 25 hours into the first leg. In Punta del Este, Uruguay, Smith took over the new W60, Intrum Justitia, before the start of Leg 2, replacing her injured skipper, Roger Nilson.

On the second leg, skippers reported sighting plenty of icebergs as the fleet sailed deeper into the Southern Ocean. Nevertheless, hard-pushing Lawrie Smith headed farther south than any other boat, risking it all. Ignoring the iceberg threat, he logged a blistering 425 miles in a single day.

There was also plenty of tension between the new kids on the block — the W60s — and the older Maxi boats. Halfway through the race, Smith lashed out at Grant Dalton at a press conference. "They're supposed to be faster, but they're not," said a peeved Smith, who had been leading until Dalton edged him out just before crossing the line. "All Dalton is doing is getting in the way," complained Smith. "He was covering my wind all the way in."

At the end of the race the W60s had proven themselves. While the Maxis had performed better in light airs, the W60s seemed to thrive in the heavy weather that so often marked the two Southern Ocean crossings. These new boats proved they could take anything the Roaring Forties could hand out, and were even friendly with the Furious Fifties.

The 1997-98 Whitbread

The seventh Whitbread Round The World Race would mark a coming of age for the event. First, the number of stopover ports increased to nine with the additions of Sydney, Australia; São Sebastião in Brazil; Baltimore/Annapolis, Md., in the United States; and La Rochelle, France. The additional ports, sponsors and organisers hoped, would increase both public awareness of the event and media coverage.

While there had been television coverage of the last two races, fans, more often than not, continued to get their news days or even weeks late. This time, the race would employ the latest in satellite and Internet technology to bring the competition home to fans, quite literally.

Using satellite uplinks from each boat, GPS position reports, email, audio reports and video could be sent directly from the boats to the fans via the official Internet Web site. For the first time in the race's history, enthusiasts would be able to follow their favorite teams almost in real time, using their home or work computer. Quokka Sports, a small startup company with a big idea, pulled together the elements needed to make this happen. It not only revolutionised this race, but would change forever the way fans follow sporting events.

More on that later. For now, on to the 1997-98 Whitbread.

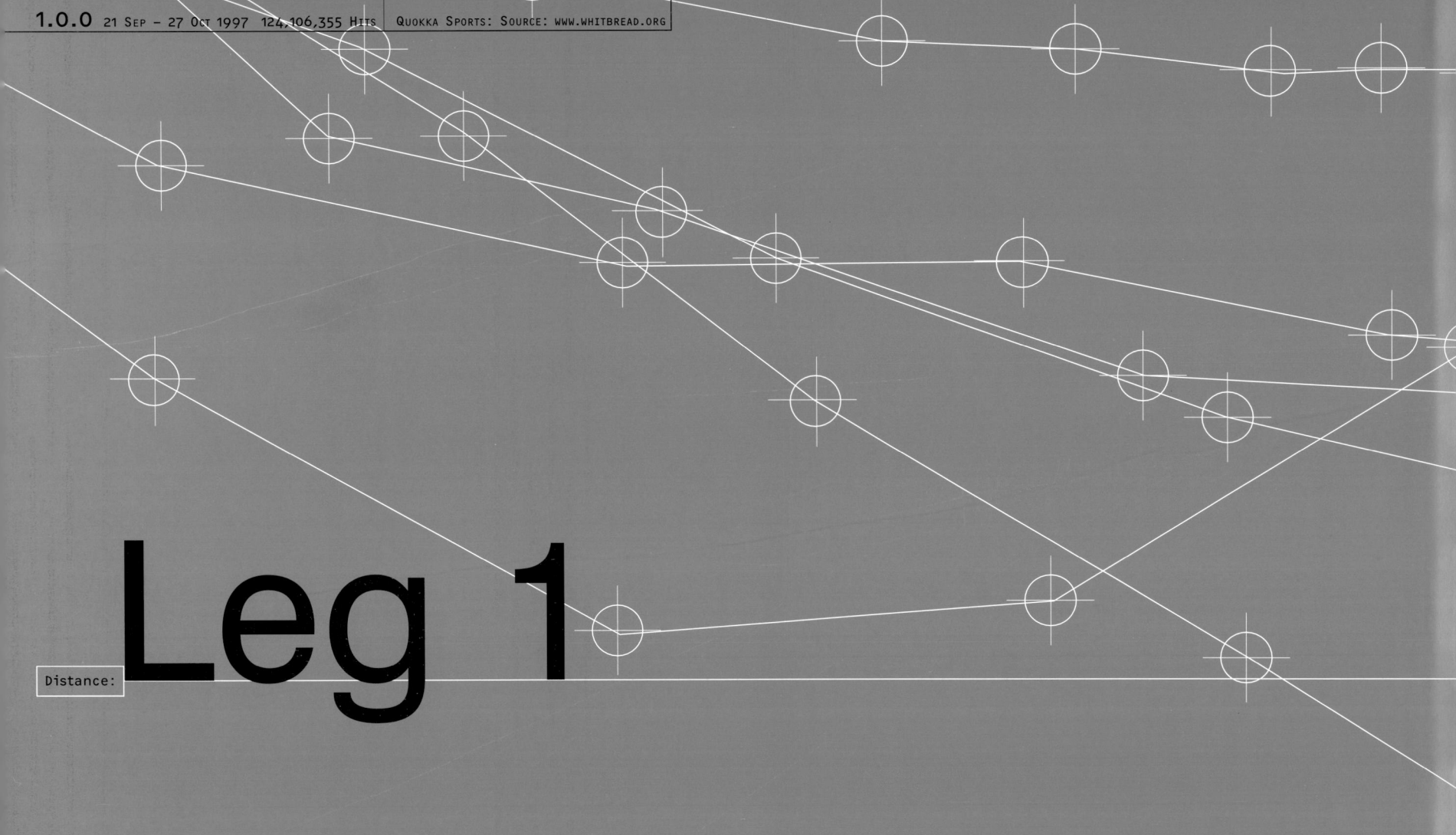

1.0.0 21 Sep – 27 Oct 1997 124,106,355 Hits Quokka Sports: Source: www.whitbread.org

Leg 1

Distance:

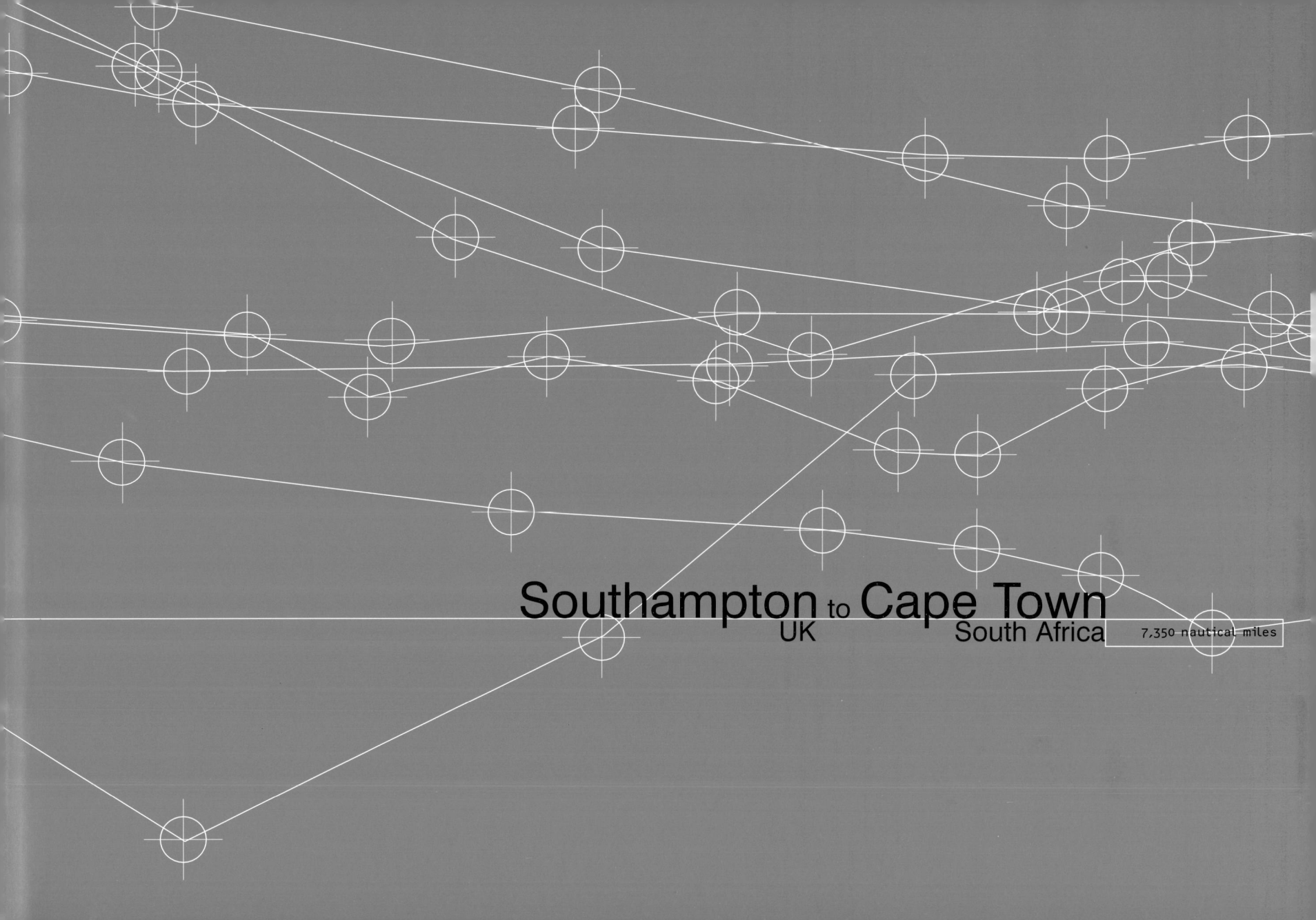

Leg 1: Prelude

"It's things like this that continuously make me realize and respect the abilities and courage of the 11 guys that surround me on this crew. Each person may have his own area of specialization but they all share a common drive to give 110% all the time. This is a good feeling to have about your crewmates, especially when you are the farthest from land anyone could ever be on Earth ... as we are right now."

Josh Belsky, EF Language

Getting to the start is one of the most difficult parts of a Whitbread race. While 42 syndicates registered to compete, only 10 actually made it to the start line.

Early on, certain teams began to capture the spotlight, with odds-makers calculating their chances. Toshiba seized the most attention thanks to the two men who were to act as co-skippers. Both were infamous to sailing fans: the irascible America's Cup legend, Dennis Conner, and the hot-tempered Whitbread vet, Chris Dickson. While everyone acknowledged that both Conner and Dickson were extraordinary sailors, they also shook their heads at the notion that these two enormous egos could cooperate amicably for the duration of the race. Critics of the arrangement were quick to recall that it was just four years prior that the same two men were exchanging vicious barbs during the last Whitbread. However, there was also no question that the Toshiba team was well financed, and had assembled a formidable crew who would have a new, state-of-the-art W60 under them.

EF Language was the other team to attract pre-race attention. The yacht was to have been skippered by British Whitbread veteran Lawrie Smith. Signing on early with the Swedish EF team, Smith had participated heavily in both boat design and crew selection decisions. Late in the game, Smith suddenly resigned, accepting an offer by cigarette brand Silk Cut to run his own British campaign — something he had always wanted to do. With just a few months to go before the start, Team EF began a frantic search for a skipper who could fill Smith's seaboots.

As fate would have it, the timing of Smith's departure could not have been better for an America's Cup skipper, Paul Cayard. From his San Francisco offices, Cayard had been struggling to round up major sponsors for his AmericaOne America's Cup challenge. Competition from other American hopefuls, principally Dennis Conner and Dawn Riley, was making it tough for Cayard to sign a key corporate sponsor. Most professional sailors will tell you that racing is easy compared to the competition for sponsorship money. Around the time Smith jumped ship from EF, one of Cayard's major sponsors withdrew from his campaign.

The loss of a deep-pocket sponsor was a body blow to Cayard's America's Cup hopes. However, just when things were looking their bleakest, Team EF asked if he would consider taking over the EF Language yacht in the upcoming Whitbread. The offer was a risk for EF, since Cayard was best known for his skill racing around buoys, not in the open ocean. When he accepted, many wondered if both he and EF were making a terrible mistake. Was EF thinking clearly, or just picking up Cayard on the rebound after being jilted by Smith? Meanwhile, the danger for Cayard was obvious; if he was having trouble convincing corporations to finance his America's Cup campaign now, imagine how hard it would be if he performed poorly in The Whitbread.

These were gambles both the EF syndicate and Cayard were willing to take. EF needed a big-name skipper, and Cayard needed a dramatic way to prove that he represented the new face of professional United States sailing.

In England, Lawrie Smith quickly took charge of the Silk Cut entry. Together with Toshiba, Silk Cut was among the top three teams odds-makers were putting their money on. The other frontrunner was Merit Cup, skippered by another old Whitbread hand, Grant Dalton.

The other entries attracted less media attention since they did not have 'rock star' skippers at their helms. Regardless, this would clearly be a strong field. Gunnar 'Gurra' Krantz would skipper the other Swedish entry, Swedish Match, a team that would surprise the 'favourites' on nearly every leg of the race. A youthful Knut Frostad would head the Norwegian team, Innovation Kvaerner. The Dutch yacht, BrunelSunergy, was led by a Whitbread novice, Hans Bouscholte.

Two American entries would also be at the starting line. America's Challenge was the darkest of dark horses. The team was being almost entirely financed by Dr. Neil Barth, a southern California oncologist. While Barth was looking for sponsors, he was paying all the team's bills out of his own bank account, including the cost of his new Alan Andrews-designed W60. As the start approached, Barth had found no major sponsors, yet one thing was on his side. Ross Field, who had won the W60 class in the last Whitbread aboard Yamaha, had signed on as the team's skipper.

The second American team was the Baltimore, Md.-based Chessie Racing. Like America's Challenge, its founder, George Collins, was financing this team. Collins had just retired after a spectacular stint as head of the Wall Street securities firm, T. Rowe Price. Under Collins' stewardship the company had blossomed; Collins, then 56, decided to step out at both the top of the market and the top of his career. With savings and investments approaching the triple-digit millions, Collins was well able to indulge his long-standing passion for sailing with the formation of the Chessie Racing team.

One great difference separated America's Challenge from Chessie Racing: money. With the average cost of fielding a team around US$10 million, Collins had more than enough to finance the entire challenge. Barth only had enough to get his team to the starting line, and he needed to find a major sponsor soon.

Finally, there was EF Education, sister entry to EF Language — literally. EF Education would field an all-woman team, the third such team to sail in a Whitbread. As had been the case in earlier races, fans lined up on both sides of the argument over whether an all-woman team could be competitive in this brutal race. The EF Education team would change more than a few minds — and hearts — before this race was over.

Last-Minute Changes

Through the spring and summer months, 10 teams trained furiously. As they sailed together, the inevitable winnowing process began. The biggest surprise came in August when EF Language performed poorly in the Fastnet race. When Cayard replaced Lawrie Smith, he inherited few crewmembers, as Smith had taken most of his recruits with him. Slowly, he built a solid crew from his America's Cup contacts, as well as Whitbread veterans.

Nick White had remained in the key post of navigator; he had won instant fame in the previous Whitbread when his weather and navigation decisions were credited with pulling Yamaha through the Doldrums first and onto the podium.

Cayard and White's personalities were so different a clash was inevitable. Cayard was a hard driver who wanted clear-cut decisions and wanted them fast, while White was more of a meteorological advisor than a decision maker. When EF Language finished a disappointing sixth in the Fastnet that summer, the relationship between the two men unraveled within days. White resigned. Before the ink was dry on his resignation, Cayard announced that this critical post would be filled by his long-time friend and sailing companion, Mark Rudiger. Rudiger had never sailed in a Whitbread race, but had performed brilliantly during California to Hawaii TransPac races. More importantly, Cayard and Rudiger worked as a single unit. They understood and complemented one another perfectly.

Rather than silencing his critics, Cayard's last-minute actions only fuelled doubts. "The EF shuffle is bad news for a team," wrote sailing commentator Andrew Preece. "Whether or not the new incumbent will do a better job, it shows that Cayard may be getting twitchy as the start of the race approaches."

Leg 1: Southampton, UK, to Cape Town, South Africa

"This is my first real taste of The Whitbread and it is a cross between really scary and really fun."
— EF Language skipper, Paul Cayard

Flags snapped in the breeze; the atmosphere was one of anticipation. Crowds lined the docks looking down on the fleet tied to pontoons. The W60s looked impossibly small to negotiate 32,000 miles of the world's toughest waters.

Multicoloured figures in electric yellow, lime green, purple and red wove in and out among the spectators, carrying kit bags and wet-weather gear, loved ones trailed behind trying to catch last-minute instructions and conversations. Then there was no more time. Leaving the docks, the crews had only their hopes, fears and dreams to sustain them.

As the W60s danced their way through the enormous spectator fleet to the starting box, the Red Arrows, the Royal Air Force's aerobatic jet team, paid tribute to the fleet with an awe-inspiring display of speed, agility and raw power.

At 1 p.m., HRH The Duke of York fired the starting cannon, and there was no turning back. An 18-knot breeze sent the fleet on their way with a perfect spinnaker start. Thousands of spectator boats clogged the Solent with a forest of masts. Seas became confused as the W60 fleet headed into the spectator craft, causing the first incident of the race: a scrape between Toshiba and a press boat. No one was injured, and Toshiba carried on.

With the breeze blowing down the Solent, the fleet had an easy run nearly all the way to the English Channel — easy for everyone but Innovation Kvaerner. Bad luck struck early for the Norwegian yacht when her genniker exploded and the crew had to scramble to pull its dragging remnants aboard. EF Language pulled into an early lead, leaving the more favoured boats astern. In what

If Cayard was getting 'twitchy,' he wasn't alone. As 21 September approached, skippers and their crews were all tight as drums. There was no longer time for small talk or joking around. A stroll down the docks at Hamble village was all even the casual observer needed to know something extraordinary was about to happen.

As the days to the start counted down to the single digits, crews could be seen unpacking their boats, weighing food packets, and deciding, literally one ounce at a time, which ones to take and which ones to leave on the dock. It was a dangerous game, because no one could be sure how many days lay between Southampton, UK, and Cape Town, South Africa. The Whitbread Race Office (WRO) was estimating a 31-day passage. Many crews believed their sailing skill and hot new W60s could beat that time by at least two days. That opened them to additional risk: If too many provisions were left behind and the Doldrums proved unusually stubborn, a team could face starvation rations before they reached Cape Town. Several teams decided a few pounds less aboard was worth the risk.

There's never enough time to get ready for such a race. As the clock ticked off the final moments, it was too late to make any further team, sail or provisioning changes.

It was time to race.

must have seemed sweet irony to the EF crew, their former skipper Lawrie Smith, now at the helm of Silk Cut, was bringing up the rear of the fleet.

On EF Language's heels were Toshiba and Merit Cup. As the boats approached the Needles, the point where the boats enter the English Channel, they would have to turn into the wind. Soon jibs would have to replace spinnakers. Toshiba took a chance and made the switch early. This allowed Chris Dickson to steer a course that would put him in a much better position to head upwind than EF Language.

Cayard saw Dickson's move, but resisted the temptation to follow suit. Instead, he held off until his spinnaker was going slack before dropping it and hoisting a jib. This longer downwind run paid off. Toshiba simply could not make up the ground she had lost to Cayard, so EF Language led down the Channel to the open sea. The significance of the moment would only show itself with time.

The first 11 hours of racing produced spectacular speeds, with the fleet managing to record around 200 miles, sailing at an average of 16 knots. However, frustration quickly set in as the fleet approached the northwest corner of France, as winds dropped and the fog invaded. Arend van Bergeijk on BrunelSunergy reported, "'Exhilarating fast sailing,' it said on the brochure. Well, for the last day and night The Whitbread has not lived up to its expectations on that front. However, right from the start it has been close sailing, with large penalties on small errors throughout the fleet."

The fleet struggled for speed in the light conditions. Then, sweeping far to the west and all alone, Innovation Kvaerner suddenly took the lead. Skipper Knut Frostad and his experienced navigator, Marcel van Triest, made a calculated guess that they could find more wind to the west. That guess proved right as they pulled three miles ahead of the other yachts.

After 48 hours of slow sailing, the three boats behind Innovation Kvaerner — EF Language, Merit Cup and Silk Cut — were duelling it out on a track farther east, remaining nearly stalled. Toshiba, which had been trailing badly, began to catch up to the pack. As all the lead boats save Innovation Kvaerner remained stalled, the boats in the rear of the fleet were able to close the gap, gaining between three and 13 miles on the rest. Even so, the all-woman yacht, EF Education, trailed 70 miles behind the lead boat.

The wind remained light and puffy and from all directions, until a northeasterly sea breeze filled in on the coast the afternoon of the third day. This meant the boats offshore were out of luck. The new leaders all came from the south, closer to shore. At midday, Swedish Match was two miles north of Innovation Kvaerner. Seven hours later, with Innovation Kvaerner well clear of Ushant, France, and heading for Cape Finisterre, Spain, the gap extended to 21 miles.

Of the inshore boats, Merit Cup and EF Language led the group around Ushant. They were followed by Silk Cut, Chessie Racing, Innovation Kvaerner, Toshiba and America's Challenge. As they streamed south along rhumb line courses toward Cape Finisterre, the fleet escaped the land effect and got into a southeasterly gradient wind. As they headed south, the winds pulled around behind them to the left.

After a few hours of modest winds, the leaders were the first to nose into what would prove to be another stubborn area of light winds. By midday of the fourth day, Innovation Kvaerner (back in the lead), Toshiba and Merit Cup saw their speeds drop to a gut-wrenching two to three knots. The boats behind them were still sailing in fair winds and logging speeds averaging around eight knots as they closed the gap. However, soon all the boats in the Bay of Biscay were contending with light winds, and navigators throughout the fleet began re-working their weather computer analyses, looking for a way out. The first hard and risky course decisions were now at hand, as teams began deciding whether to head east or west in search of stronger winds.

Aboard Toshiba, navigator Andrew Cape and skipper Chris Dickson could not seem to make up their minds on a course. Toshiba crossed from west of the leaders to east of them, then back to the west over the next 20 hours. The indecision cost them dearly as they trailed the new leading pair, Merit Cup and EF Language, by 20 miles.

Swedish Match headed east, only to find herself languishing in eighth position as the boat found only fluky winds. Toshiba finally decided to head farther to the east, moving closer to shore than any boat in the fleet. Aboard the boat, the mood was downbeat. It was eight days into the leg and Dickson, an early favourite, was barely holding onto sixth.

"Obviously we didn't expect to be sixth," wrote Dickson. "And I'm sure Swedish Match didn't expect to be eighth."

Meanwhile Innovation Kvaerner, EF Language and Merit Cup were racing together at the head of the fleet, trading places regularly. After nine days of sailing, the fleet was scattered across 200 miles of ocean, running in light northerly winds, and sailing nearly parallel to the coast of Morocco. Behind them Silk Cut and Chessie Racing were having their own private match race over fourth and fifth position. Toshiba was paying a high price for her radical inshore strategy and had lost another 80 miles. She was now 100 miles behind the leader.

As the boats sailed just north of the Tropic of Cancer, heading south toward the Cape Verde islands, Innovation Kvaerner stubbornly held to the lead. Fifteen miles behind her in second was Merit Cup; EF Language was 10 miles farther back in third. As the boats dived south, temperatures were on the rise and wind conditions continued to be fluky. Squalls swept the fleet, turning winds in strange and unpredictable directions. "Another frustrating day," reported Grant Dalton on 30 September, after sailing through a squall. Dalton said the squall "was running its own weather system, the wind coming from the opposite direction than that which we entered with — and there we sat knowing one thing for sure, that the other boats were most likely sailing away."

The Cape Verde islands ahead posed a tactical dilemma for navigators. The shortest distance was a course straight through the island chain. Of course, passing through these land masses meant risking unpredictable wind effects. Leaving the islands to the east meant being in their lee. Going west was a longer course, yet avoided the risk of being downwind of the islands.

Leader Innovation Kvaerner and Merit Cup decided early on to pass to the west of the islands. Paul Cayard struggled with his decision until the last possible minute. His instincts tugged him toward the down-the-middle short course. In the end, it was his boat's nighttime ETA amongst the islands that changed his mind. The fear of darkness bringing unpredictable local land effects turned EF Language away; Cayard dropped in behind Innovation Kvaerner and Merit Cup. Behind Cayard, Silk Cup followed, with Toshiba finally clawing her way out of her disastrous far-easterly position to follow Silk Cut. Swedish Match, America's Challenge and EF Education also took the safer westerly route.

Chessie Racing's navigator, Juan Vila, plotted a course straight through the island chain, keeping Porto Grande on his leeward bow. Only Brunel-Sunergy headed east of the islands. The easterly route was the most radical of all possible courses, forcing a subsequent undesirable easterly entry into the rapidly approaching Doldrums.

The Atlantic decided to hand the leaders a couple of days of perfect sailing before plunging them into the Doldrums. With Innovation Kvaerner 37 miles ahead of second-placed Merit Cup and 53 miles ahead of EF Language, the three leaders raced along at 12 to 13 knots in the hot 14-knot trades.

Two days later, on 4 October, the 14th day of racing, the leaders hit the outer edge of the Doldrums. This is the area where the northeast tradewinds of the North Atlantic meet the southeast trades of the South Atlantic. When these two bodies of air interact there is nowhere for the opposing air flows to go except up, a direction that does sailors no good whatsoever. "I think we have just been welcomed to the Doldrums by black clouds and a violent squall," reported Grant Dalton on Merit Cup.

After days of clipping along in the double-digits, the leaders hit the well-known 'wind vacuum' and briefly slowed to a crawl. A frustrated Frostad saw his hard-won gains slipping from his grasp as he sat without wind, watching the boats he had passed one by one over the last two weeks close on him. "The boats behind have started to eat up quite a bit of our lead," wrote Frostad. "It's very hard in these conditions to predict the right changes ... and to keep the boat going — somewhere."

Finally, though, the Doldrums failed to live up to their advance billing. Different years bring different conditions. Some years the Doldrums cover a wide area, other years they are weak and narrow. To everyone's delight, 1997 turned out to be latter case. "Hardly any Doldrums," reported Innovation Kvaerner skipper Frostad on 5 October. "It felt a bit unfair when we realised being the first boat would mean that we might have been the only boat to get a taste of what was left of the Doldrums before the fresh wind filled in from behind."

On EF Language, Paul Cayard reported that while the charts told them they were in the Doldrums, he was still getting wind, though with squally and unpredictable conditions. His navigator, Mark Rudiger, saw similarities between these conditions and conditions he had experienced on several TransPac races. It was, he conjectured, "just like rounding Catalina on the L.A. to Honolulu TransPac. Everyone jockeys for position and adjusts slightly to cover or evade." Rudiger and Cayard scrambled to find ways to evade, if not cover, and the two men took turns running back and forth between the navigation station and cockpit, plotting a hopscotch path through wind-producing squall lines. The intense sailing paid off. EF Language moved past Merit Cup into second and put Innovation Kvaerner in her sights.

While things were going well for the leaders, trouble was reported from the back of the fleet. Brunel-Sunergy skipper Hans Bouscholte radioed that his boat had hit a whale. The collision had stripped away a hunk of the boat's rudder and, he reported, they were having trouble steering the boat. If they sailed on and the rudder failed completely, they would have to use the small emergency rudder, forcing the boat to sail slowly. After a couple of days consulting with the crew and shore staff, Bouscholte decided not to risk a rudder failure. He radioed race officials to inform them that he was diverting to Recife, Brazil, to effect repairs.

By Day 16, the fleet was halfway to Cape Town. Innovation Kvaerner continued to lead, EF Language was second and closing, and Merit Cup was third. Behind them lined up in order were Silk Cut, Chessie Racing, Toshiba, Swedish Match and America's Challenge. EF Education was bringing up the tail end of the fleet, now 573 miles behind the leader, while BrunelSunergy headed into Recife for a rapid rudder replacement.

Over the next two days Merit Cup would close in on EF Language again, snatching back second place. As each boat crossed the equator and headed farther south, temperatures began to drop; shorts and T-shirts were replaced by pants and jackets. The boats were now heading down the coast of Brazil toward the leg's second waypoint, Ilha da Trindade. Still holding a healthy lead, it did not appear that either Merit Cup or EF Language could catch Innovation Kvaerner before she rounded the island.

Cayard and his navigator Mark Rudiger were biding their time. Thanks to prevailing weather patterns in the South Atlantic, they thought they saw a breakaway opportunity once they rounded Ilha da Trindade. "It looks like the western lobe of the South Atlantic high is moving east, so we may, in fact, be able to sail toward Cape Town when we get to Trindade," Cayard speculated. "This means a longer route around the bottom or a tricky route trying to cut to the north of the high."

Sure enough, on 11 October, the 21st day of the race, EF Language made her break and snatched the lead from Innovation Kvaerner. To add insult to injury, Merit Cup had followed Cayard's course and passed as well, shoving Frostad and his crew into third position. No sooner had the deck been shuffled than fluky wind conditions settled once again over the three leaders, locking them in place. Aboard Merit Cup, a frustrated Dalton moaned, "It's a cruel race! Black clouds, rain and calms have interrupted our tropical cruise." Aboard Innovation Kvaerner, Frostad reported, "We are parked ... no wind. What more can I say?"

While this leg was occasionally punctuated by fast conditions, the repeated periods of fluky winds were stretching the duration of the leg beyond original expectations. By Day 24, those teams who were seen leaving food on the dock back in Southampton were having second thoughts. Race organisers had estimated that the leg would take about 31 days to complete. With the winds down and some boats still facing over 2,000 miles to Cape Town, estimated leg lengths for the boats trailing EF Language now ranged from 30 to 36 days. Food rationing began immediately on many of the boats.

As the meals got smaller, dark humour began on several boats. Aboard America's Challenge, Campbell Field, the son of skipper Ross Field, cut the end of his index finger off on a running backstay. After reporting that he was on the mend, his father joked that they were saving the bit of finger on ice for a later meal.

Meanwhile, well in the lead, Cayard reported his team had logged 370 miles in the last 24 hours. He was back into good winds gusting to 35 knots, and EF Language had maintained a steady 15 to 16 knots all night. Cayard called it his "first real taste of The Whitbread," describing the sensation as "a cross between really scary and really fun." By Day 28, Cayard had extended his lead over Merit Cup to 113 miles.

The food situation was getting quite serious for certain crews. On Chessie Racing they ran out of powdered milk for the tea and began substituting Gatorade. On Innovation Kvaerner, Day 28 marked the last day of regular meals. The crew reported that from then on they "were living on savings and leftovers from the previous week."

Dwindling food supplies were a good enough reason to sail fast — Silk Cut skipper Lawrie Smith reported on Day 28 that his team recorded an impressive 417.2-mile 24-hour run.

On Merit Cup, Grant Dalton ordered all sail hoisted as he fought off a fierce challenge from Innovation Kvaerner, which briefly retook second place, and tried to catch up with EF Language. "No one has slept for 24 hours," Dalton reported. "We've been on deck for all that time. At least it has temporarily stopped them moaning about food! But Cayard is sailing well and he will be difficult to catch."

Dalton was right about that. Cayard not only held his lead, he extended it. On 21 October, EF Language crossed the finish line in Cape Town first. The winner of Leg 1 had been at sea for 29 days, 16 hours and 54 minutes. Behind EF Language followed Merit Cup in second, with Innovation Kvaerner hot on her heels less than two hours behind.

Dockside, all the attention was focused on Cayard, the man so many doubted had the right stuff for this race. It appeared this America's Cup skipper was not a one-trick pony after all.

At a dockside press conference after his win Cayard remained cautious. "We have the yellow jersey for now," the unshaven skipper said. "It will not be easy to hold on to."

How right he was.

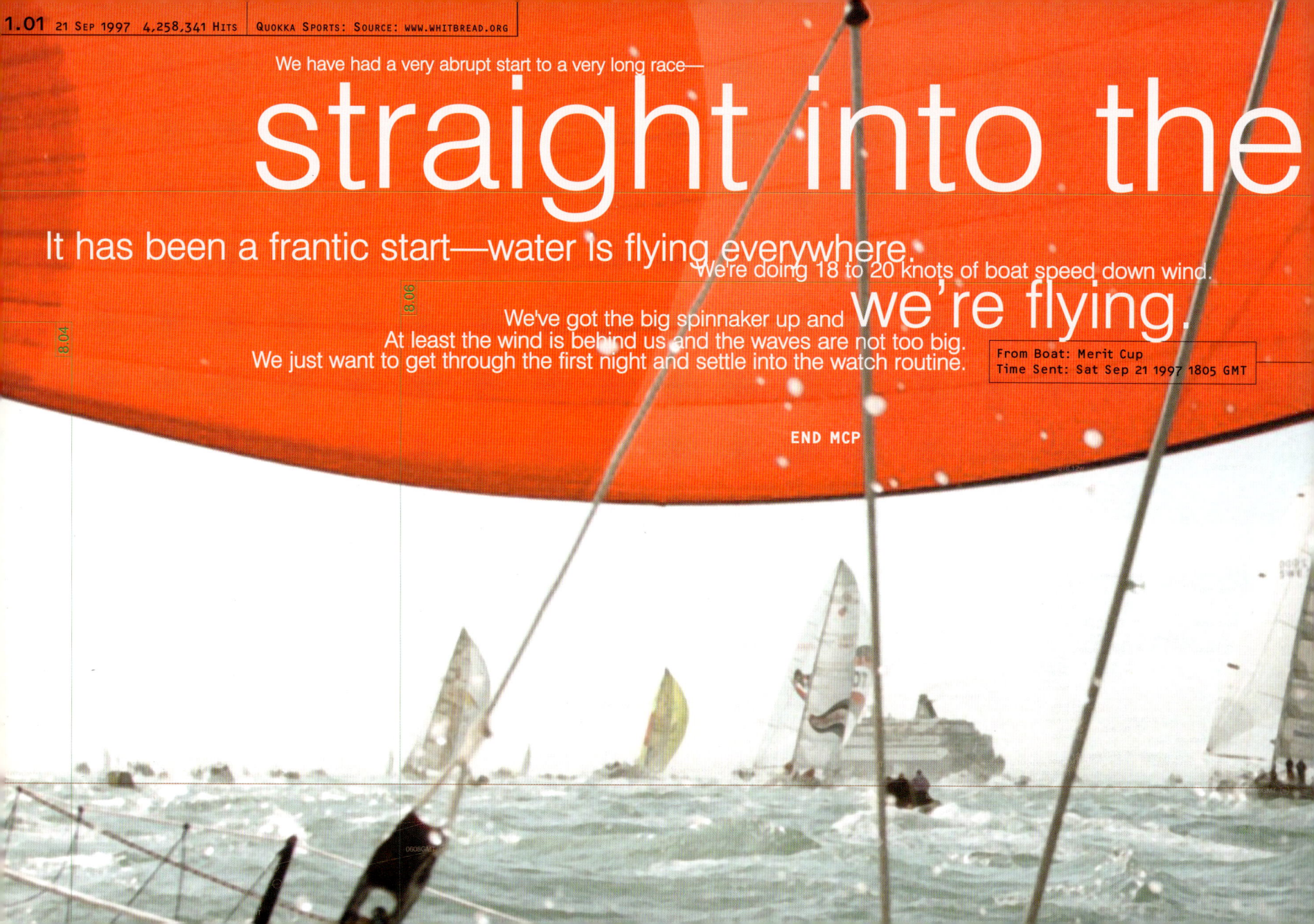

1.01 21 Sep 1997 4,258,341 Hits | Quokka Sports: Source: www.whitbread.org

We have had a very abrupt start to a very long race—

straight into the

It has been a frantic start—water is flying everywhere.

We're doing 18 to 20 knots of boat speed down wind.

We've got the big spinnaker up and **we're flying.**

At least the wind is behind us and the waves are not too big.
We just want to get through the first night and settle into the watch routine.

From Boat: Merit Cup
Time Sent: Sat Sep 21 1997 1805 GMT

END MCP

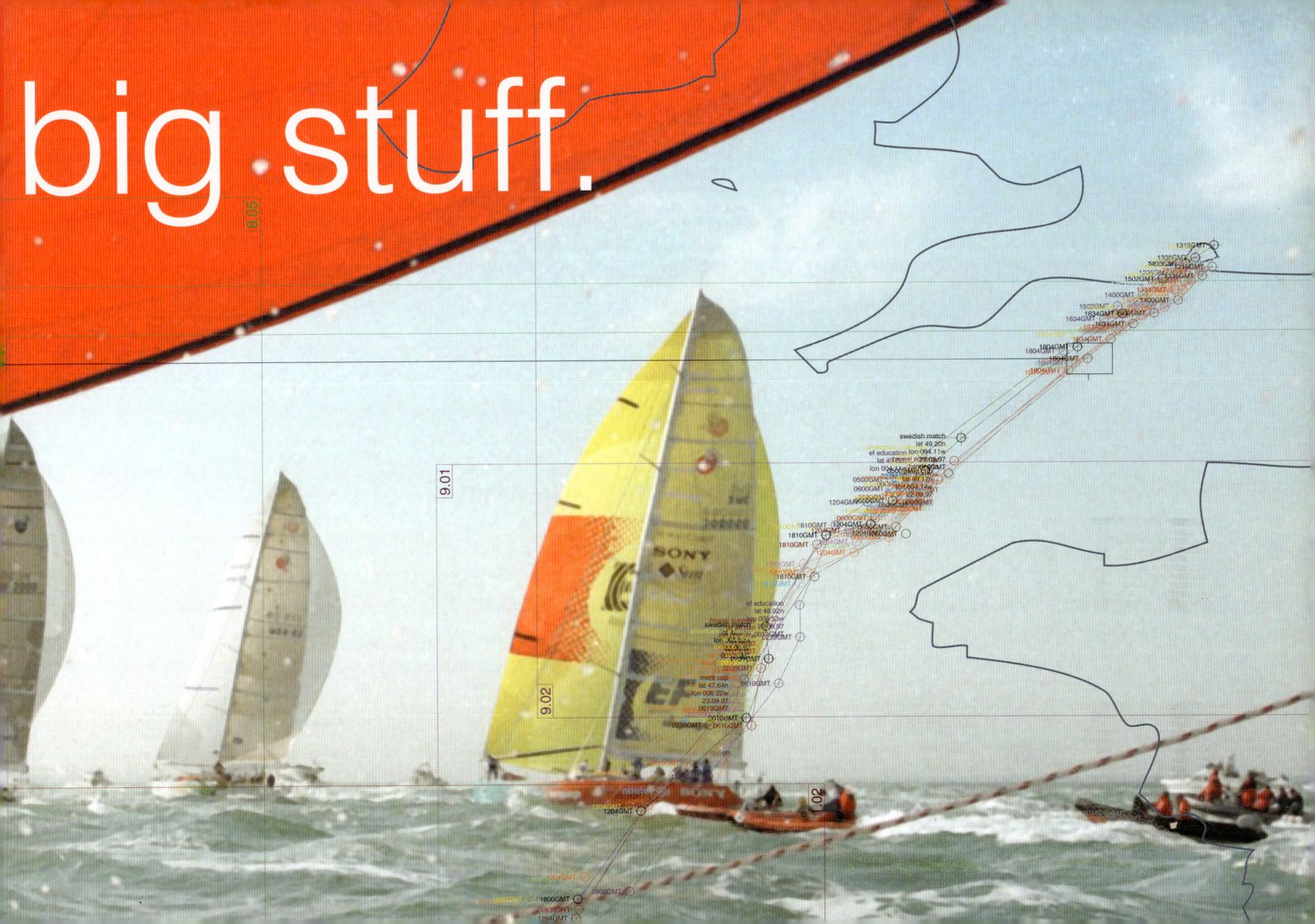

1.02 22-23 SEP 1997 8,321,321 HITS QUOKKA SPORTS: SOURCE: WWW.WHITBREAD.ORG

1.01

From Boat: Chessie Racing
Date Sent: 22 Sep 1997

We have been side by side by boat with Silk Cut and Merit Cup.
 ...have been as close as 3 boat lengths.

...we can only see the
tops of the rigs
sticking out
It's a rather amazing sight

From Boat: EF Education
Date Sent: 23 September 1997

After the wind died yesterday morning the fog came rolling in. Around midday it lifted briefly and we could see 7 boats strung out around us. Unfortunately we sailed ourselves into a frustrating windless hole about 15 miles north of Ushant with 0-2 knots of breeze coming from all over the place. We lost out badly to the boats inside of us who managed to keep the breeze and get around Ushant before the tide turned foul. We bucked the tide last night and now this morning are sailing with spinnaker up and the sun is shining too!

We've had to slow down several times to get seaweed off the rudders. We've also used the light winds to go up the rig to check that all is well. Have had two visits by schools of dolphins.

Bye

END EFEDU

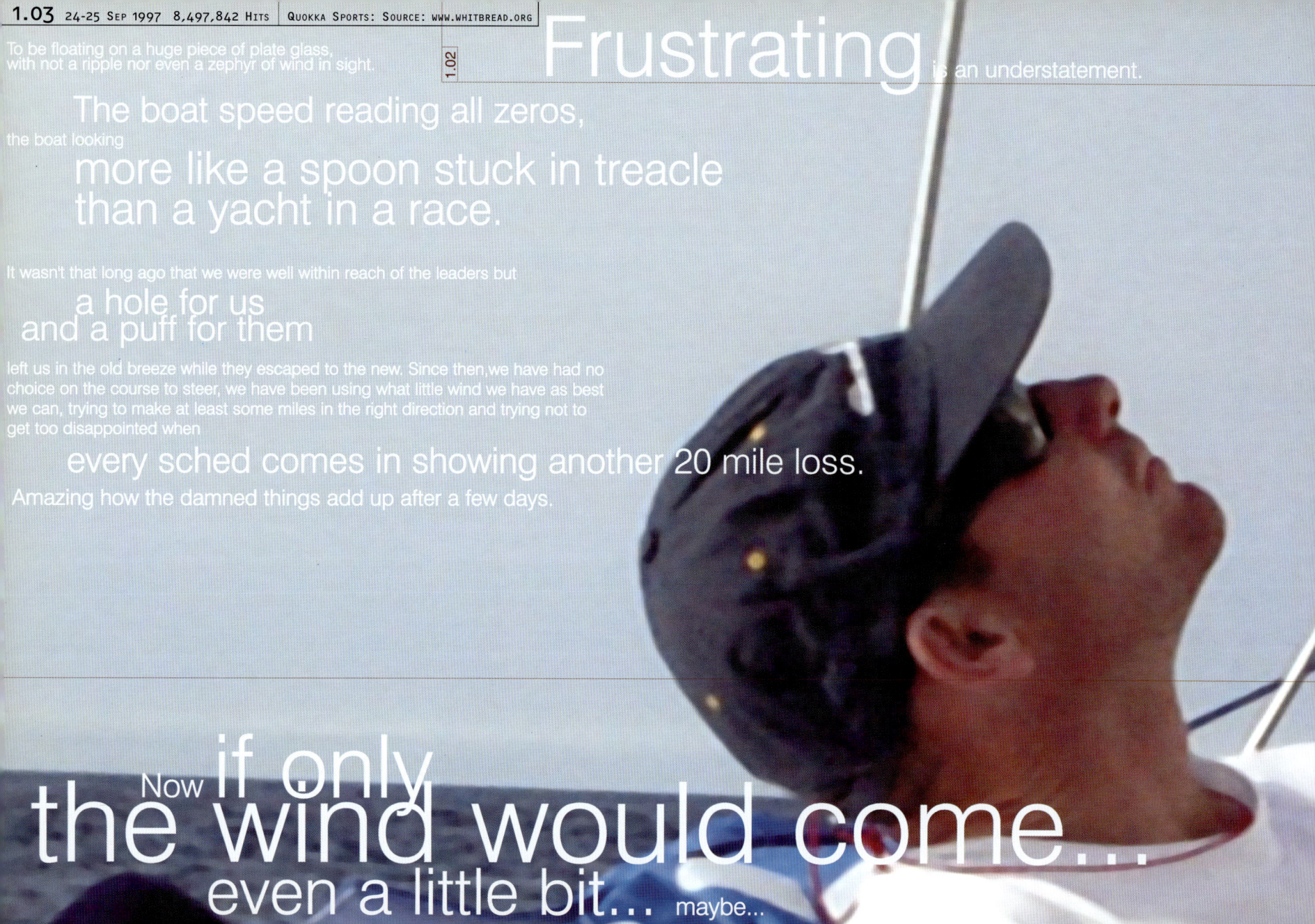

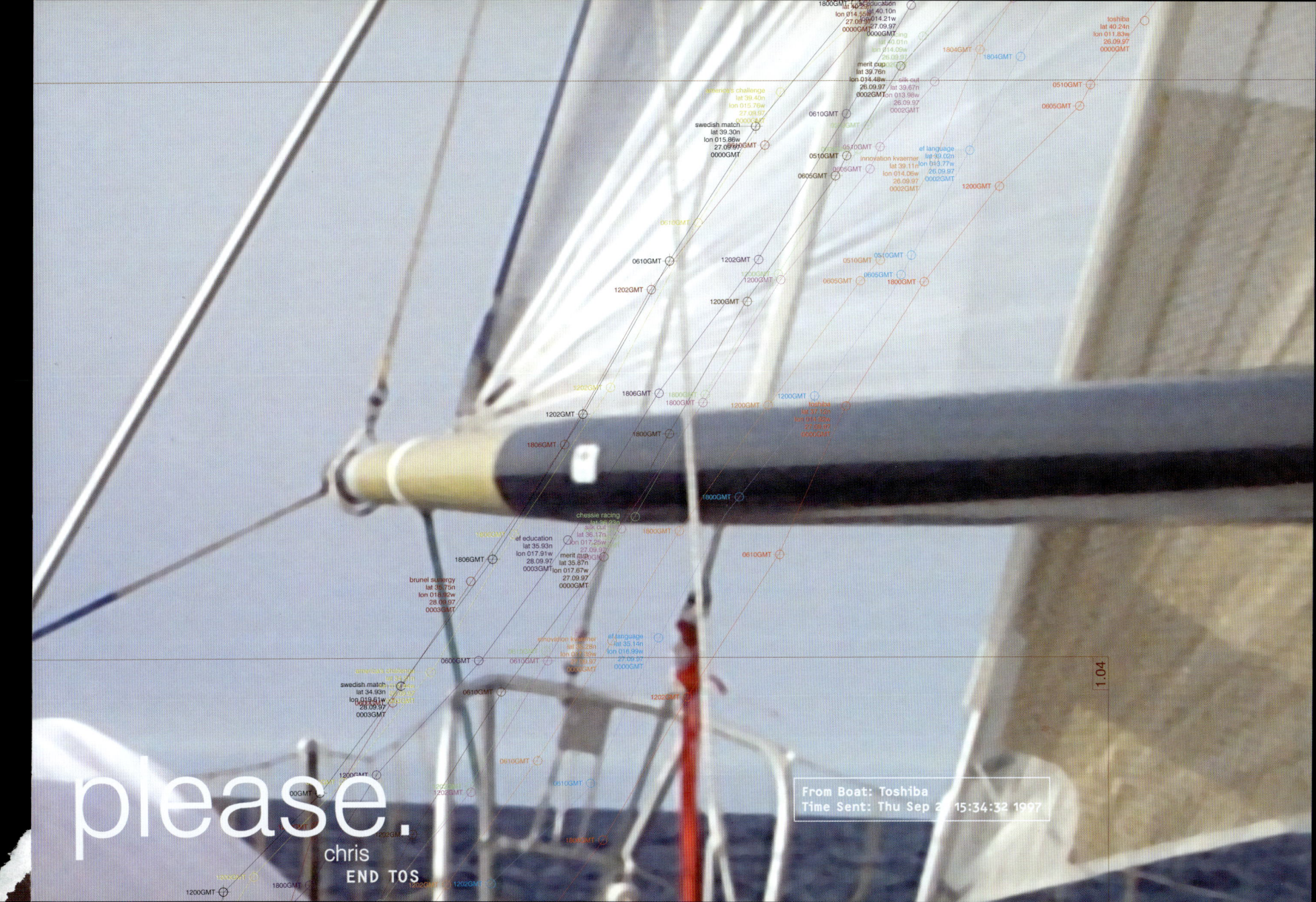

1.04 26-27 SEP 1997 8,730,881 HITS QUOKKA SPORTS: SOURCE: WWW.WHITBREAD.ORG

From Boat: Chessie Racing
Time Sent: Fri Sep 26 13:39:58 1997

During the last 12 hours we've been having a preview of the tropics.

Sailing in warm conditions with **clouds coming at us like balls in a bowling**

Each cloud brings either **heavy rain** and/or large changes in the wind's direction and velocity.

The crew has been working hard changing sails to each changing condition.

Regards from Grant Spanhake Watch Captain "Chessie"

END CHR

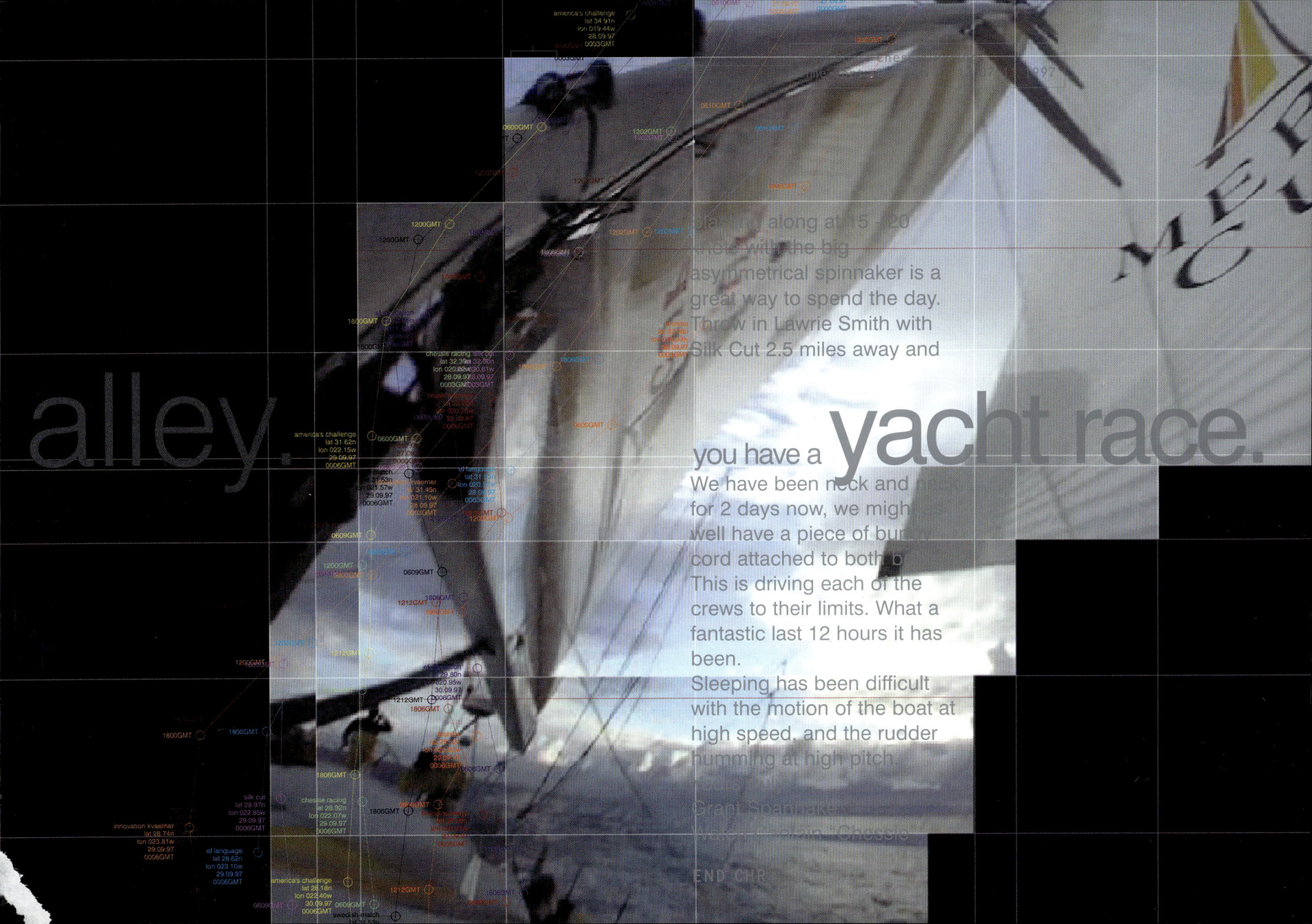

alley.

...along at 15-20 knots with the big asymmetrical spinnaker is a great way to spend the day. Throw in Lawrie Smith with Silk Cut 2.5 miles away and you have a yacht race. We have been neck and neck for 2 days now, we might as well have a piece of bungi cord attached to both. This is driving each of the crews to their limits. What a fantastic last 12 hours it has been.
Sleeping has been difficult with the motion of the boat at high speed, and the rudder humming at high pitch.

Grant Spanhake
Watch Captain Chessie

END CHR

1.05 28-29 SEP 1997 7,051,411 HITS QUOKKA SPORTS: SOURCE: WWW.WHITBREAD.ORG

From Boat: Merit Cup
Time Sent: Sun Sep 28 15:07:54 1997

AN IMPORTANT TACTICAL DECISION NOW WHICH IS WHEN TO GYBE ONTO PORT AND START TO HEAD SOUTH OR STAY ON THE UNFAVORED STARBOARD GYBE LONGER AND END UP IN 1 WEEKS TIME WITH A BETTER ANGLE TO THE DOLDRUMS. A YACHT GYBING FIRST WILL INITIALY LOOK GOOD ON PAPER WHEN LOOKING AT MILES TO GO BUT THIS COULD QUITE QUICKLY CHANGE. THIS MOVE IS ONE OF THE MOST IMPORTANT OF THE FIRST LEG AND GIVES NAVIGATORS DEEP FURROWS IN THEIR BROW WE HAVE OPTED TO HEAD WEST AND TAKE THE INTIAL LOSS HOPEFULLY FOR THE LONGER TERM GAIN— WHO KNOWS!

CERTAINLY THERE WILL BE WINNERS AND LOOSERS AS USUAL. STILL IN LIGHT WINDS WITH THE ODD RAIN SQUALL AND NOW IT IS STARTING TO GET HOT ESP DOWN BELOW. WE ARE COMING TO THE CONCLUSION QUICKLY THAT THE PORTIONS FOR EACH MEAL THAT WE HAVE ARE TOO SMALL SO WE WILL BE LOSING A LOT OF WEIGHT.

PASSED CLOSE TO A LARGE FENCE POST TODAY WITH A LARGE FISH STUCK ON WHAT APPEARED TO BE A NAIL- ROTTEN LUCK. GRANT DALTON

END MCP

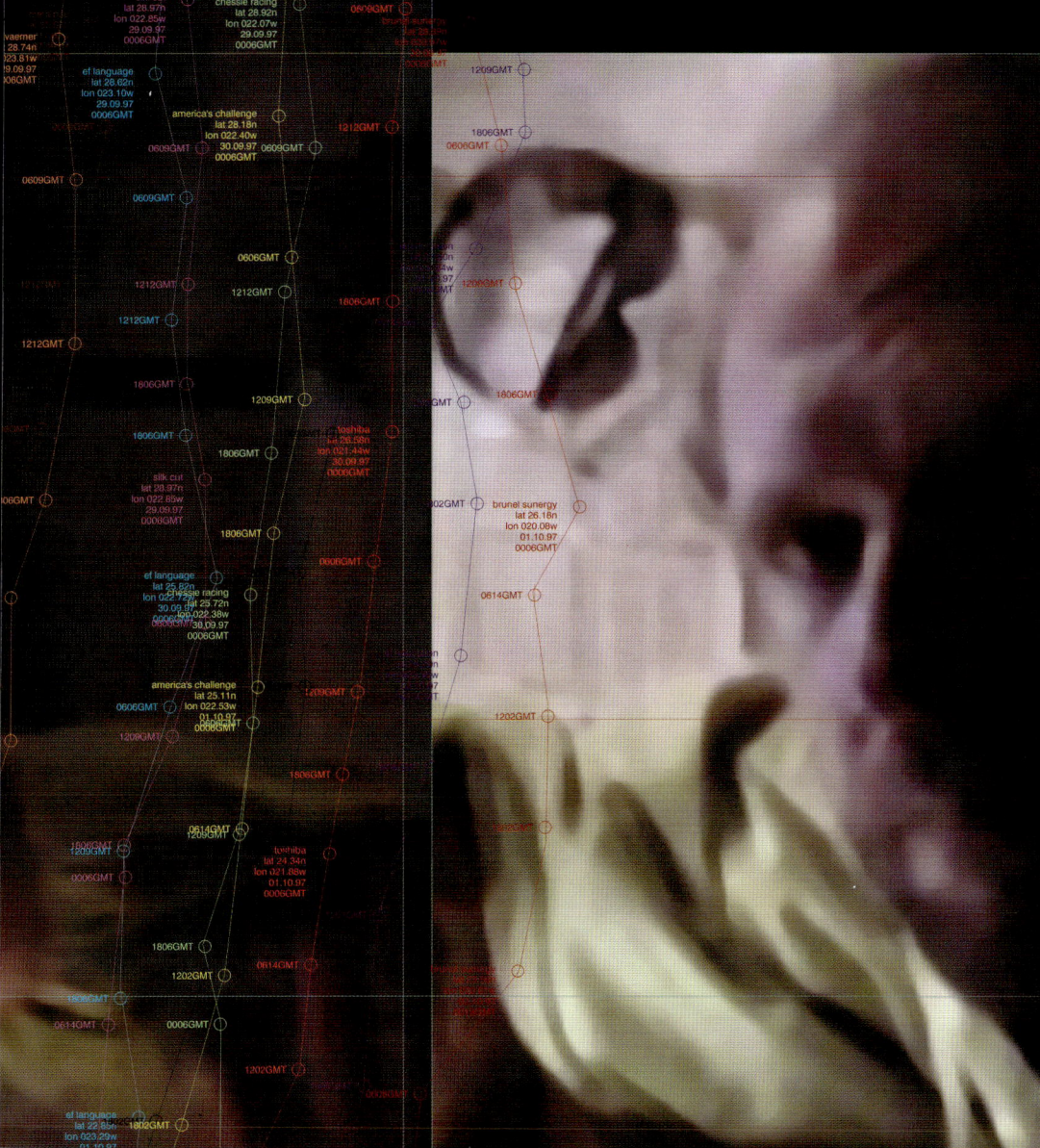

1.06 | 30 Sep–01 Oct 1997 | 8,671,608 Hits | Quokka Sports: Source: www.whitbread.org

From Boat: Chessie
Time Sent: Tue Sep 30 17:06:07 1997

The wind, over a period of 6 hours, has turned 360 degrees around the compass. Twice!

Spinnaker, jib top, headsail, wind seeker and

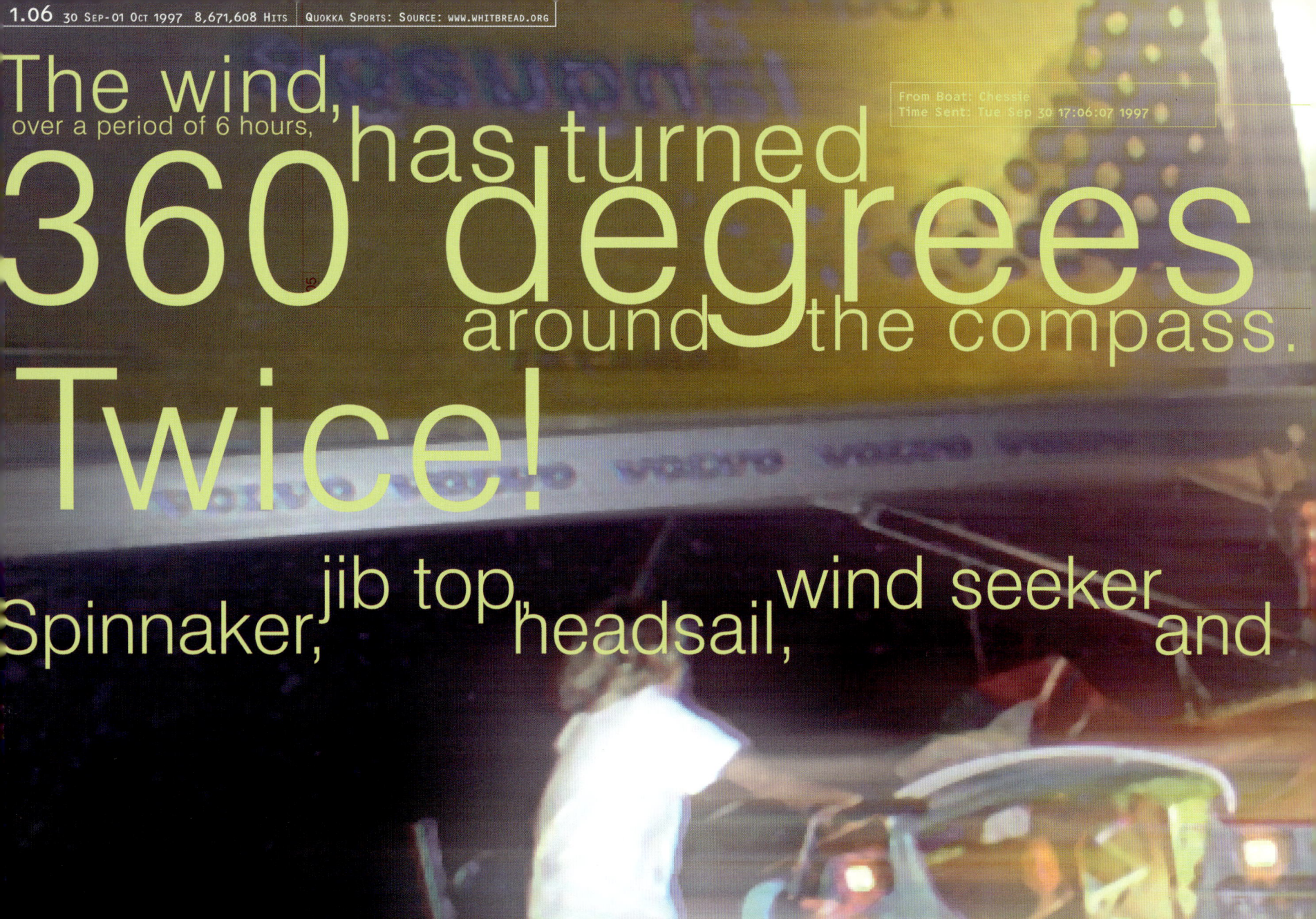

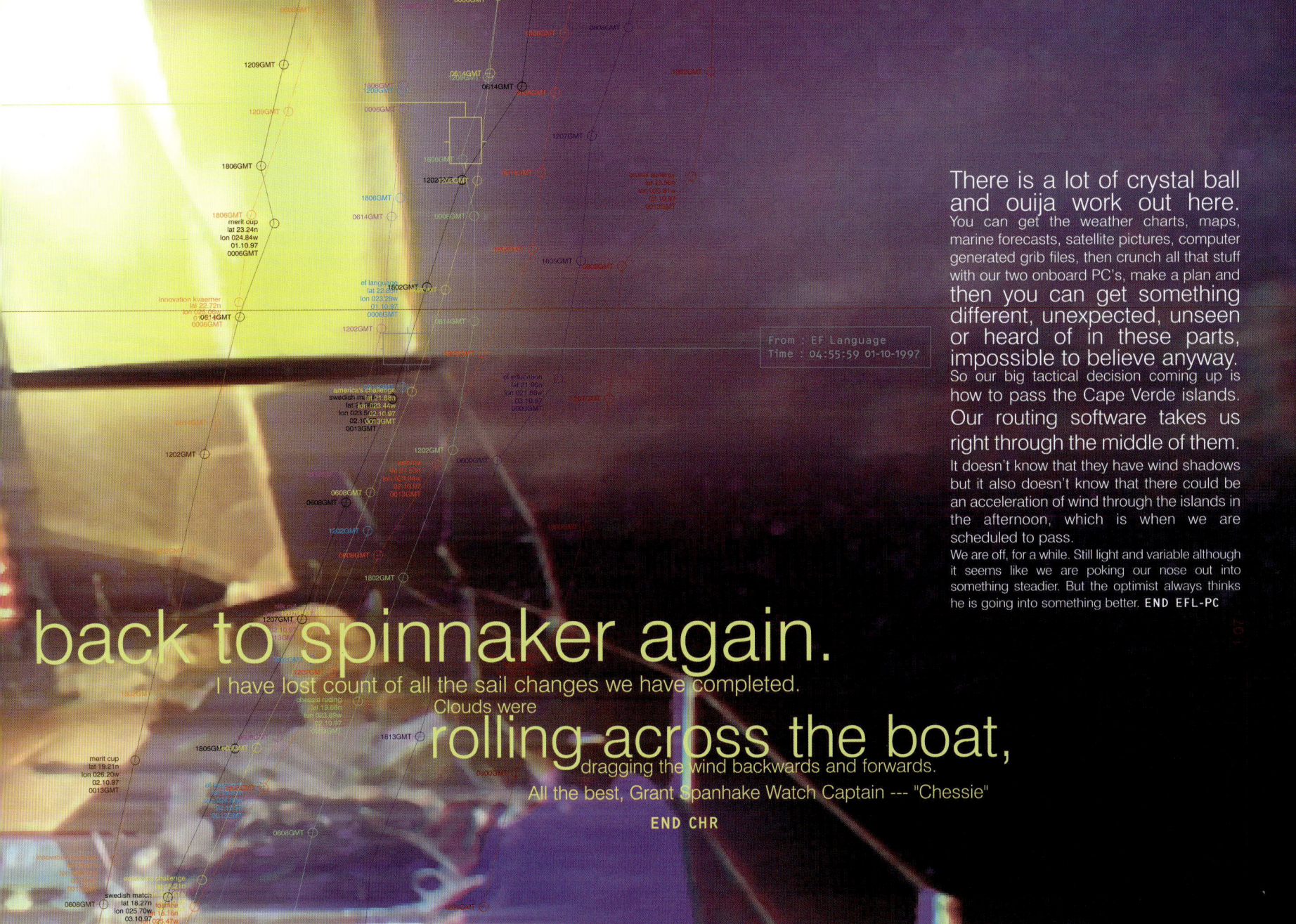

There is a lot of crystal ball and ouija work out here. You can get the weather charts, maps, marine forecasts, satellite pictures, computer generated grib files, then crunch all that stuff with our two onboard PC's, make a plan and then you can get something different, unexpected, unseen or heard of in these parts, impossible to believe anyway. So our big tactical decision coming up is how to pass the Cape Verde islands. Our routing software takes us right through the middle of them. It doesn't know that they have wind shadows but it also doesn't know that there could be an acceleration of wind through the islands in the afternoon, which is when we are scheduled to pass.

We are off, for a while. Still light and variable although it seems like we are poking our nose out into something steadier. But the optimist always thinks he is going into something better. END EFL-PC

back to spinnaker again. I have lost count of all the sail changes we have completed. Clouds were rolling across the boat, dragging the wind backwards and forwards. All the best, Grant Spanhake Watch Captain --- "Chessie"

END CHR

1.07 02-03 OCT 1997 4,086,782 HITS QUOKKA SPORTS: SOURCE: WWW.WHITBREAD.ORG

From Boat: Toshiba
Time Sent: Thu Oct 2 02:03:06 1997

Real distractions have been minor such as watching the **bright luminescent trails of dolphins** around the boat at night time. They

Early this morning we passed about 75 Nm west of Cape Verde Islands. We positioned ourselves two days ago to have good clearance, and it paid off compare to the boats which gybed too early and ended up These Islands are very high.

 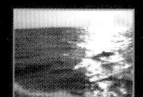 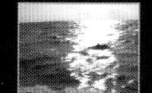 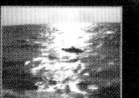 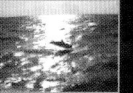 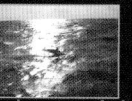 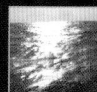

With just under 5000 miles to go, one can conclude that the fleet is spread out in a way nobody could predict. It is over 500 miles between first and last boat. The close encounter is of course there,

From Boat: Swedish_Match
Daily Report 02/10/97

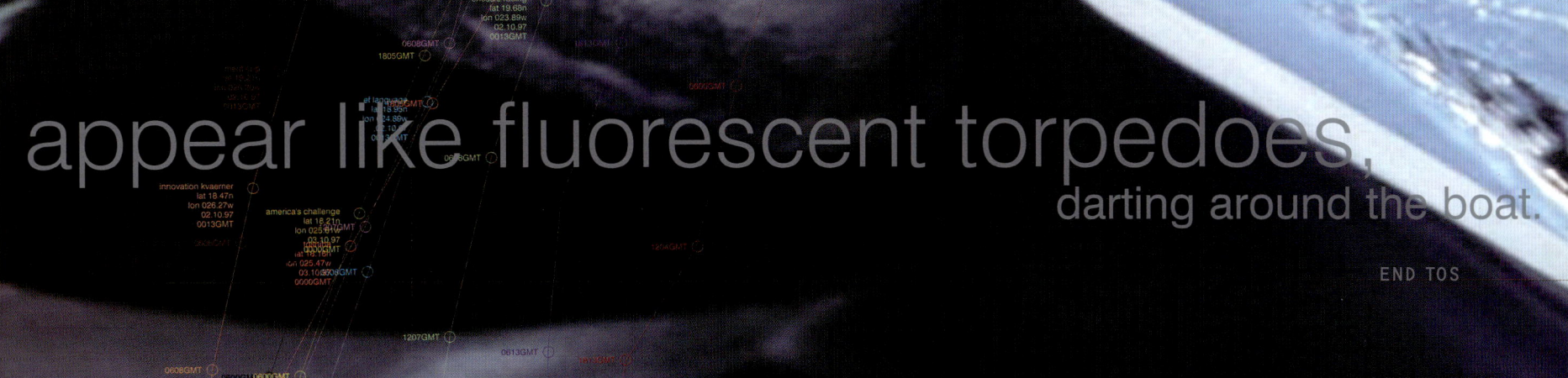

appear like fluorescent torpedoes,

darting around the boat.

END TOS

From Boat: Kvaerner
Time Sent: Thu Oct 2 20:29:40 1997

too close to the Islands.
Up to 2.900 m., and we have estimated they leave a wind shadow up to 30 Nm to leeward. The next couple of days will show a lot more unstable wind speed and direction for us, with potential squalls and calms.

We are definitely having a drag race with Merit Cup at the moment. END KVA

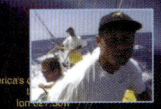 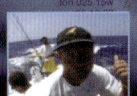 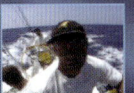 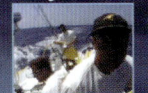 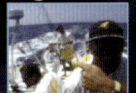 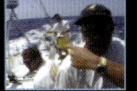 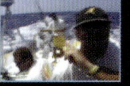 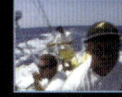

Video: Merit_Cup 02/10/97

we have been neck to neck with America's Challenge for days now
and Kvaerner and Merit Cup are battling for first place.
Regards Gurra END SWE

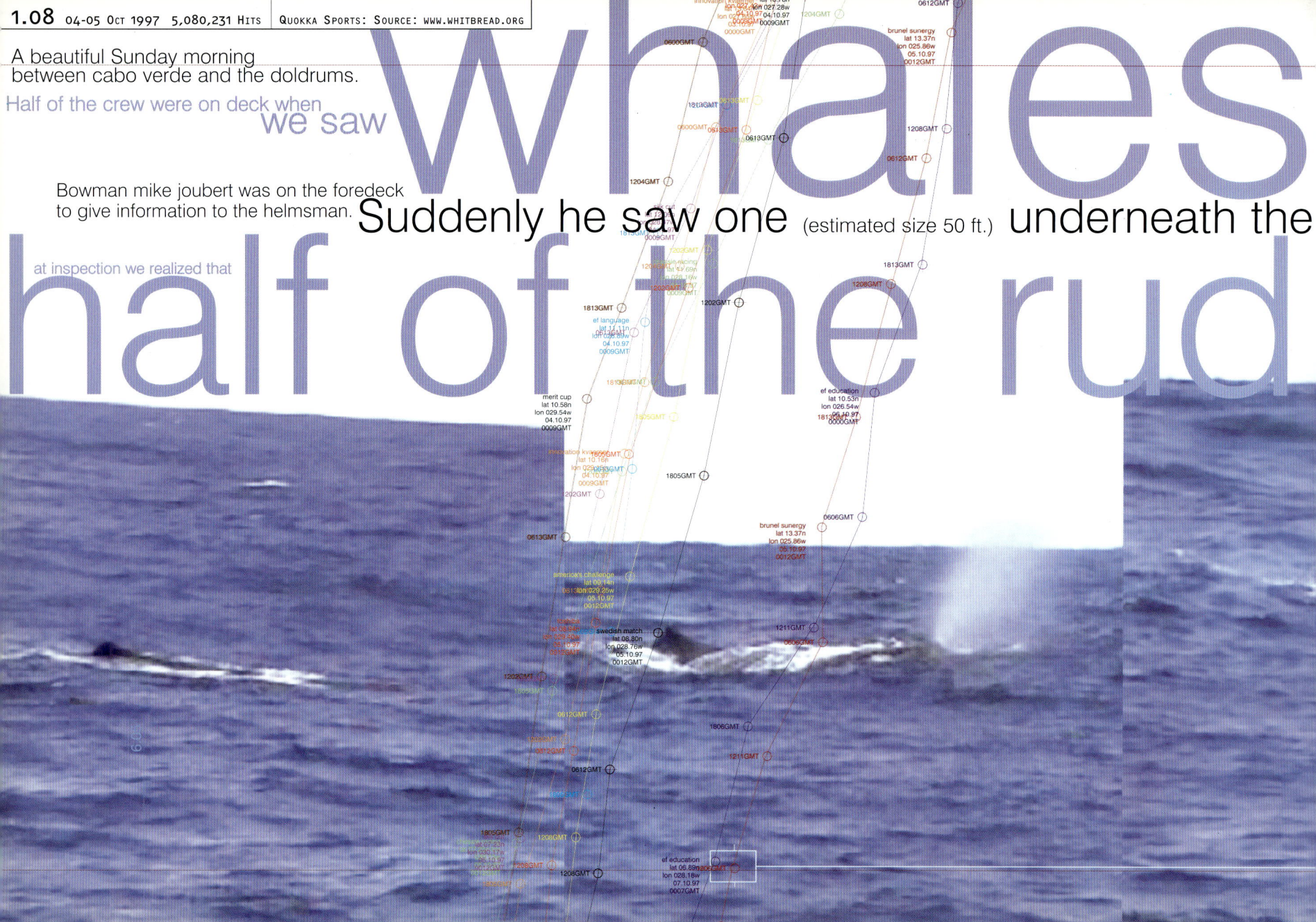

1.08 04-05 Oct 1997 5,080,231 Hits | Quokka Sports: Source: www.whitbread.org

A beautiful Sunday morning between cabo verde and the doldrums.

Half of the crew were on deck when we saw whales

Bowman mike joubert was on the foredeck to give information to the helmsman. Suddenly he saw one (estimated size 50 ft.) underneath the

at inspection we realized that half of the rud

in front of us. We bore off to give them a wide berth, They were jumping out of the water in front of us.

boat on portside. Directly after that we heard a loud bang. and because we were doing 10-knots,

der was gone

WHAT NOW?

If there is not too much pressure on the helm, we can still drive the boat, but we can not go to fast.
We have 2-options.
1-Sail on and if this rudder breaks completely, put the emergency rudder on, but with this emergency rudder you only can go at low speed.
2-Find a harbour and put in a new racing rudder so that we can continue in normal racing mode. We will take a decision together with our Brunel Sunergy shorebase in holland.
Best regards—Hans Bouscholte

END BRS

From Boat: Brunel_Sunergy Time Sent: Sun Oct 5 21:26:51 1997
Latitude: 10 05.62 N Longitude: 027 03.10 W Course: 172 Speed: 09 knots

PS. the whale said he would report to GREENPEACE about careless driving of brunel sunergy.

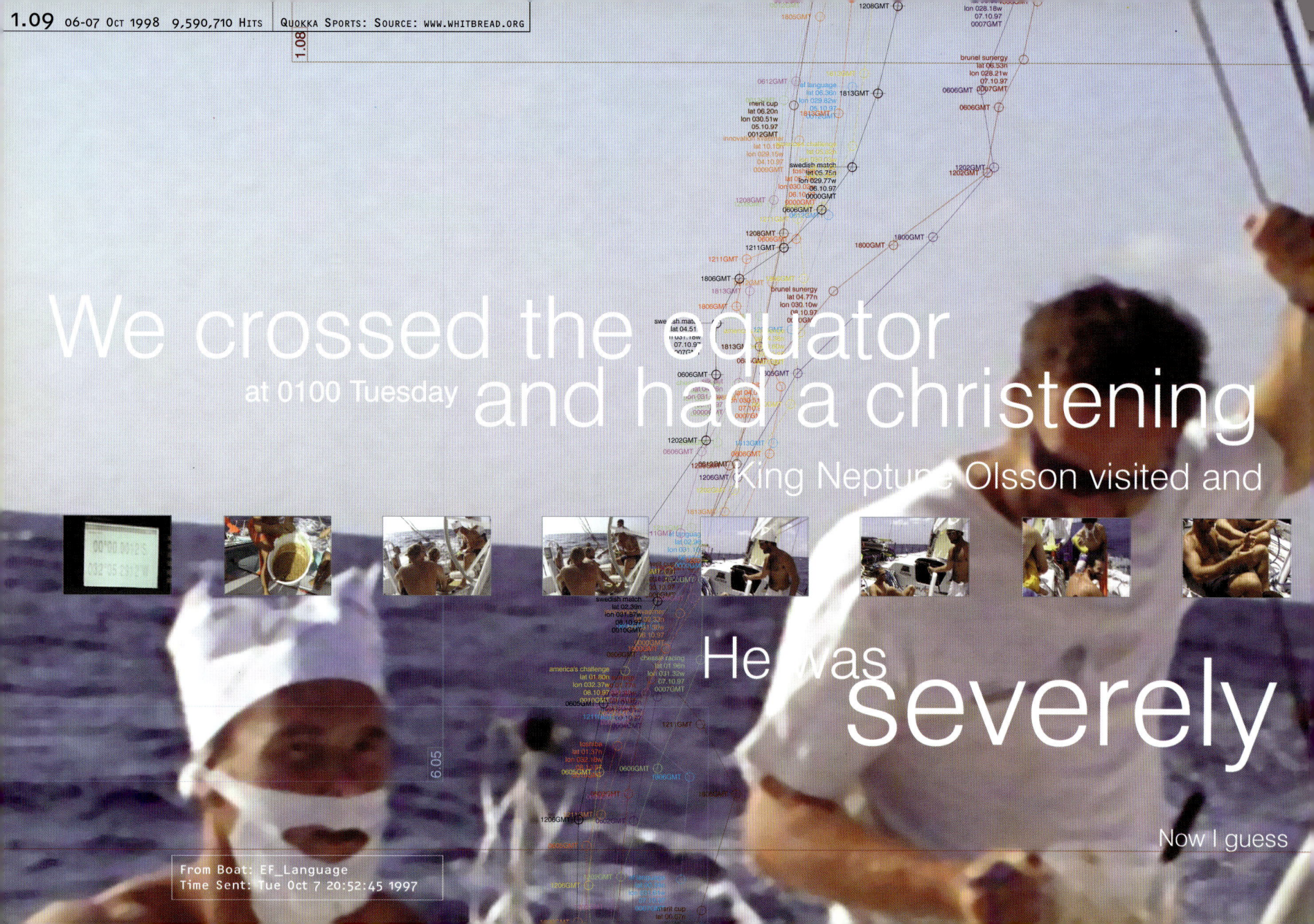

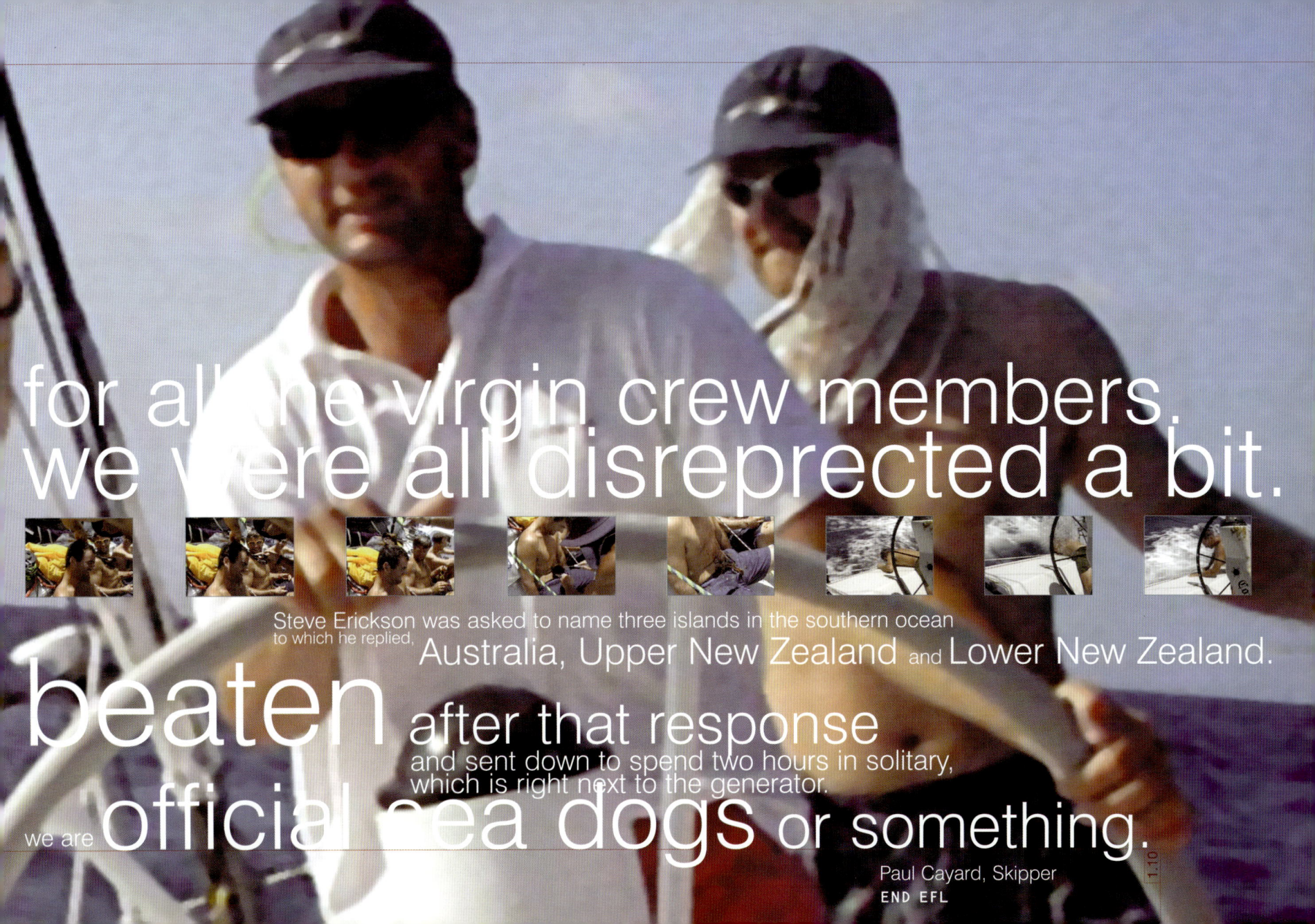

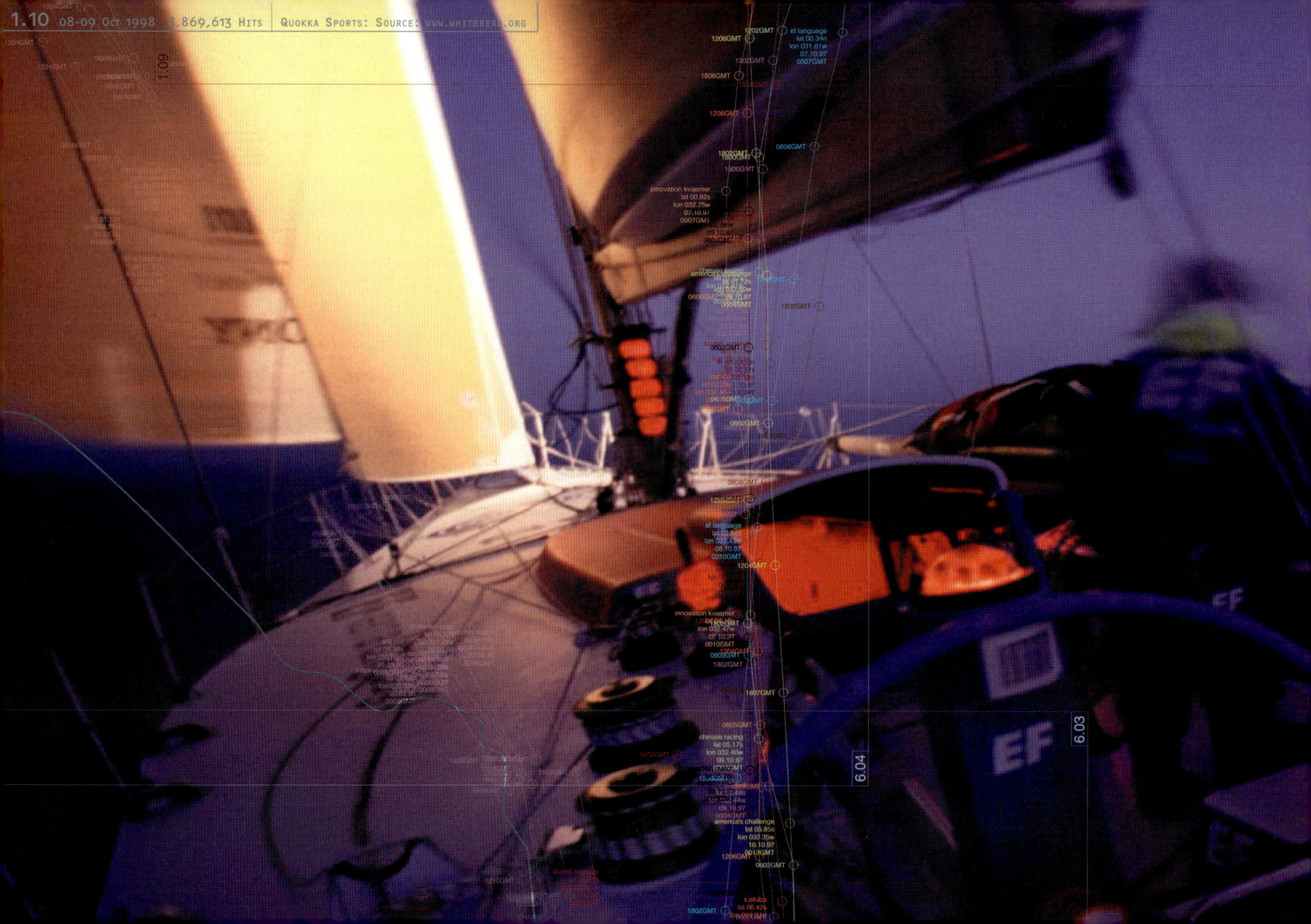

From Boat: Chessie Time Sent: Thu Oct 9 20:49:43 1997
The Whitbread "Why"? By Rick Deppe

By any definition the WRTWR would easily rank as one of the world's most physically challenging sports/adventure events. For sheer duration, this race outlasts many such as the Iditarod or Ultrasmarathons by a significant time factor. The extremes in weather conditions would make most undertakings this side of the Himalayas or the Sahara seem like a nice day out.

I think a race like this, and all the hardships that go with it, can change you in many ways. Taking a deep breath before heading out to that pitch dark deck as the wind howls through the rigging, or going up the mast for the fifth time that watch are the moments that you live for. After such hardships returning home is the best feeling of all. It makes you appreciative of the small things in life, the joy derived from a day spent with your child or loved ones is magnified by these other moments encountered in such undertakings as the WRTWR. The lessons learned from going toe to toe with your rivals both externally and in your own head for such an extended period of time will stay with you all your life.

When you live the Whitbread you live big.

END CHR

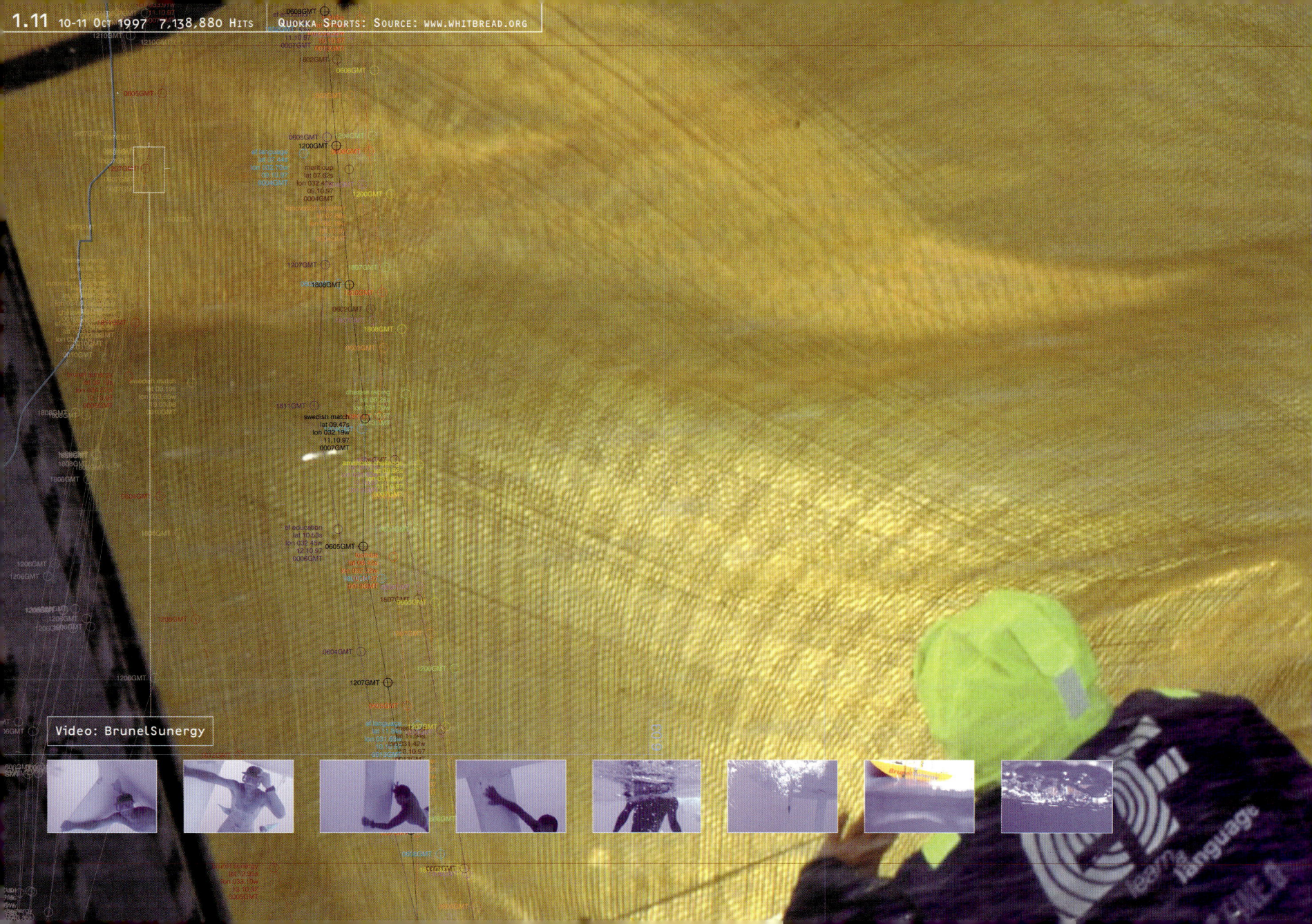

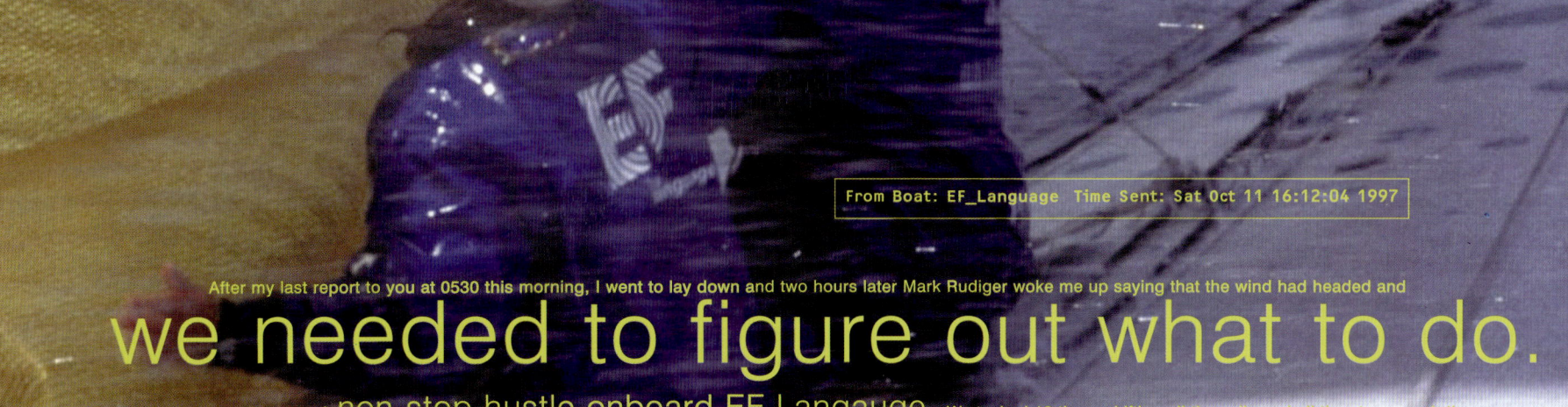

From Boat: EF_Language Time Sent: Sat Oct 11 16:12:04 1997

After my last report to you at 0530 this morning, I went to lay down and two hours later Mark Rudiger woke me up saying that the wind had headed and

we needed to figure out what to do.

What ensued was 6 hours of non-stop hustle onboard EF Langauge. We tacked 10 times shifting all the sails and all the stores each time, we changes sails seven times using everything from our lightest jib to our heaviest spinnaker. We were running in a wind from 020 and beating in a wind from 020.

We could see the squall clouds all around us and

we just tried to keep on the good side of them

and not let any of them run over us. We were in a miniature low pressure system that didn't even show up on the satellite pictures of yesterday.

Got to go. EF Language, skipper Paul Cayard END EFL

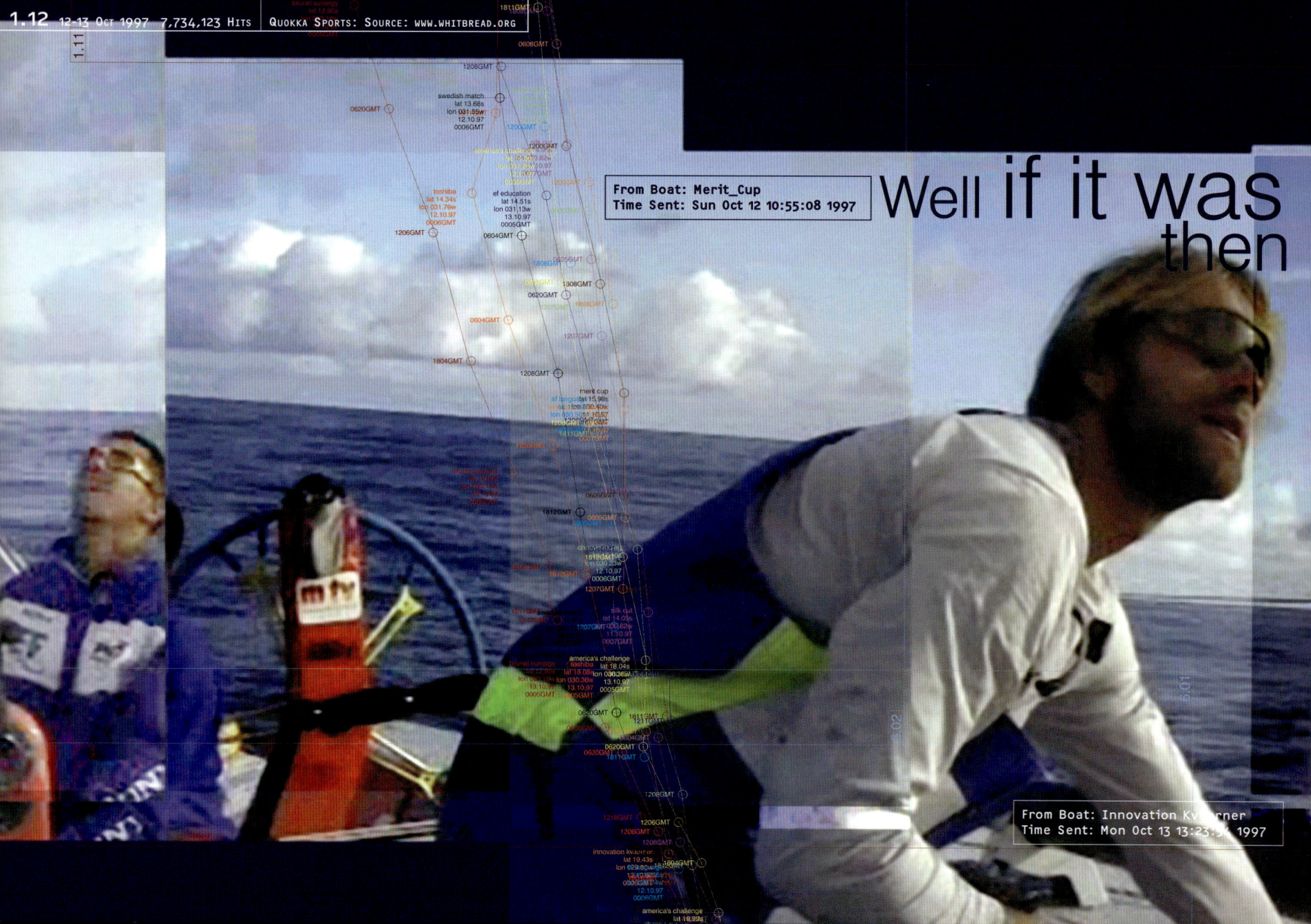

close racing you were looking for
this is it.
EF have done nice work
first round Trindade 1 mile ahead of us
with Kva about 3 miles back. But
now the race starts in earnest
and with the changeable weather ahead of us
it would be a brave man who would write off anyone
even those well behind at this stage.
So the sprint begins,
we are looking forward to it
Grant Dalton
END MCP

EF made a jump yesterday, but we are holding her and Merit even though it should be some more pressure in the south. We can still see Merit ahead of us. This morning we have soaked down a bit to end up a bit to the west of her, and all three boats are now in line. The ETA for Cape Town was on December 3rd yesterday night, and we started the discussion about who to eat first when we run out of food. Unfortunately for him and his family, Barney ended up on top of the list. However after considering his pretty unhealthy past, we might end up with Alby's spare ribs as a starter and maybe a French entrecote from Pierre as main course. Luckily for our tall, skinny navigator, he was not even on the top ten list. Rgrds Knut F. and Crew Innovation Kvaerner END KVA

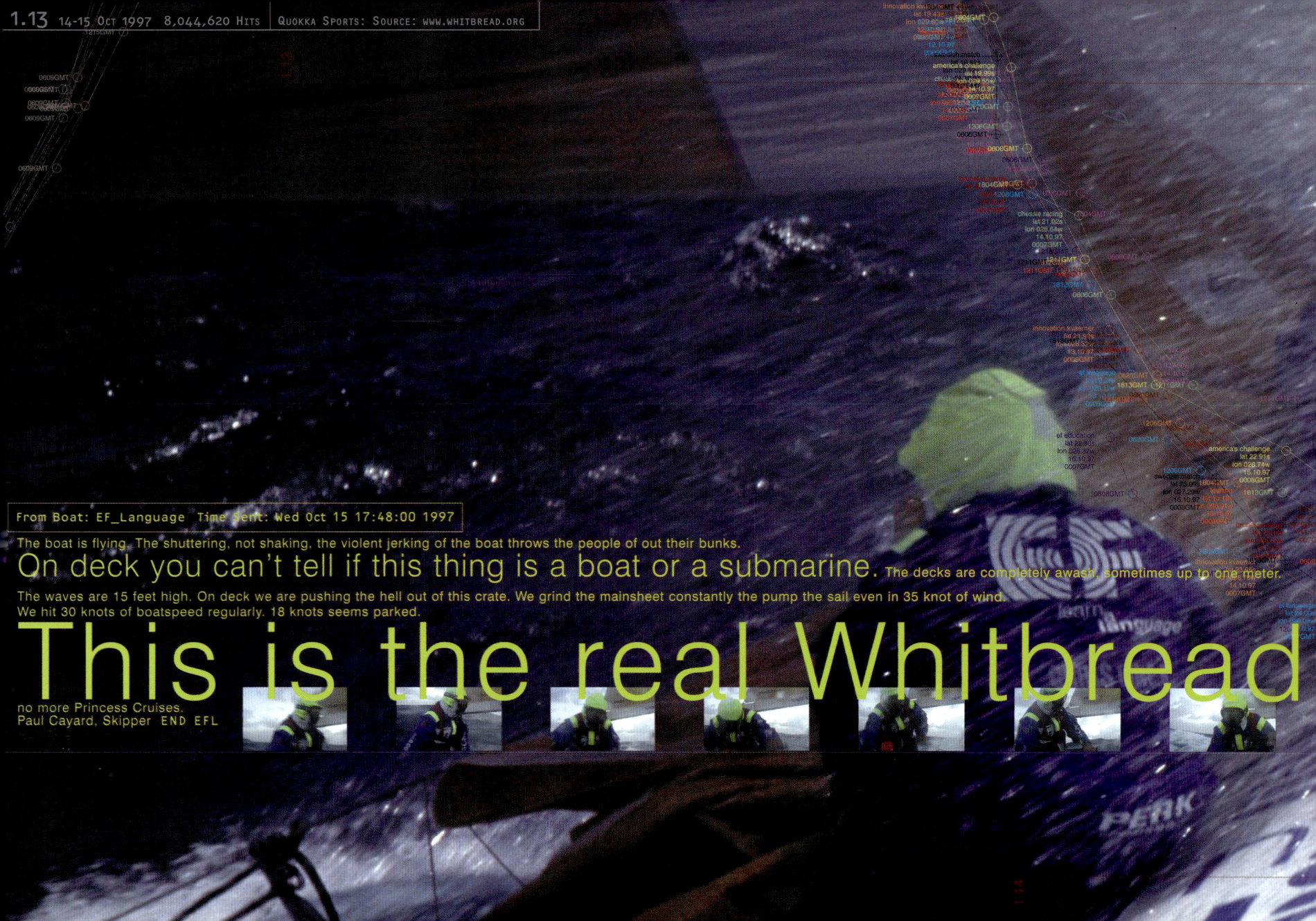

1.13 14-15 Oct 1997 8,044,620 Hits Quokka Sports: Source: www.whitbread.org

From Boat: EF_Language Time Sent: Wed Oct 15 17:48:00 1997

The boat is flying. The shuttering, not shaking, the violent jerking of the boat throws the people of out their bunks.

On deck you can't tell if this thing is a boat or a submarine. The decks are completely awash, sometimes up to one meter.

The waves are 15 feet high. On deck we are pushing the hell out of this crate. We grind the mainsheet constantly the pump the sail even in 35 knot of wind. We hit 30 knots of boatspeed regularly. 18 knots seems parked.

This is the real Whitbread

no more Princess Cruises.
Paul Cayard, Skipper END EFL

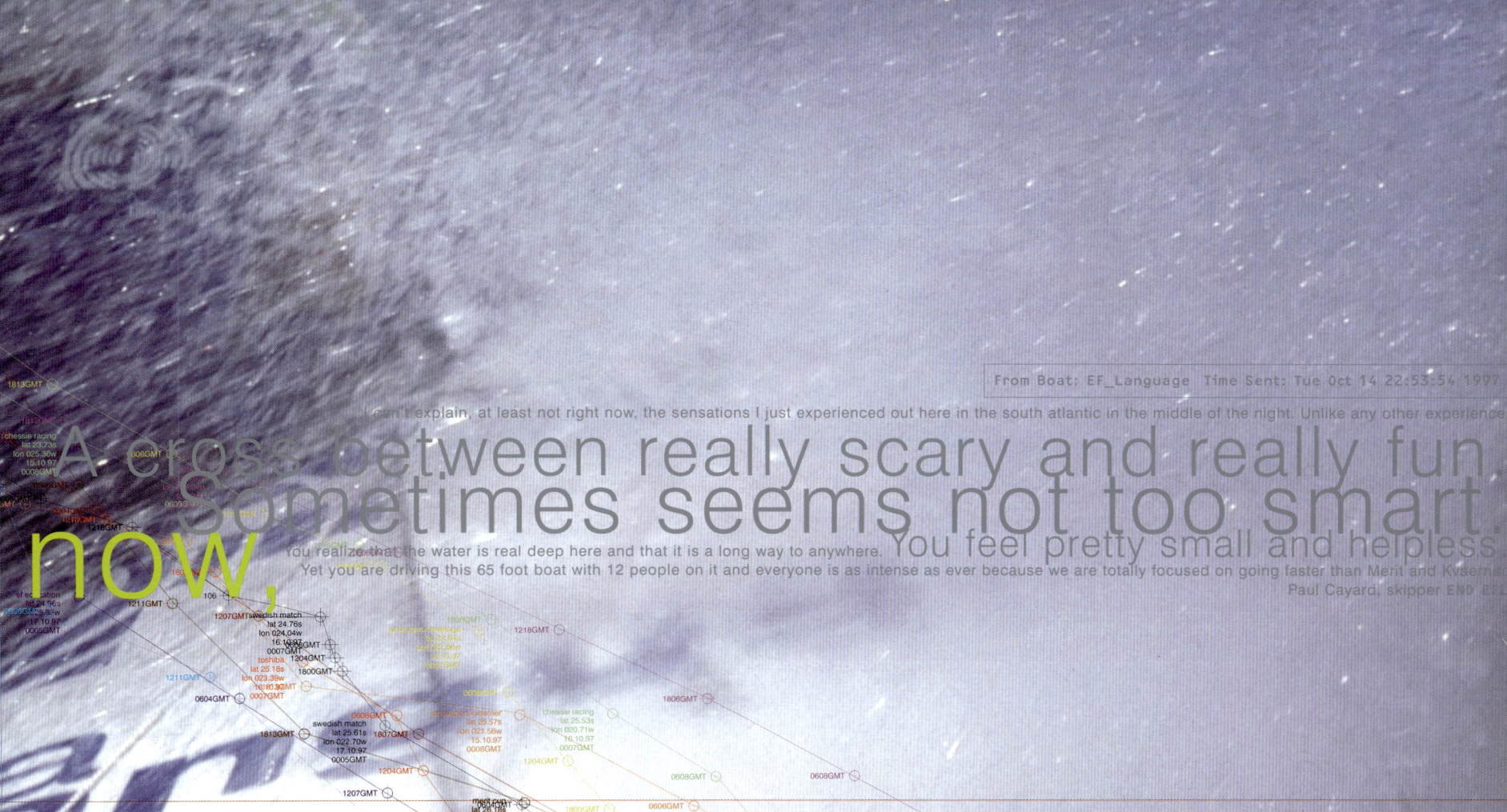

From Boat: EF_Language Time Sent: Tue Oct 14 22:53:54 1997

I can't explain, at least not right now, the sensations I just experienced out here in the south atlantic in the middle of the night. Unlike any other experience. A cross between really scary and really fun. Sometimes seems not too smart. now, You realize that the water is real deep here and that it is a long way to anywhere. You feel pretty small and helpless. Yet you are driving this 65 foot boat with 12 people on it and everyone is as intense as ever because we are totally focused on going faster than Merit and Kvaerner.

Paul Cayard, skipper EF9 EF

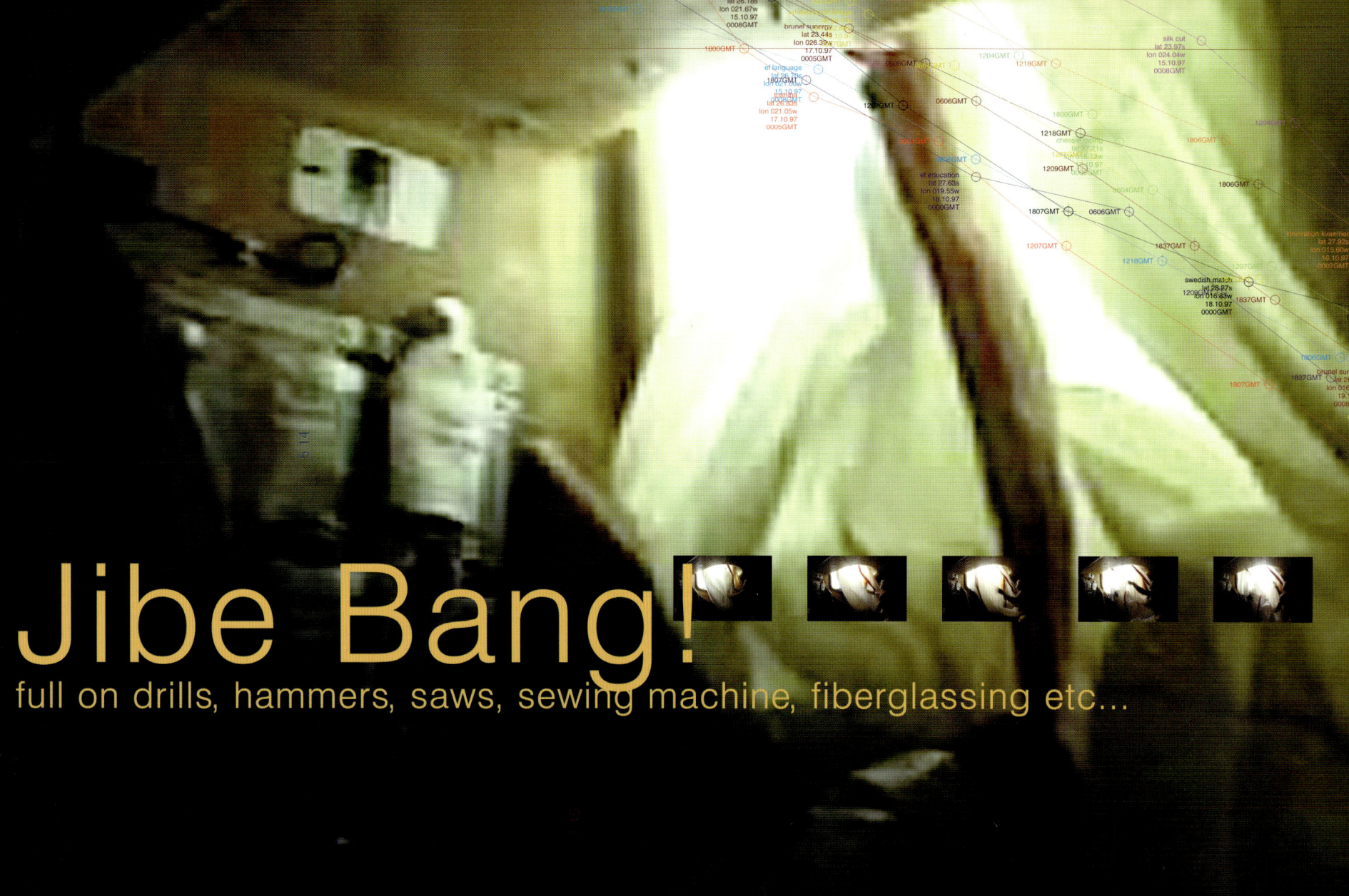

1.13

From Video: Merit_Cup

The demolition derby just has slowed down for a while and, ah, just for the last 6 hours we actually haven't broken anything.

I've got with me a jib halyard clip –
10,000 kilo breaking load.
Sheared right off, right there.
Cost us a lot of time – spinnaker in the water –

Up here I've got a backstay clip
– 10,000 kilo clip –
sheared off right there
– damn near cost us our mast.

These boats are producing a lot more load than anybody has thought.
Certainly as first-time Whitbread competitiors or Whitbread 60 competitiors, more than we had expected.
And we've broken a lot of gear.
All of which we'll be able to fix and into the Southern Ocean but, uh,
it's been a frenetic pace the last few days.
We just managed to hold on to Kvaerner – I don't know how

we've broken everything

but we'll certainly get it fixed and be ready to go into leg two.   END MCP

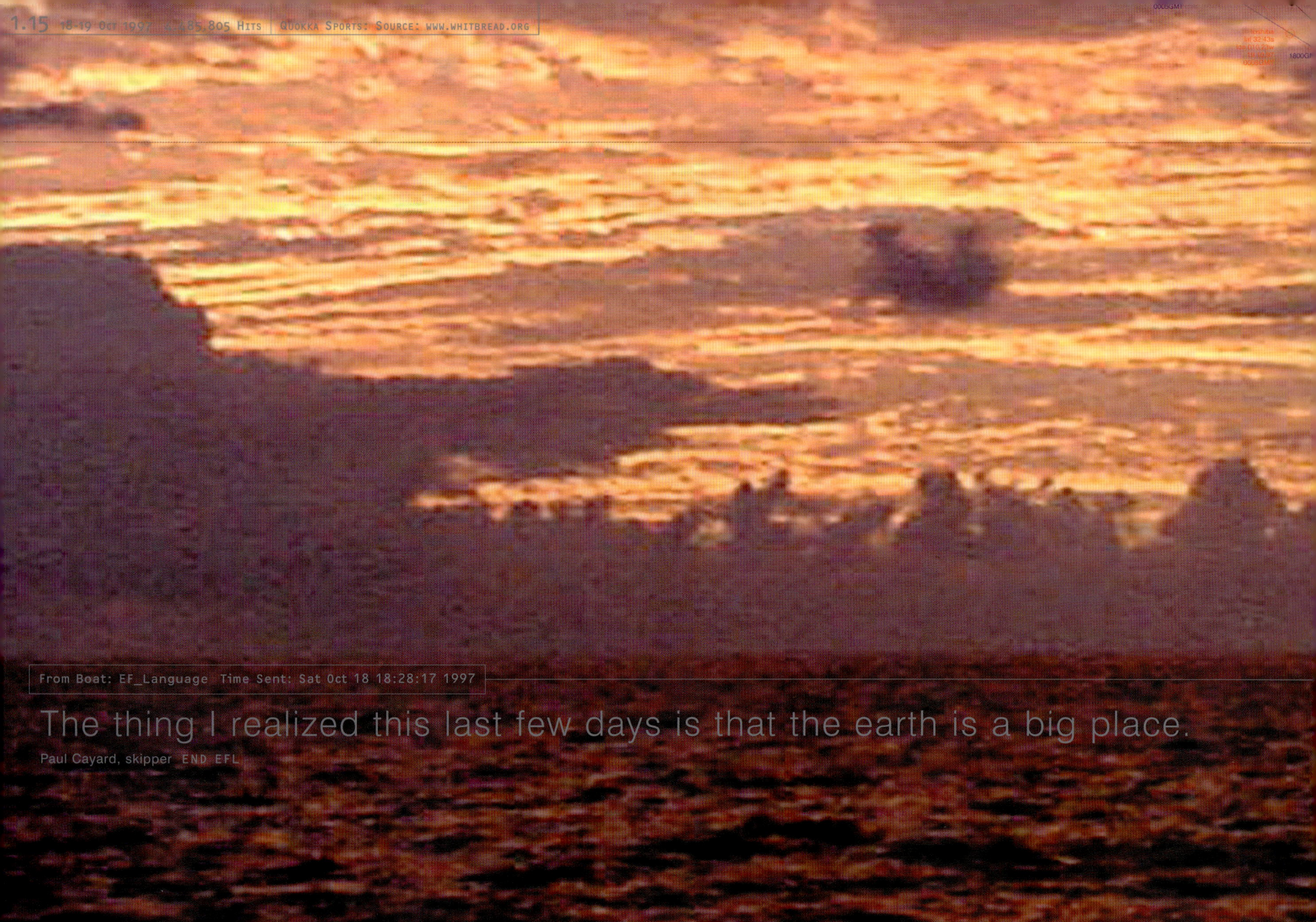

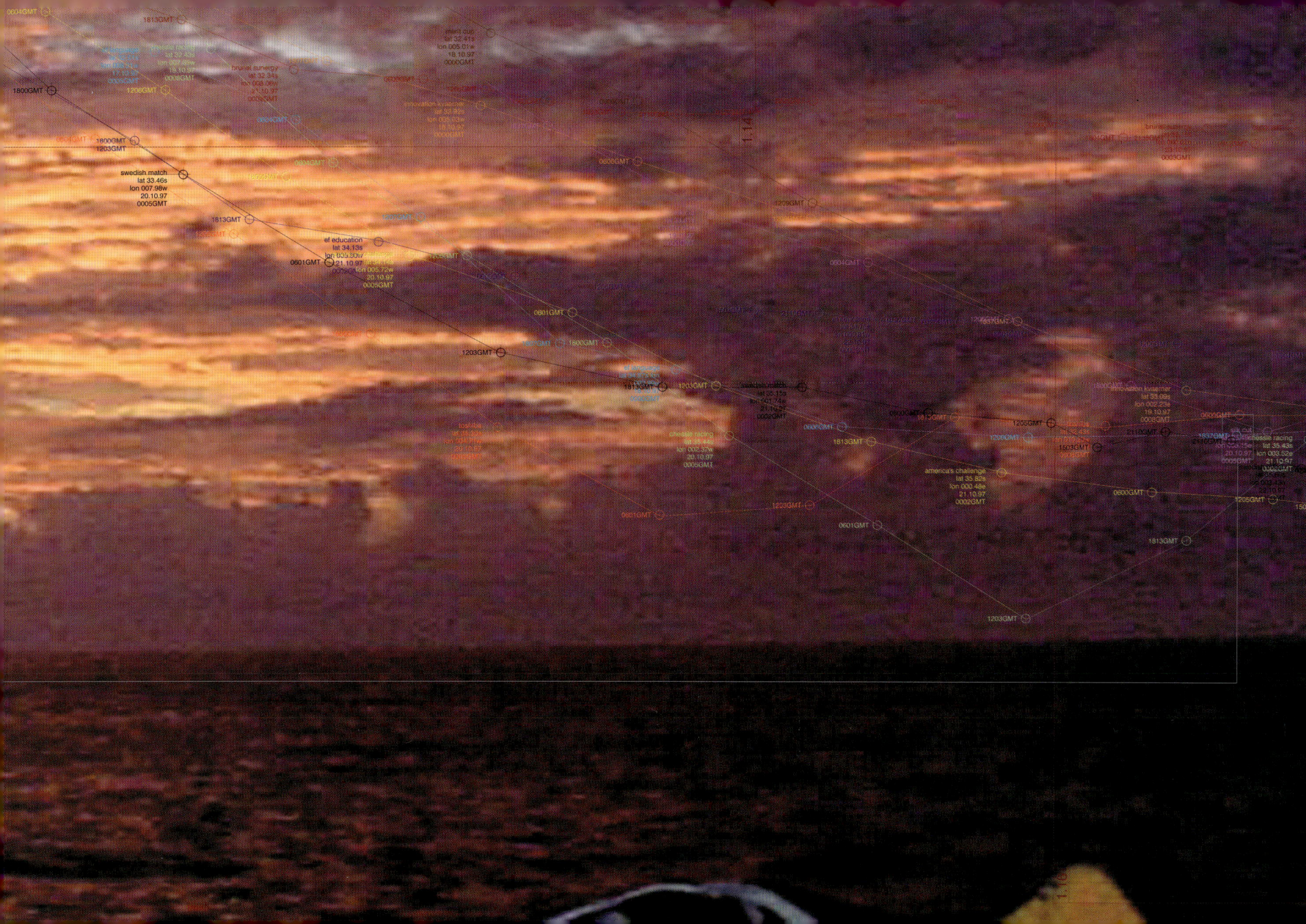

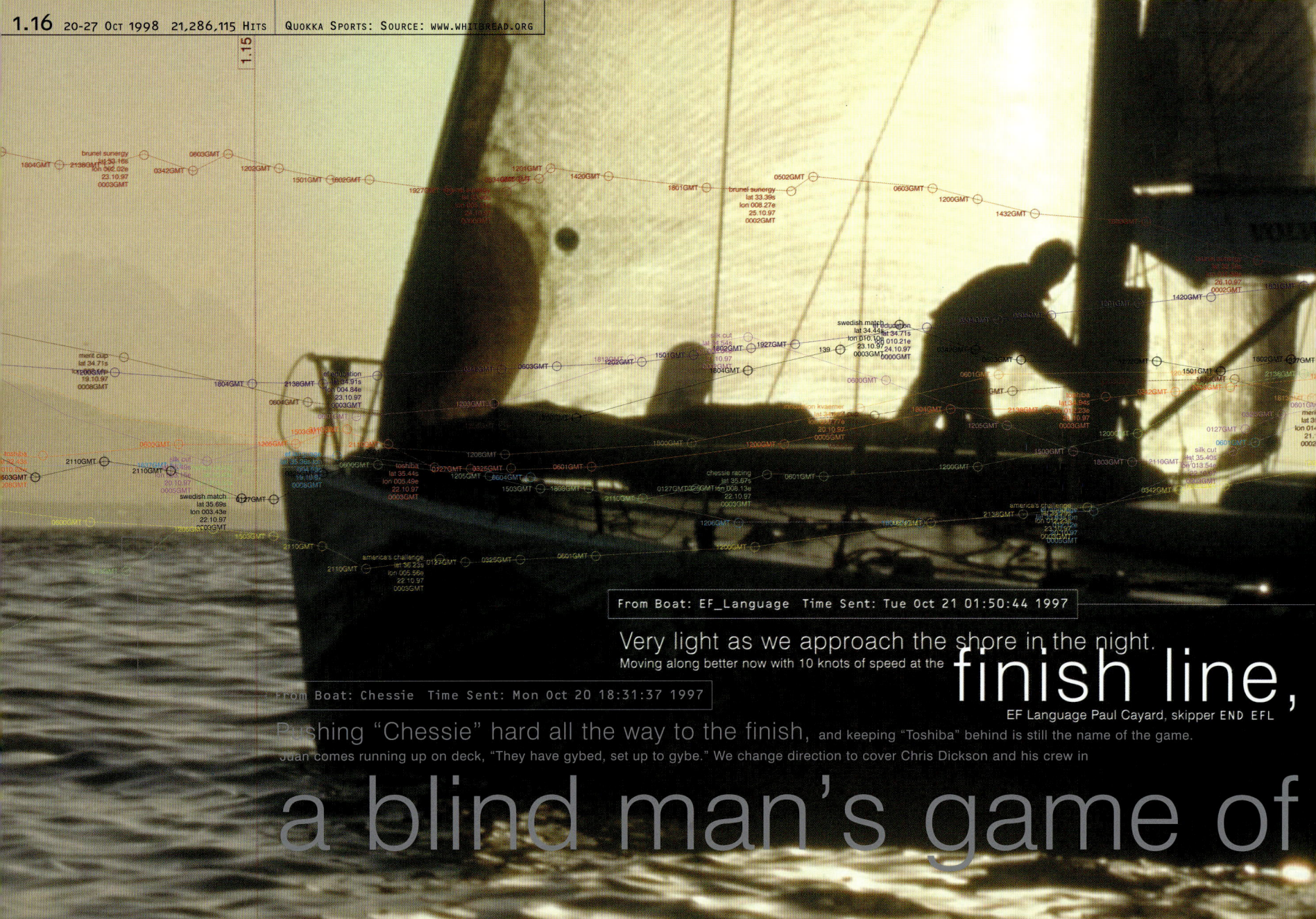

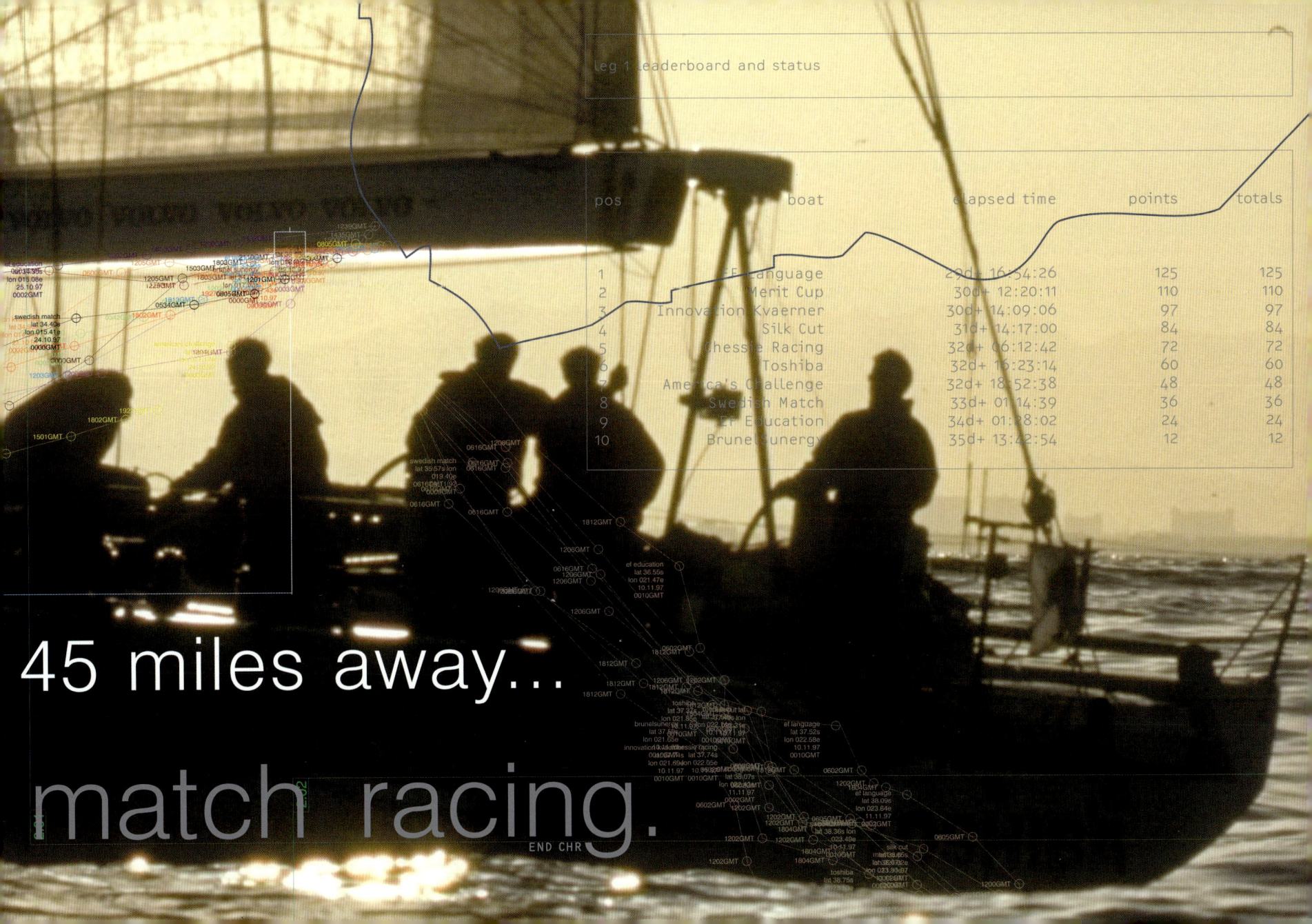

45 miles away...
match racing.

leg 1 leaderboard and status

pos	boat	elapsed time	points	totals
1	EF Language	29d+ 16:54:26	125	125
2	Merit Cup	30d+ 12:20:11	110	110
3	Innovation Kvaerner	30d+ 14:09:06	97	97
4	Silk Cut	31d+ 14:17:00	84	84
5	Chessie Racing	32d+ 06:12:42	72	72
6	Toshiba	32d+ 15:23:14	60	60
7	America's Challenge	32d+ 18:52:38	48	48
8	Swedish Match	33d+ 01:14:39	36	36
9	EF Education	34d+ 01:28:02	24	24
10	BrunelSunergy	35d+ 13:42:54	12	12

2.0.0 08 Nov – 27 Nov 1997 89,727,344 Hits | Quokka Sports: Source: www.whitbread.org

Leg 2

Distance:

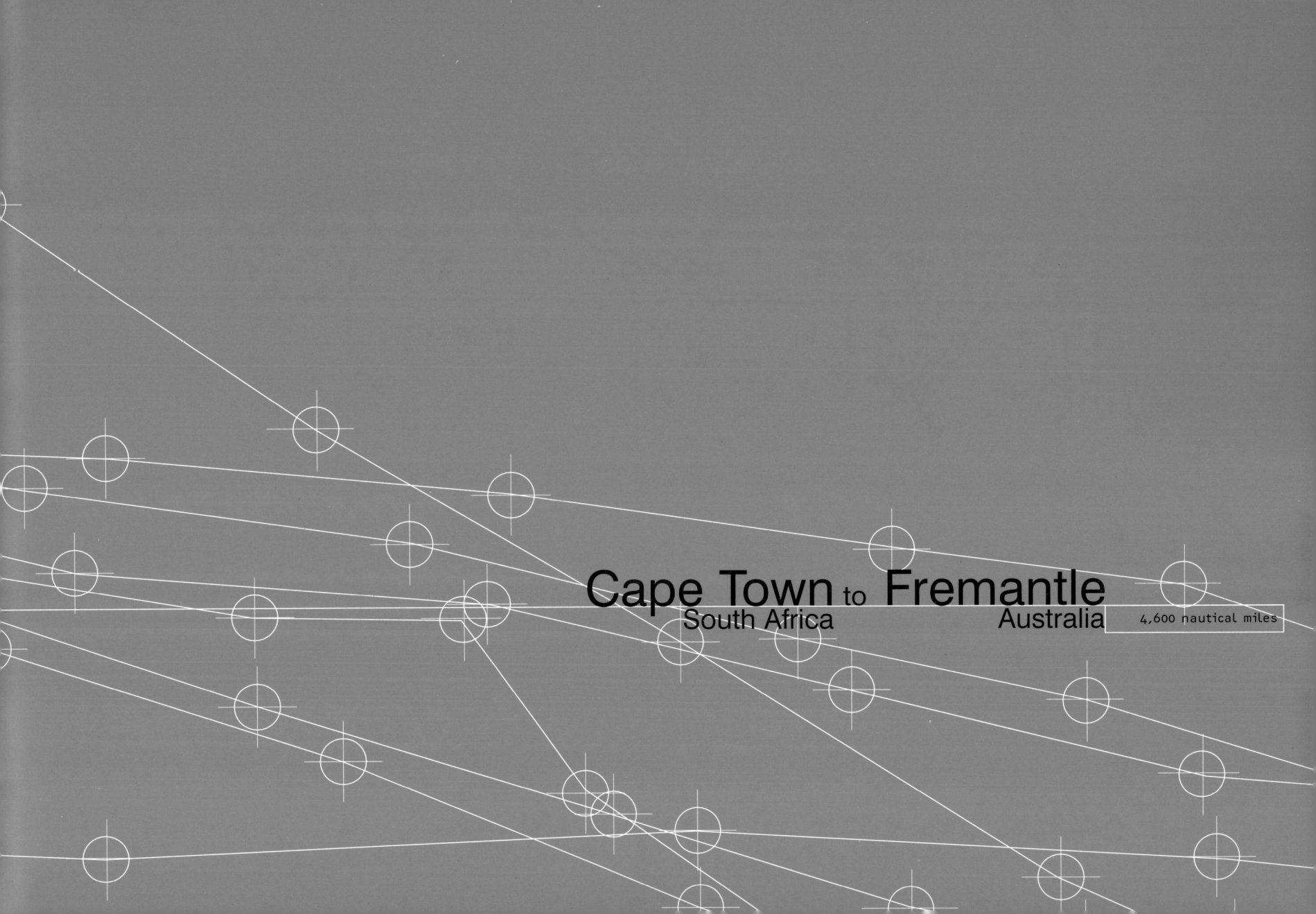

Leg 2: Prelude

BrunelSunergy was the last boat to struggle into Cape Town, South Africa, at the end of Leg 1, six days behind the winner, EF Language. The Dutch boat had been forced to divert to Brazil for repairs to her rudder after a collision with a whale halfway through the leg.

Once all the teams were ashore, the Toshiba team announced shocking news: co-skipper Chris Dickson had resigned. For the record, the team played down rumours that friction between Dickson, his crew and Dennis Conner had promoted the action, noting only that Dickson's decision "was a personal one."

Because Toshiba had left Southampton the favourite of odds-makers, her disappointing sixth-place finish, three full days behind EF Language, had everyone wondering what had gone wrong aboard the boat. When asked directly why he was leaving, Dickson was vague. "I would be letting myself down by continuing the campaign," he said, without explaining how or why that was the case.

Others close to the team said that Dickson felt the crew and boat had not performed up to his standards. Dickson demanded that changes be made in both the crew and on the boat during the stopover. Conner, sources said, did not agree with Dickson's assessment and refused his request. Without the changes Dickson felt were needed, he said he could not sail a competitive race, so he resigned.

This marked the second trip down a Whitbread dead end for Dickson. In the 1993-94 race, he was at the helm of Tokio. He drove her hard for four legs, amassing what looked to be an unassailable 10-hour lead. Eventually, his yacht could not take the stress — her mast came tumbling down on Leg 5.

His announcement this race was met with a good deal of anger and dismay from fans, reflected in a flood of email to the Whitbread Web site. After the terse announcements from both camps, Dickson slipped quietly out of Cape Town and headed north on a safari. No sooner was he gone than the team announced his place would be filled by Toshiba watch captain and four-time Whitbread veteran, Paul Standbridge. It was a glassy-eyed Standbridge who met with reporters later that morning. "The first I knew about it was at 7:30 this morning when I called the lads," he said, when asked how he learned of his sudden elevation to skipper.

Life had begun to settle back to normal around the Cape Town Race Village in the wake of the Dickson bombshell when a second round landed. The unthinkable happened — an entire syndicate was forced to withdraw. Dr. Neil Barth announced that he was withdrawing his America's Challenge team from the race. While everyone was shocked by the announcement, none were more so than skipper Ross Field and his crew. Suddenly, the winner of the last Whitbread had no boat to race. The crew knew that Barth had been having trouble finding a major sponsor, but they had been told just before The Whitbread began that three Mexican beer and food companies had joined together to sponsor the team. In his withdrawal announcement, Barth would only say there had been "unforeseen circumstances involving a third party in Mexico." The bottom line was that the money never materialised.

It was a bitter disappointment for the team. But it was also a disappointment for sailing fans anxious to see how the America's Challenge yacht performed. Of the ten boats in the race, only two were designed by someone other than Bruce Farr. One, America's Challenge, was drawn by another American designer, Alan Andrews. The boat differed in many respects from the Farr boats, and her crew said she sailed remarkably well. They believed the boat could beat her Farr-designed competitors. Now, no one would know whether they were right: America's Challenge would sit out the race tied to a dock.

The unexpected Leg 1 victory by EF Language, Dickson's sudden departure, and the withdrawal of America's Challenge sent the bookies back to their calculators. When they finished weighing the changes, EF Language was suddenly the new co-favourite, ranking alongside Merit Cup. Silk Cut and Innovation Kvaerner shared second, while Toshiba had slipped to third.

Leg 2: Cape Town, South Africa, to Fremantle, Australia

"Whatever the programme, whoever it is, no matter how much it is worth to you, DON'T EVER COME DOWN HERE AGAIN!"
Chessie Racing Watch Captain
Grant Spanhake on the Southern Ocean

On 8 November 1997, the nine remaining boats left Cape Town to begin one of the most difficult legs of the race. Leg 2 would take them deep into the cold and treacherous Southern Ocean, where gales are the norm, sleet covers sails and lines, and the deck is often slick with snow.

None of this was apparent that first sunny afternoon. The start was a picture postcard: Table Mountain with her cloth on acted as a backdrop to the unfolding drama. With a light westerly breeze blowing, Merit Cup was first across the starting line. Twenty-five minutes later it was Silk Cut in the lead, as the boats rounded the final buoy and began to chart a course south. The conventional wisdom among the fleet was to stick close inshore, and it seemed to be what everyone was doing. Then abruptly, Swedish Match broke from the fleet and pointed her nose out to sea. The others watched in amazement.

The decision to go offshore had been unplanned. Swedish Match skipper Gunnar Krantz made a split-second decision that would seal his team's fate for the duration of the leg. Co-skipper Erle Williams had spotted a freighter far offshore. He could see smoke from her stack being blown briskly away. Williams pointed this out to Krantz, who, after a moment's thought, suddenly cranked the yacht's wheel and headed out to sea. "When we left Cape Town I had every intention of sticking close to the rest of the fleet as they followed the coast," said Krantz, later. Williams recalled the moment. "My legs started to shake a little as we tacked over there," he said. "Gunnar just kept driving the boat fast. I think if he had got shaky I would have bailed out and we would have trailed the whole fleet back into the coast."

It would prove to be one of those instinctual moves that distinguish born leaders. The rest of the fleet meekly hugged the shore. Their caution earned them meagre winds, averaging less than one knot of boatspeed. EF Language skipper Paul Cayard complained, "We are drifting around out here without rhyme or reason." Meanwhile, Swedish Match found the wind the freighter's smoke hinted of offshore, leaving Krantz and his crew sailing along at ten times the speed of the rest of the fleet at a healthy 10 knots.

A day into Leg 2, Swedish Match had opened up a 44-mile lead over the nearest boat, EF Language. During the night, Krantz reported enjoying near-perfect reaching conditions in 12- to 16-knot southwest winds. By Day 2, there was more than a 100-mile spread separating the fleet, with EF Education bringing up the rear.

By the fourth day out of Cape Town, EF Language skipper Cayard was receiving lessons in humility. The Leg 1 winner was stuck in eighth place, and he was not enjoying the feeling. "No more jokes," the normally upbeat Cayard wrote that day. "This is not funny anymore."

The next day, EF Language navigator Mark Rudiger located a bit of wind, and the boat clawed her way from eighth to fifth. Disdainfully, Swedish Match only continued to extend her lead. She was now 205 miles ahead of the second-place boat, Innovation Kvaerner. Just past Prince Edward Island, the two leaders were now well within the Roaring Forties, where gales are the rule rather than the exception.

Crews began preparing for the beating they knew this part of the ocean could deliver. They stowed gear below, then tied down anything that had to remain above. The precautions were not a moment too soon. Just after passing Prince Edward Island, the wind gauges aboard Innovation Kvaerner shot up. "Yes, we are in the Roaring Forties," reported skipper Knut Frostad at the end of Day 6. "It is windy, wet, cold and wet, wet, wet, wet. And we love it."

The strong winds allowed the boats to rack up impressive mileage. Swedish Match reported a 24-hour run of 420.6 miles, just 14 miles short of the monohull record set by Toshiba in July.

The boats behind the leaders had yet to reach these heady winds. Cayard and his crew on EF Language were still in fifth, four miles behind Merit Cup. Back in seventh place and stuck in a high-pressure trap was Silk Cut, whose skipper, Lawrie Smith, was clearly not happy. "There is an old saying that below forty there is no law, below fifty there is no God, and below sixty there is no mercy," wrote Smith. "We think that it should be amended to read that below forty there is no wind!"

After a week of racing Swedish Match, now nearly halfway to Fremantle, was still in the lead and still showing the fastest average speed of the fleet, 15.6 knots. She held firmly to a 300-mile lead over Innovation Kvaerner, leaving Toshiba in third, 452 miles back. Overall, the fleet was now strung out across 900 miles of the Southern Ocean.

As boat after boat traversed the Roaring Forties, damage reports started pouring in. Chessie Racing reported damage to her keel after a high-speed collision with a whale. Bowman Jerry Kirby went overboard in a wetsuit to survey the damage. He announced that the whale had taken out a four-foot section of the leading edge of the keel.

Lawrie Smith reported damage to his yacht after surfing down a steep wave while being pushed by a 32-knot tailwind. The W60 was doing about 25 knots when she buried her bow into the trough of the wave. A solid wall of water swept aft, dragging full sail bags along with it. As this frigid stew of water and sails travelled the length of the yacht, it tore off every stanchion along the way.

On Merit Cup the crew began pushing the boat hard after being overtaken by the all-woman EF Education team. They hoisted a large fractional spinnaker, but Dalton at the helm lost control of the boat. The yacht twisted sideways and slammed down on her side. "We laid on our side for five minutes," Dalton said. "During all this time the boat laid on her side kicking." Other than damage to the spinnaker (and Dalton's pride), the boat was in good shape when she finally came up for air.

By Day 11, it seemed that Swedish Match could do no wrong on this leg. For 12 hours the previous day she had been the fastest boat in the fleet, averaging just over 18 knots. Meanwhile, Leg 1's golden boy, Cayard, struggled back in fifth place, unable to get traction enough to vault his team to the front of the pack. He responded by pushing his boat and crew even harder, reporting on Day 12 that he was sailing at 20 knots in 30 knots of wind. "The boat is shuddering, shaking, slamming and generally just in a state of violence," Cayard reported. On deck, he said, it was just plain freezing.

Two days after her last mishap, Merit Cup found herself on her side again, following a particularly nasty broach in high seas. The boat lay flat on the water, pinned down by a succession of icy waves that crashed, one after the other, on her. It took fast work of shifting water ballast to finally bring the boat upright. This was two soakings in a row for the Merit Cup's crew, at a time and in a place where being wet was not recommended. "It is now cold, it snowed on deck today and none of this adds to our feeling of well being," a despondent Dalton reported.

For Silk Cut, Day 13 proved a rare lucky one. The Race Office recorded that Smith and his team had logged 449.1 miles in 24 hours, smashing the record Toshiba had set in July by 15 miles. Silk Cut averaged 18.7 knots during the period. Later that day she averaged a blistering 19.4 knots in one six-hour period, proving this new breed of W60 not only could handle brutal Southern Ocean conditions, but thrived on them.

Silk Cut's record run aside, Swedish Match maintained her chokehold on the lead. Innovation Kvaerner held stubbornly to second. Frostad radioed in to report winds gusting over 50 knots, snow and high waves, conditions that would have most cruising sailors sailing under bare poles. But these were not ordinary sailors. They had a race to win. So the Kevlar stayed up and the boats crashed mercilessly along. Frostad reported early that morning that a crewman had been slammed by a wave into the steering wheel. The crewman was fine, but the wheel was snapped completely off the pedestal. A bit later the boat nosed into a wave; when it emerged from the other side, the pulpit was gone.

Back in the pack, Cayard was fighting hard as Lawrie Smith mounted a prolonged attack on EF Language. Cayard, with his overall first position to defend, fought back furiously, pushing boat and crew harder and harder. However, the Southern Ocean had a lesson for this newcomer. Cayard would later describe it as "a night of terror." The boat was sailing through a fierce gale when she suffered a broach that damaged her mainsail and boom. Crewman Curtis Blewett had a dangerous 'front-row' seat when the boat broached: He was 60 feet up the mast at the time trying to reset the spinnaker when the sail blew open suddenly. The force threw the yacht off balance, and the helmsman lost control. The boat spun violently into the wind. "Curtis was up the rig while it was shaking violently," Cayard recalled. "I really thought he was going to die."

It was quite a different scene aboard Swedish Match, now a mere 370 miles from the finish line. It was Day 15, with Swedish Match gliding along at a pleasant 13.5 knots. As they had since Erle Williams spotted the freighter's smoke, the winds favoured this Swedish boat. Clearly, she was going to win this leg. As that reality set in, skippers from less-fortunate boats began to acknowledge the fact. On Merit Cup, back in seventh place, Grant Dalton boasted that he thought he now had sixth-placed Chessie Racing in his sights, then quickly added that of course those were little more "than the final words of a dying man."

No one took the outcome of Leg 2 harder than Paul Cayard, stuck back in fifth. He took himself to the woodshed in long, cathartic emails to shore. "I take full blame for the mistakes made," Cayard wrote as Swedish Match crossed the finish line. He acknowledged that, as critics had claimed before the race, he was new to the savage conditions of The Whitbread's Southern Ocean legs. Consequently, he had badly underestimated the debilitating effects the harsh conditions would have on himself and his crew. "Now we know how it feels to still be racing after the leader finishes."

Nineteen hours behind Swedish Match, Innovation Kvaerner crossed the line in second; the next day Toshiba followed in third. Silk Cut arrived ten hours later to capture fourth. EF Language slipped into port in fifth, a humbling setback for the skipper and crew who had dazzled everyone on Leg 1.

Was Cayard's first-leg win simply beginner's luck? He had seven more legs to answer that question.

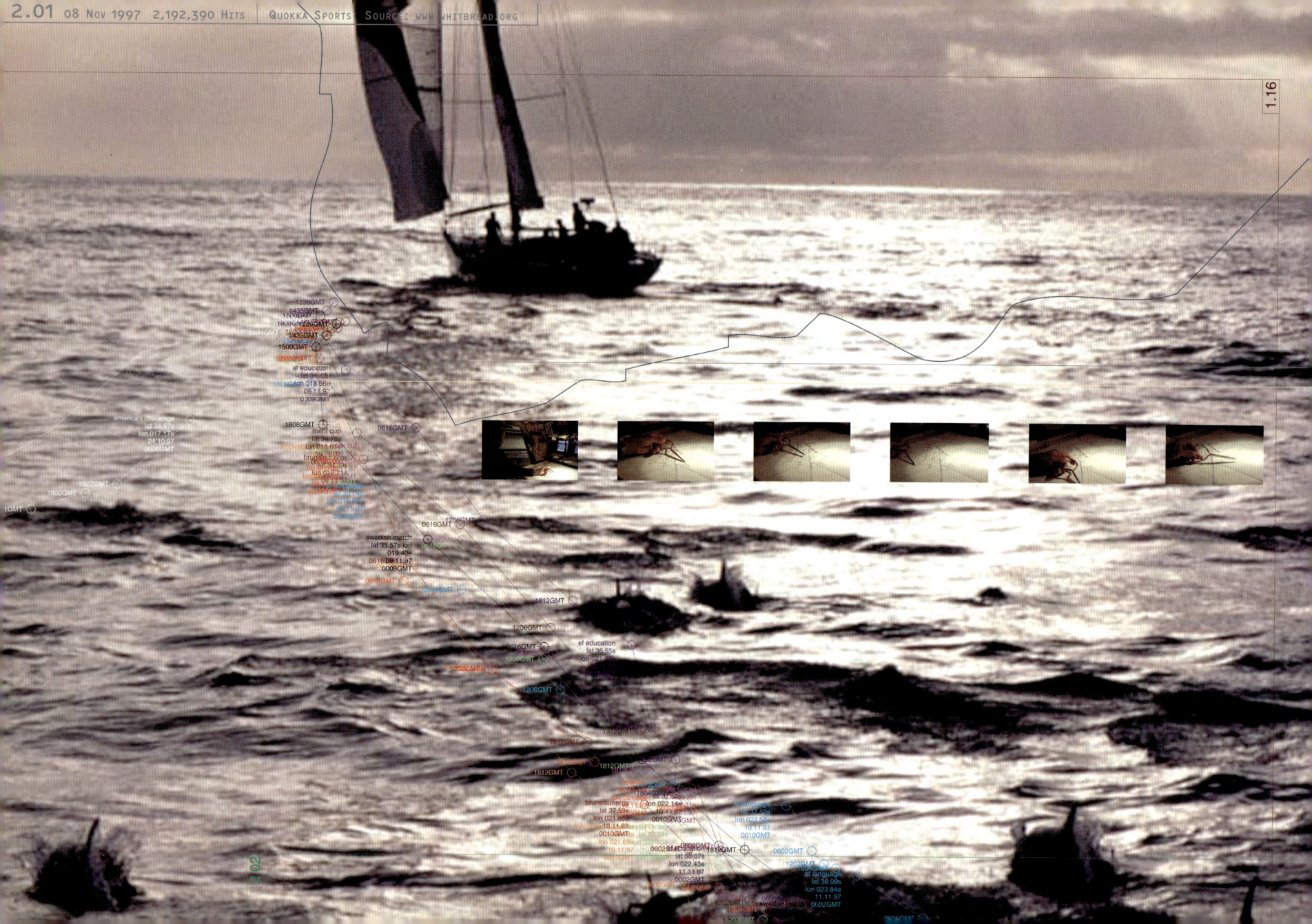

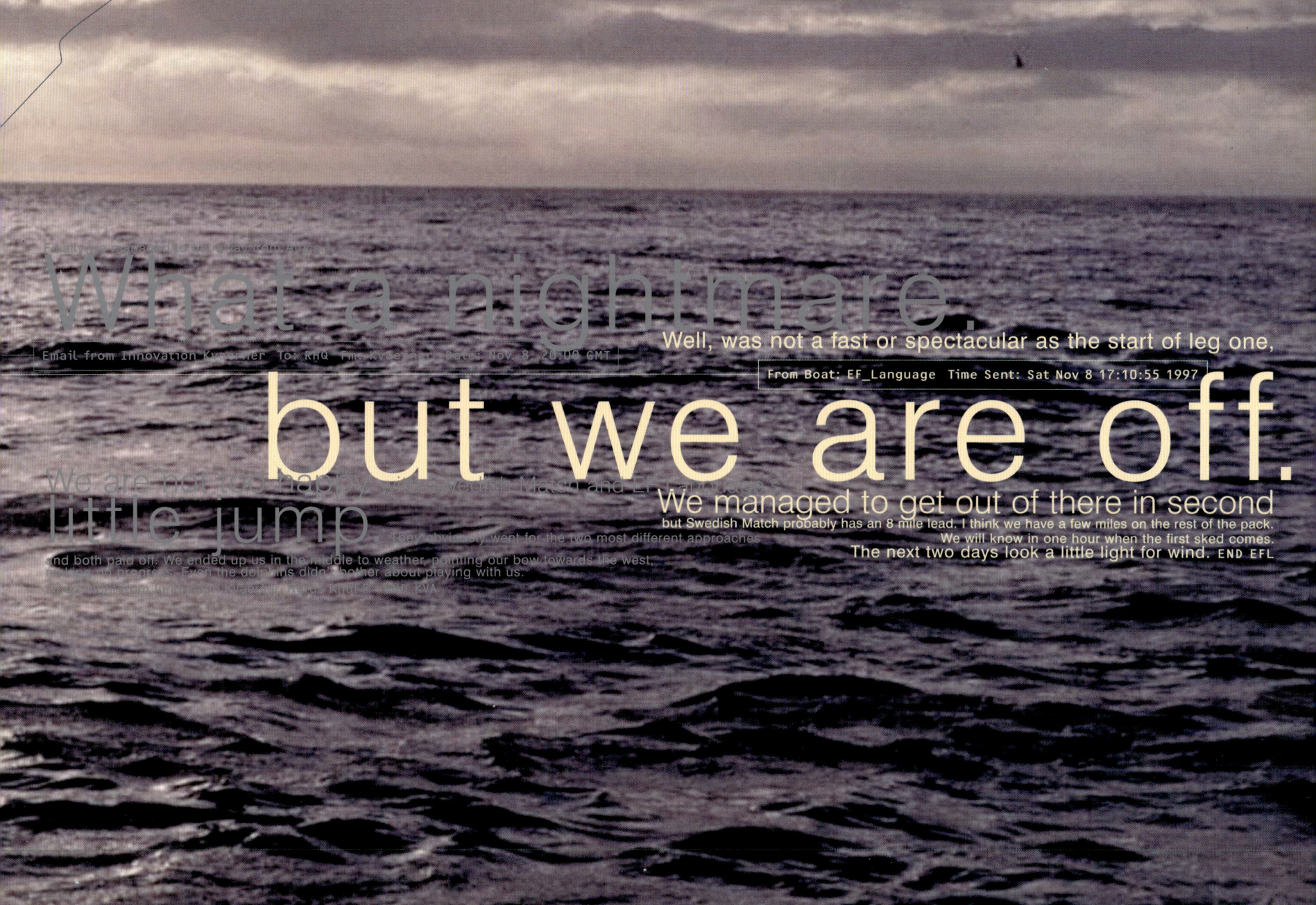

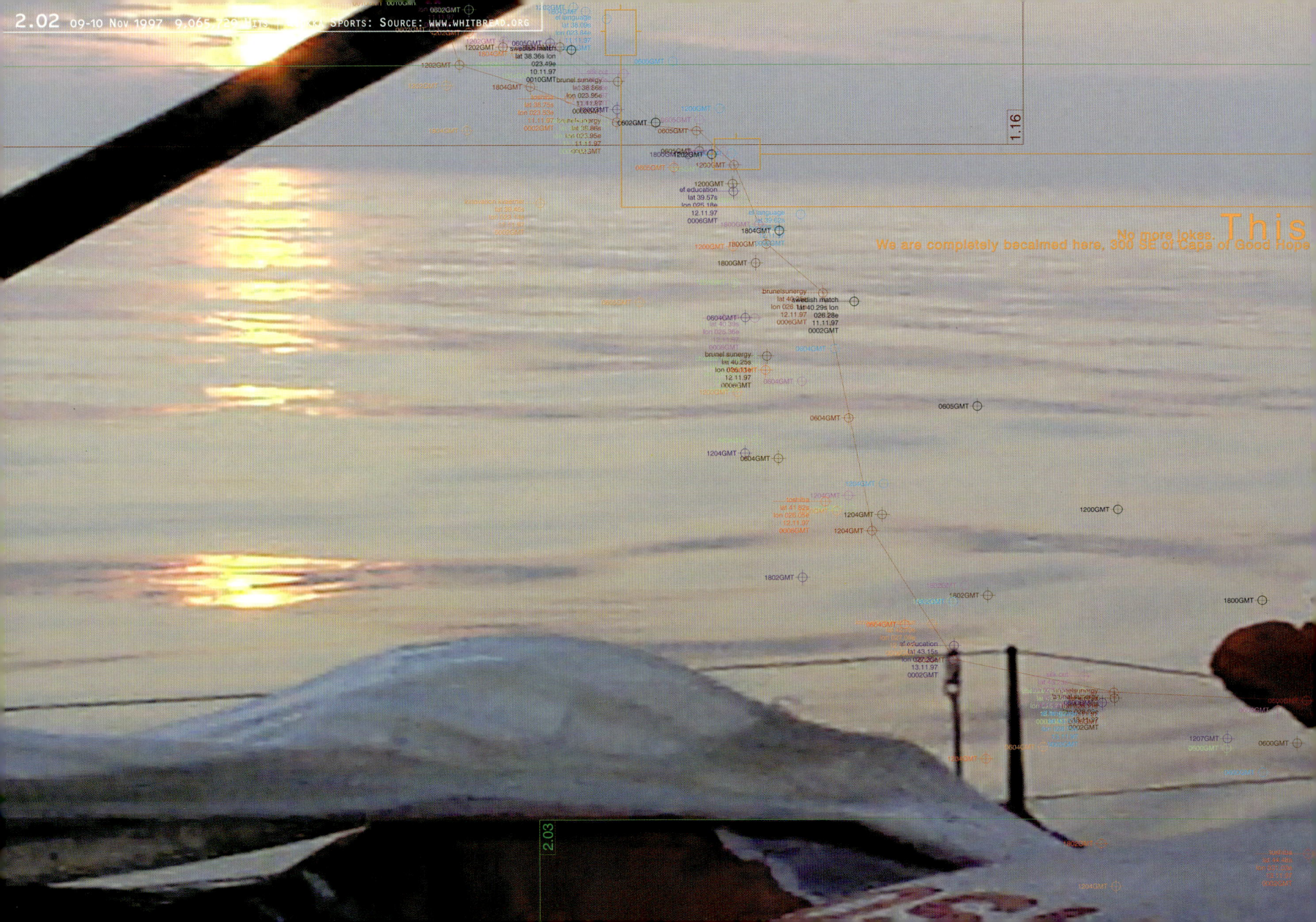

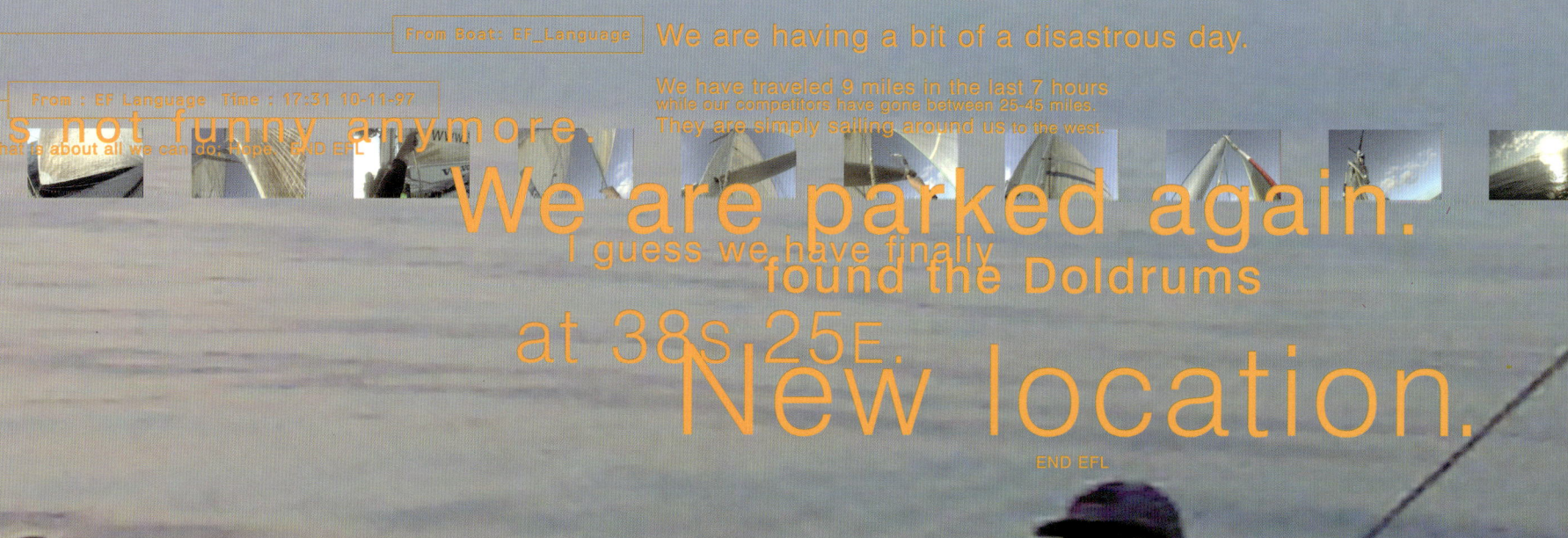

From Boat: EF_Language   We are having a bit of a disastrous day.

We have traveled 9 miles in the last 7 hours while our competitors have gone between 25-45 miles. They are simply sailing around us to the west.

From : EF Language Time : 17:31 10-11-97
is not funny anymore.
That's about all we can do. Hope. END EFL

We are parked again.
I guess we have finally found the Doldrums at 38s 25E.
New location.

END EFL

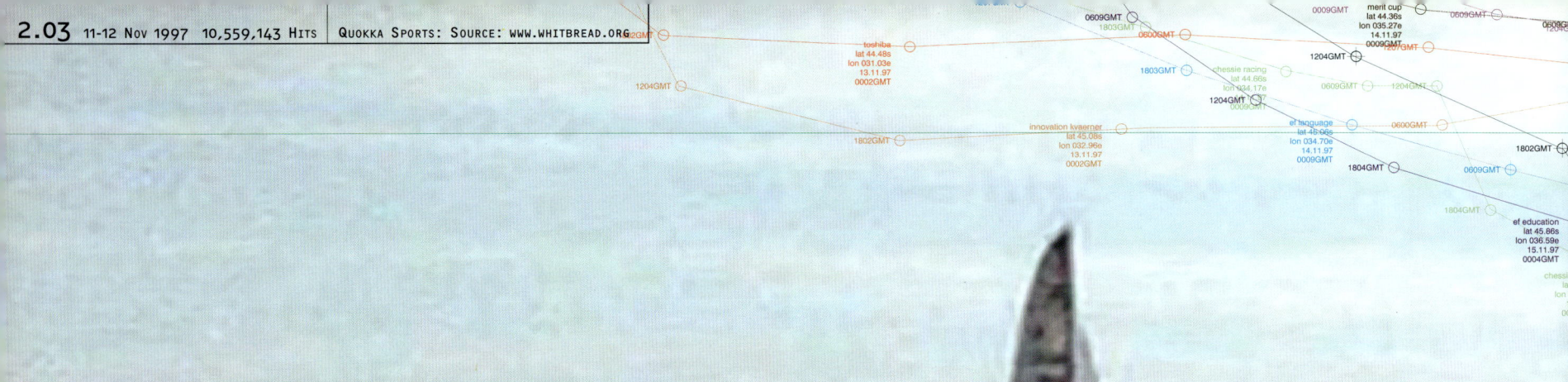

2.03 11-12 Nov 1997 10,559,143 Hits Quokka Sports: Source: www.whitbread.org

From Boat: Silk_Cut Time Sent: Tue Nov 11 21:46:53 1997

A very frustrating day.

We have ***** up in not being more protective of the south.
We let Chessie slip by us two nights ago and last night Merit slipped through leeward.

We are trying very hard to get southing on everyone at the moment
but with everyone else playing the same game it is always going to be hard.

It comes down to just how many miles you are prepared to give away in order to place your boat where you want it.
Right now we are making al

It's always very hard to do but sometimes it is the only way out.
I am confident that we can make up the miles with some slightly more aggressive tactics.
Lawrie Smith and the crew of Silk Cut

END SCT

From Boat: Chessie_Racing Time Sent: Wed, 12 Nov 1997 18:58:47 +0000
Day 4 - Chessie Wind Speed 17 knots Boat Speed 10.5 knots

During the last **24 hours** "Chessie" has gone from

The mood onboard is very quiet and sober.
The joke and story telling is down to a minimum since
Merit Cup sailed away from us yesterday which put a damper on the whole day.
We are trimming and driving as hard as we can

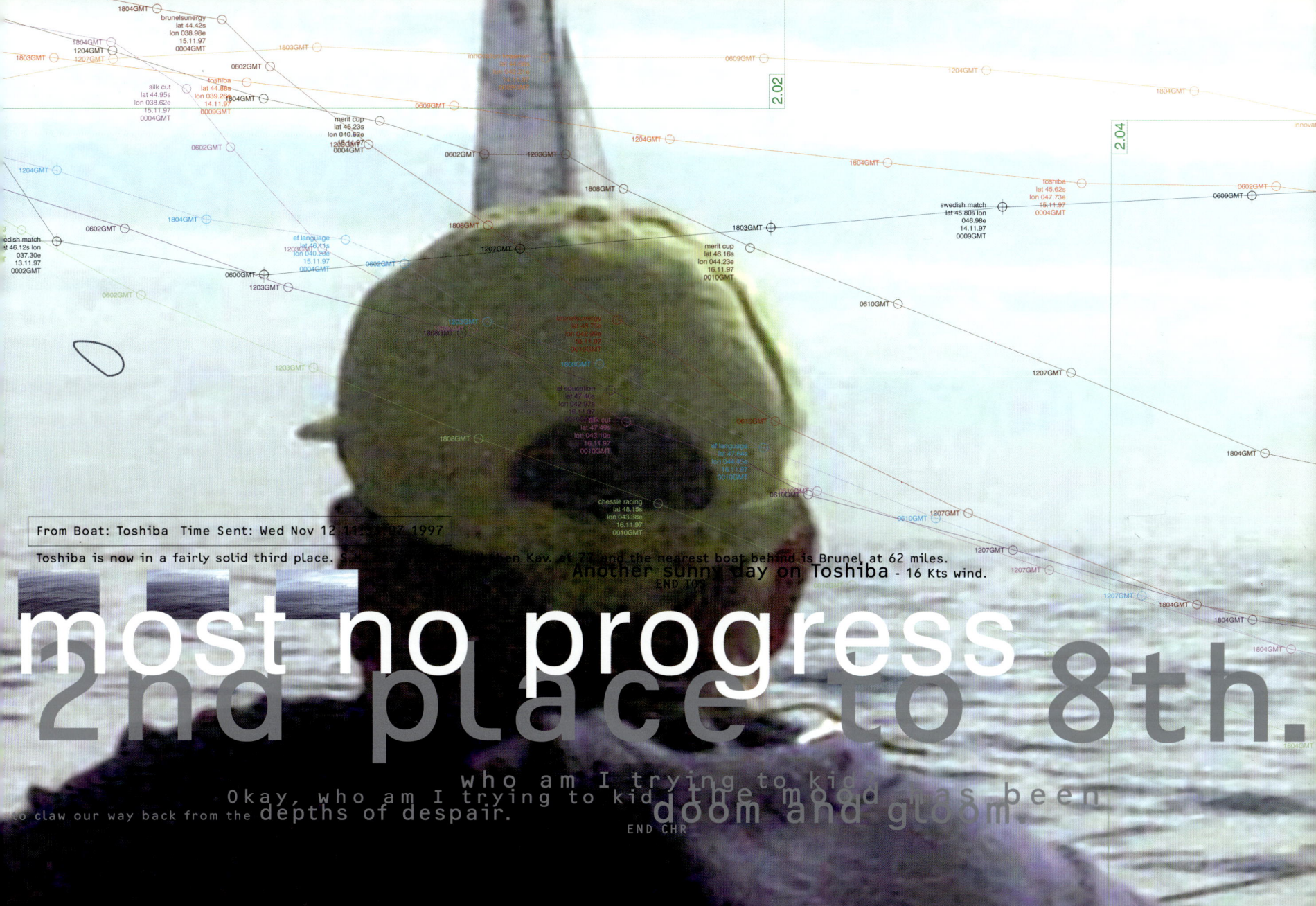

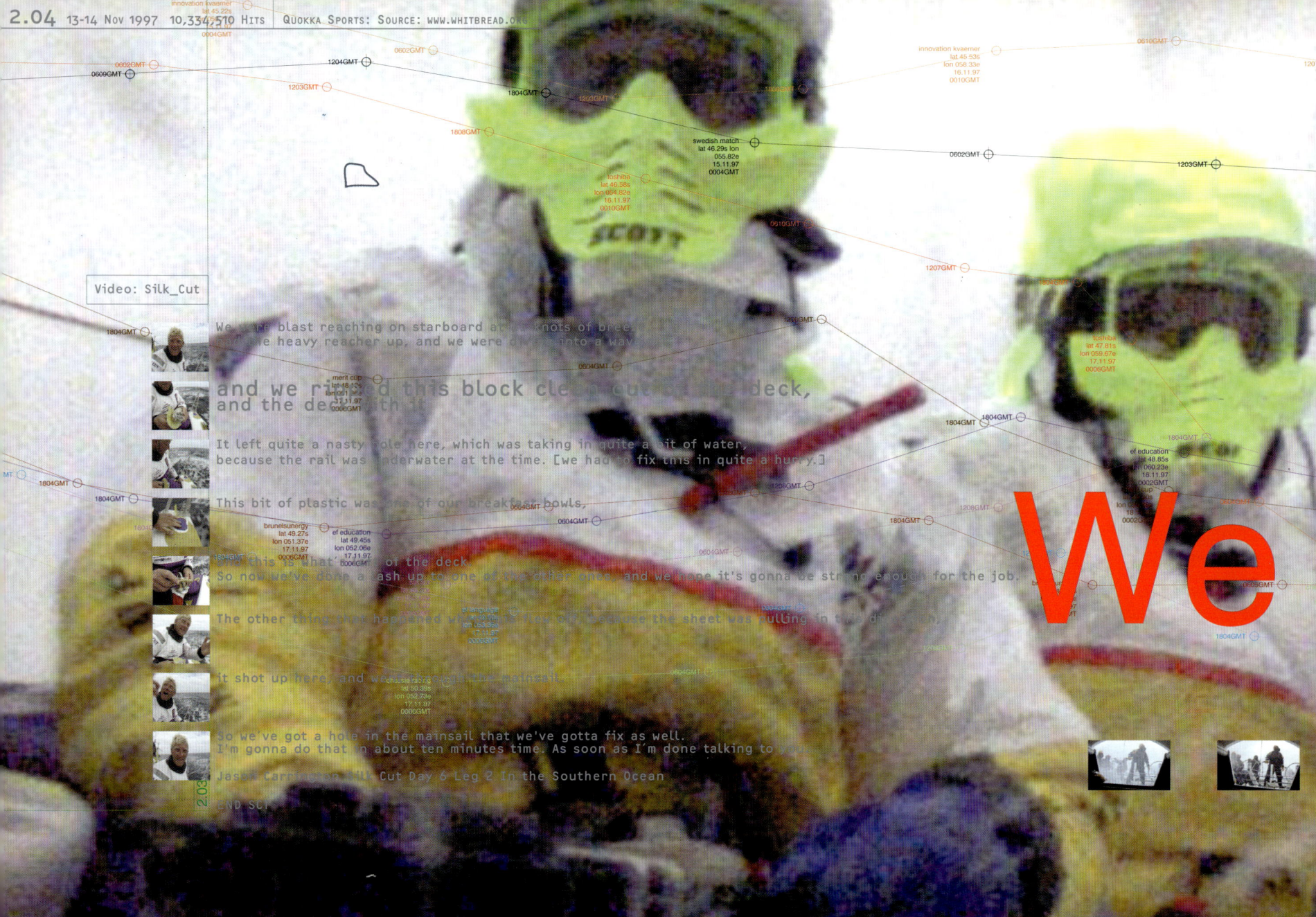

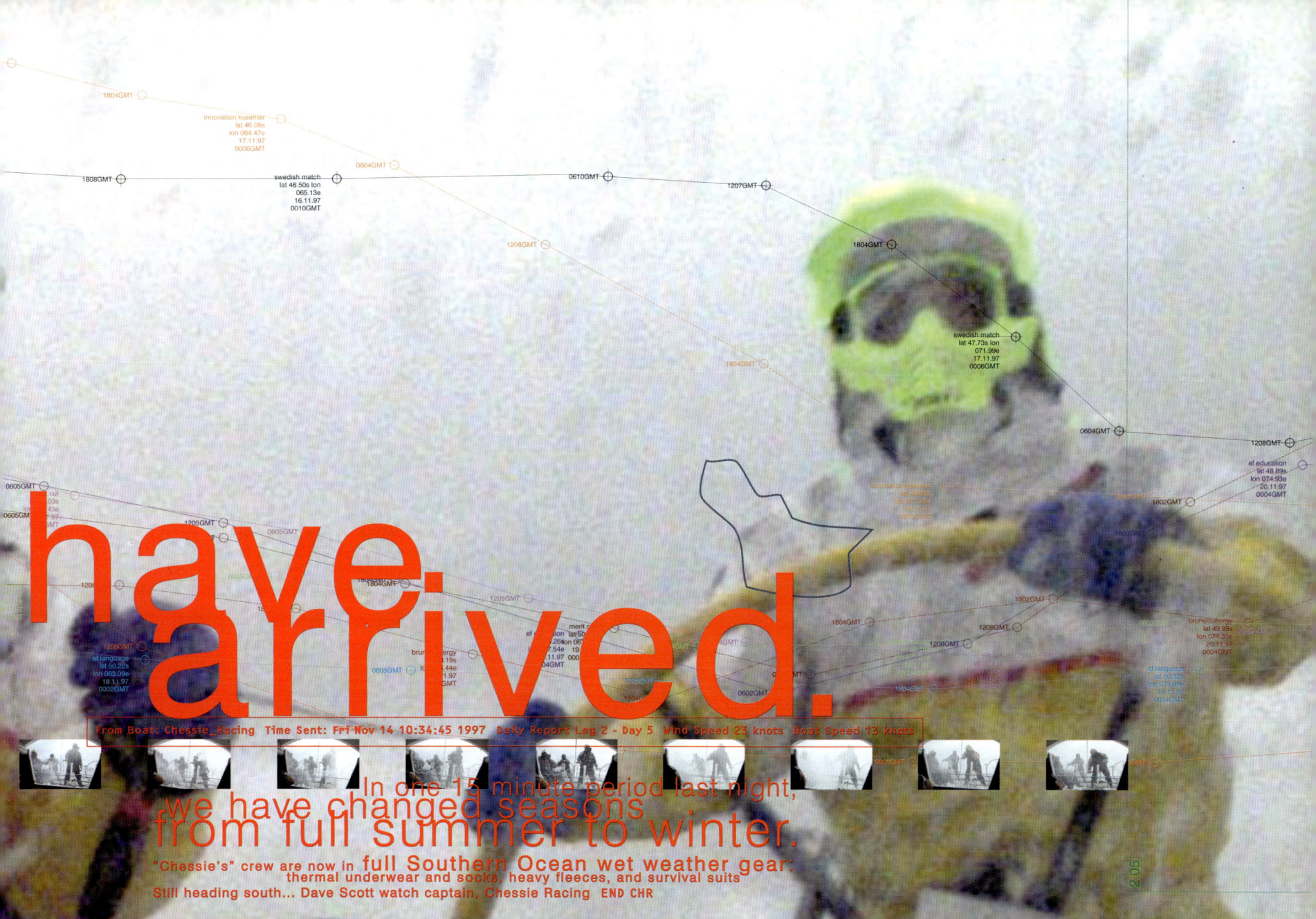

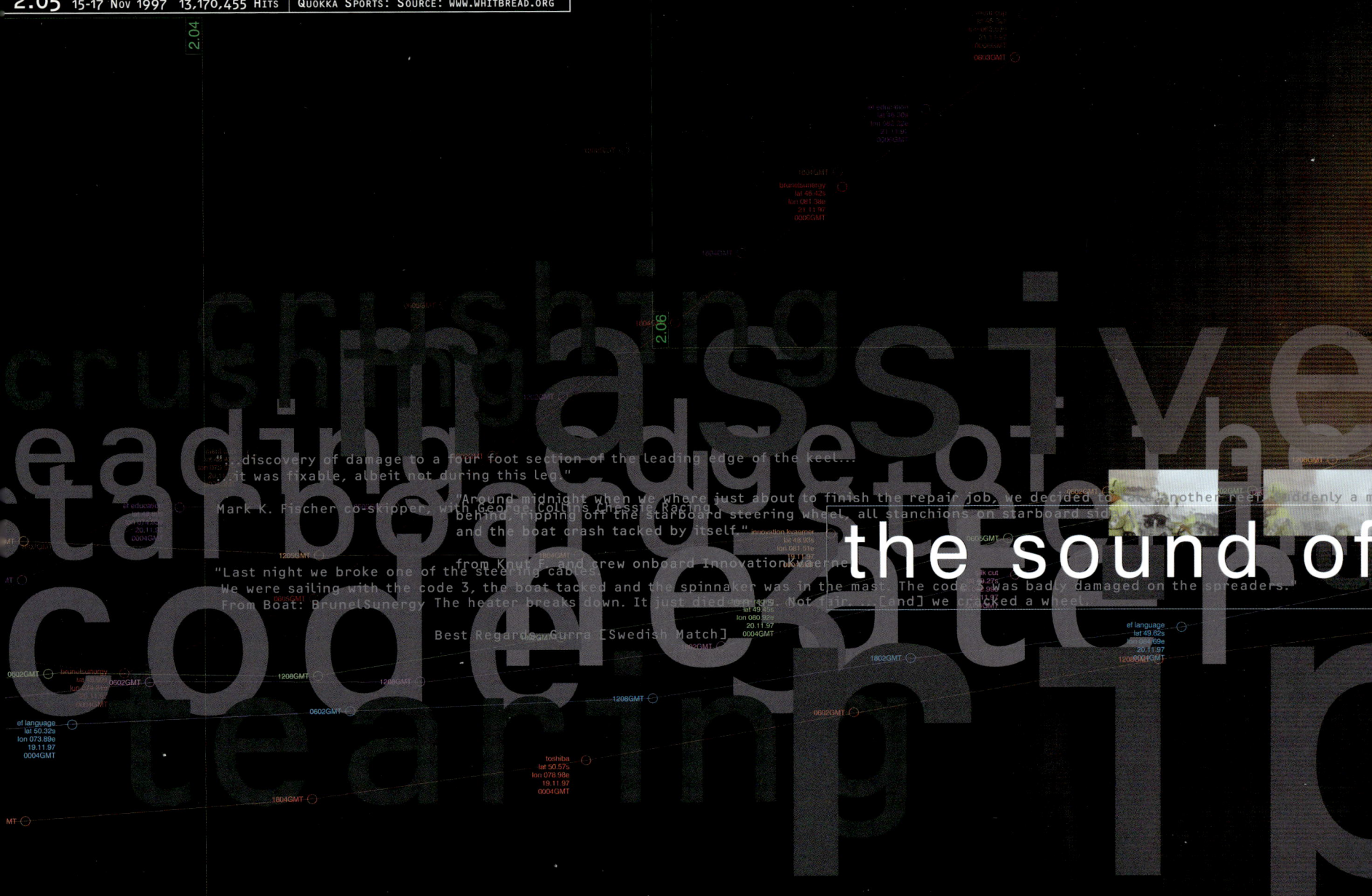

From Boat: EF_Language Time Sent: Mon Nov 17 08:58:19 1997 Daily Report #1

tearing, crushing and breaking

The wind had built to a lovely 30 knots, from 010, so we were dead running with the big Kahuna up and spinnaker stay sail. We were quite loaded. The boat came to a sudden slow down and then there was the sound of tearing, crushing and breaking.

Sails overboard hanging by their ties. Unidentifiable bodies running around trying vainly to lift these sails back onboard from over the side. A large wave had come down the deck and put so much pressure on the sails that they wiped out the back half of the lifelines and stanchions on the portside.

END EFL

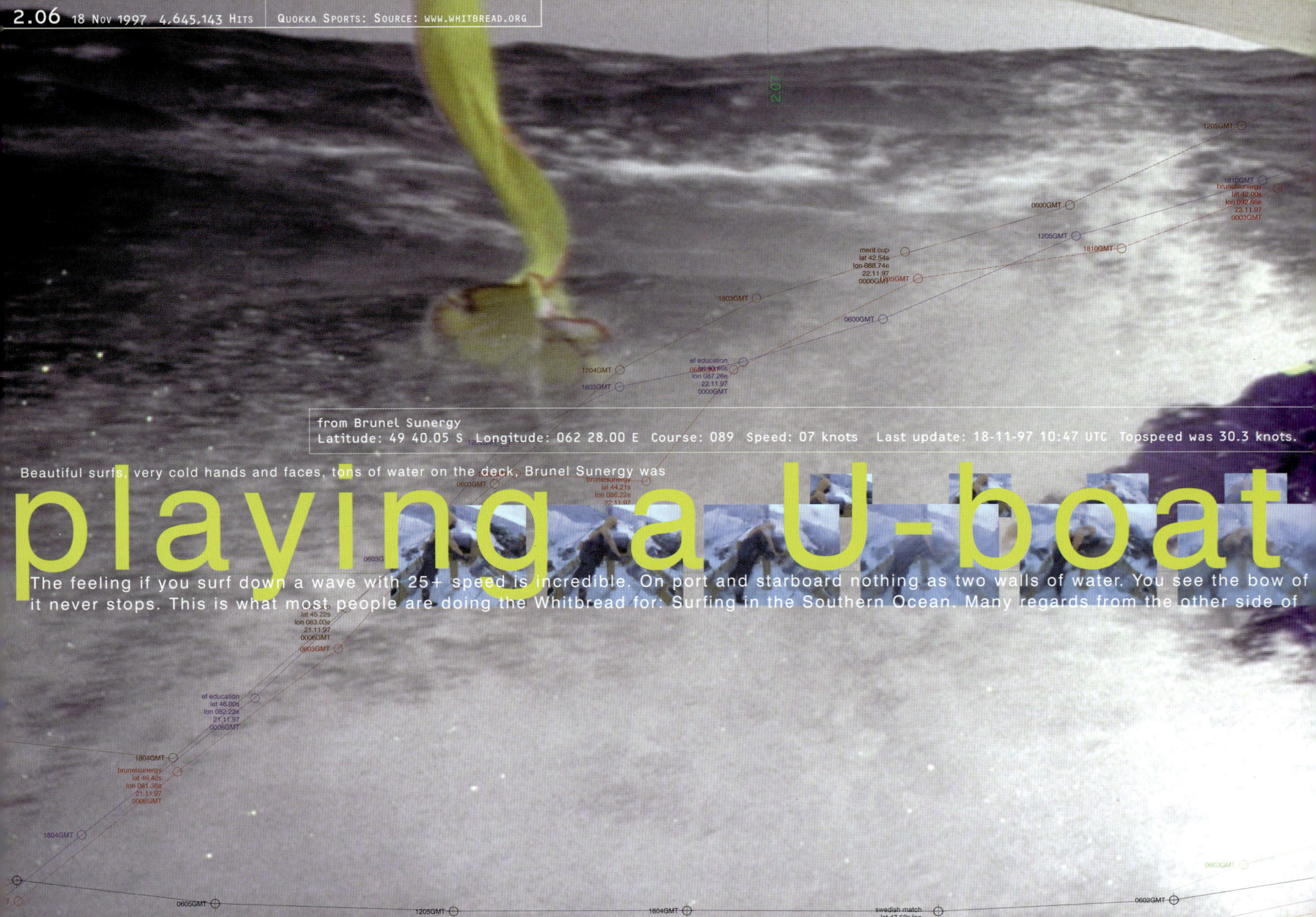

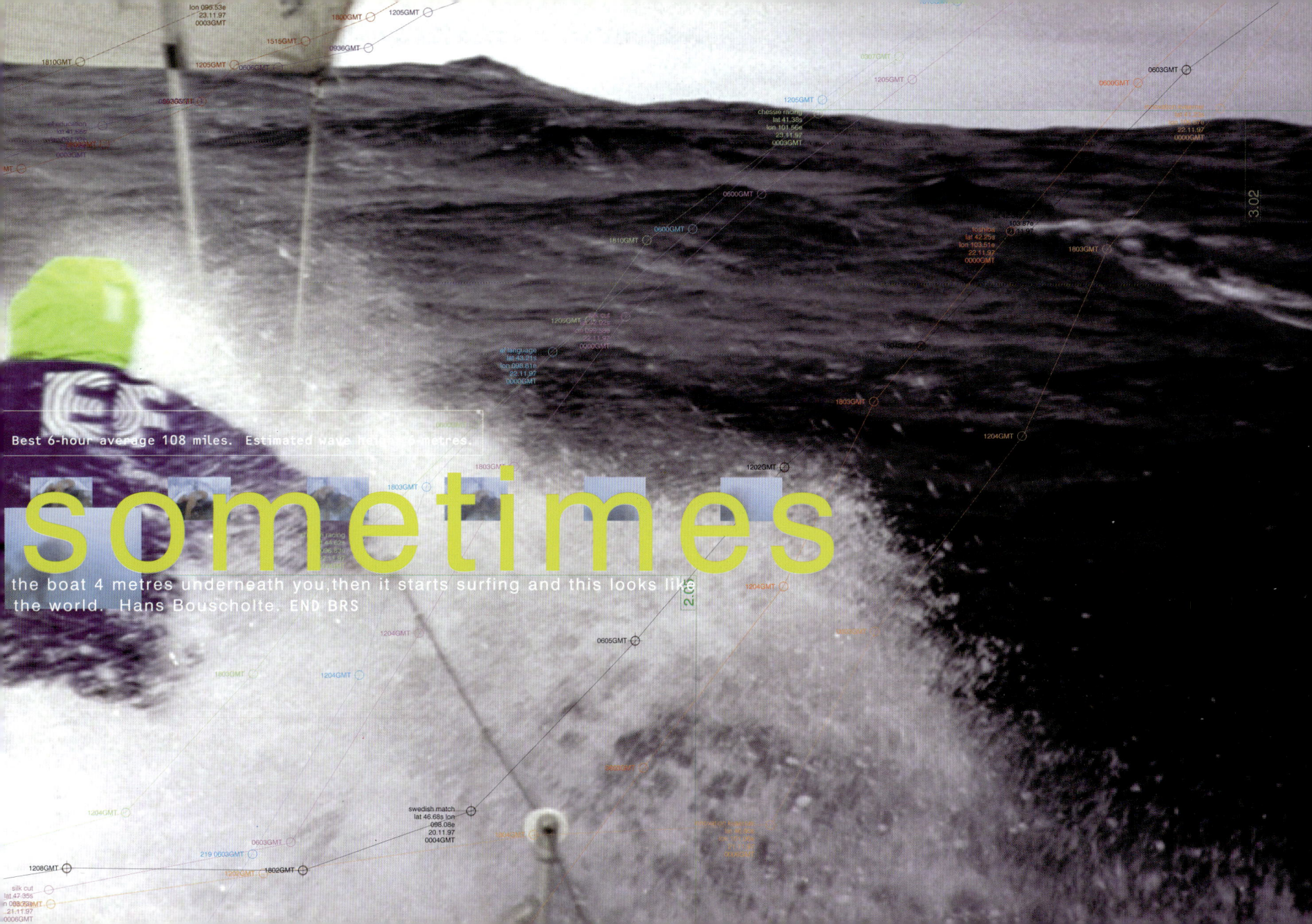

Best 6-hour average 108 miles. Estimated wave height 6 metres.

sometimes

the boat 4 metres underneath you, then it starts surfing and this looks like the world. Hans Bouscholte. END BRS

2.07 | 19-20 Nov 1997 | 11,907,968 Hits | Quokka Sports: Source: www.whitbread.org

Fm: KVA Su: DAILY REPORT NO. 12 Date: Nov. 19, 13:00 GMT

Just came down from deck.

Snow storm,

big waves and wind speeds gusting over 50 knots.
END KVA

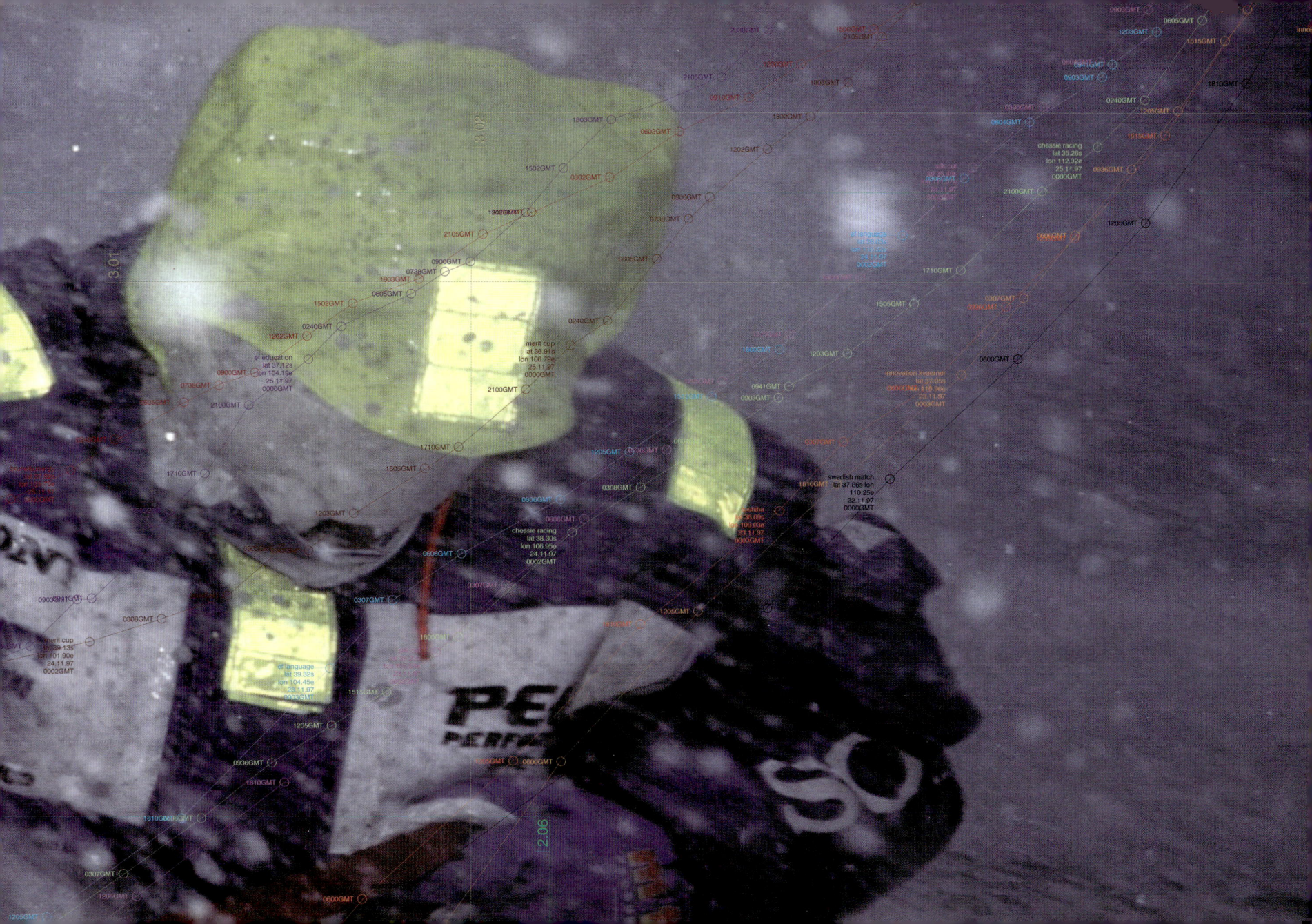

2.08 21-27 Nov 1997 16,776,325 Hits Quokka Sports? Source: www.whitbread.org

Without light, horizon, orientation, only darkness,
there is no difference between the colour of the water or the colour of the sky or clouds,

everything is dark grey.

Many regards from Hans Bouscholte onboard BrunelSunergy. END BRS

From Boat:Brunel_Sunergy Time Sent: 11:57:53 1997
Position report from MES 424519210 at 21-11-97 11:00 UTC
Latitude: 44 48.73 S Longitude: 083 55.73 E Course: 035
Speed: 05 knots Last update: 21-11-97 11:00 UTC

leg 2 leaderboard and status

pos	boat	elapsed time	points	totals
1	Swedish Match	15d+ 03:45:03	125	161
2	Innovation Kvaerner	15d+ 22:02:35	110	207
3	Toshiba	16d+ 05:27:12	97	157
4	Silk Cut	16d+ 15:03:09	84	168
5	EF Language	16d+ 20:06:25	72	197
6	Chessie Racing	17d+ 11:51:47	60	132
7	Merit Cup	19d+ 02:37:47	48	158
8	EF Education	19d+ 10:15:32	36	60
9	BrunelSunergy	19d+ 11:24:39	24	36

3.0.0 13 Dec – 22 Dec 1997   49,508,329 Hits | Quokka Sports: Source: www.whitbread.org

Leg 3

Distance:

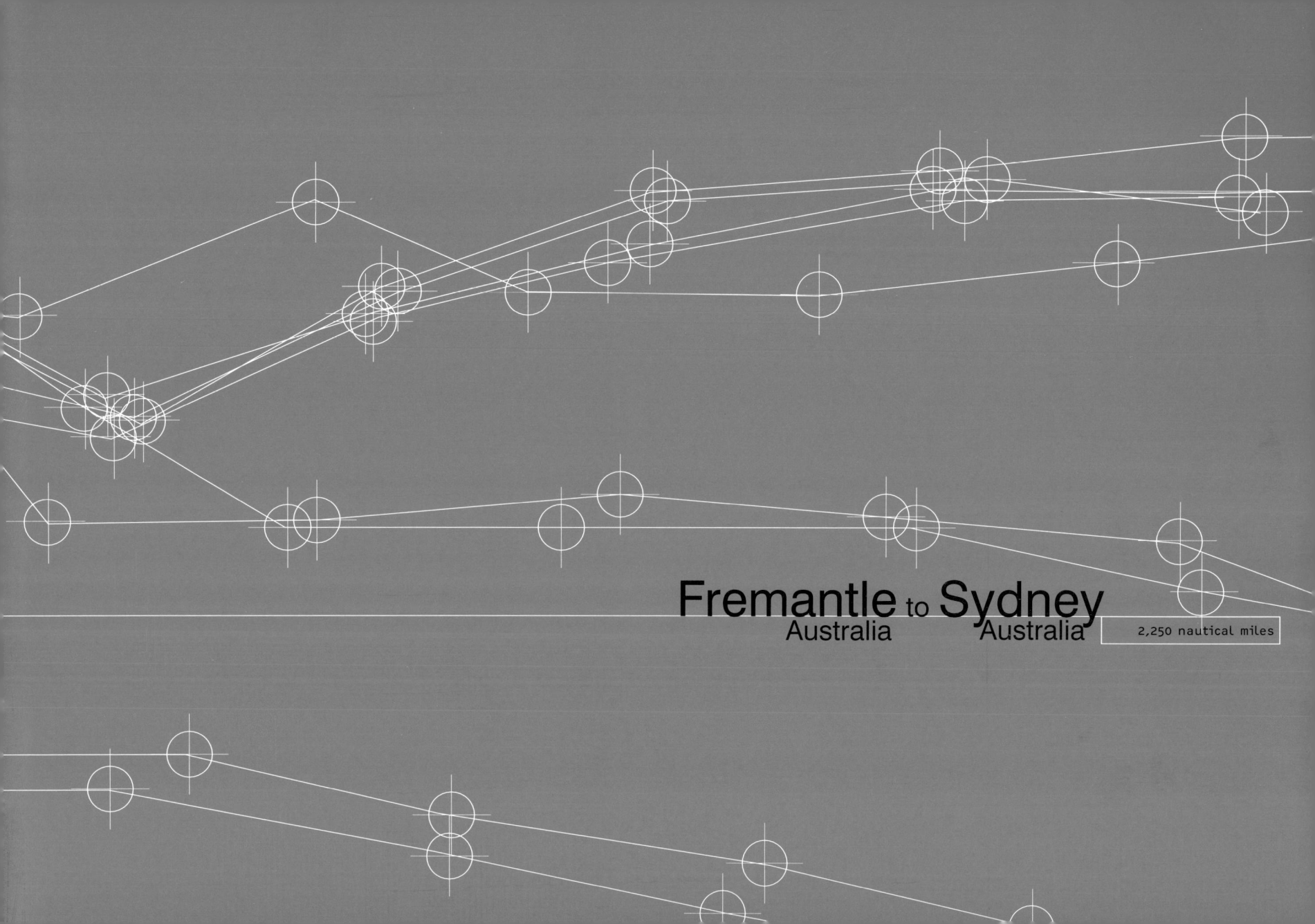

Leg 3: Prelude

The nine-boat fleet had arrived in Fremantle beaten and battered. The Southern Ocean had lived up to its fearsome reputation. The good news was no one had been seriously injured. Though everyone finished the 4,600-nautical-mile leg in under 20 days, the boats and their crews looked as if they had been at sea for months when they pulled up to the dock. Innovation Kvaerner's navigator, Marcel van Triest, a veteran of the Southern Ocean, described the leg as the wildest crossing he had ever experienced.

Besides the days on end of gale-force winds, sleet, snow and ice, the leg had a record number of collisions with whales, leaving some boats with damaged keels and all with shaken nerves. "We were sailing neck and neck with Silk Cut and EF Language," recalled Chessie Racing's skipper, Mark Fischer, "when we hit this submerged object while doing about 12 knots. It was like running into something very large ... the boat lifted and we all stumbled forward."

Hardware was not the only thing that took a beating on the leg, as egos were also badly dented. EF Language skipper Paul Cayard took every public appearance as an opportunity to blame himself for the team's dismal fifth-place showing. Cayard explained to reporters in Fremantle that he had tried to sail the leg as if it were an America's Cup race.

"I've won five America's Cup races by one second," Cayard said. "This race is a matter of hundreds of miles and hours. I did not appreciate that, and I pushed too hard and we broke too much stuff."

Grant Dalton was also nursing a bruised ego after limping into Fremantle in seventh place. "Obviously we are angry with ourselves," Dalton said. "Once my ego has corrected itself, and that will take a few days, we will be able to sit down and reflect."

Ego repair was not going to be enough for the Dutch entry, BrunelSunergy. Leg 2 marked the second leg in a row the boat had come in dead last. A week after arriving in Fremantle, the team announced that skipper Hans Bouscholte was stepping down. Bouscholte blamed his team's poor showing on a lack of adequate funds and limited training. Roy Heiner, an Olympic medallist and one of Holland's most successful sailors, would replace him. Heiner had a reputation for sailing hard and playing hard. Henceforth, winning or losing, the team referred to itself as the "Happy Crew."

Changes were also afoot aboard Chessie Racing. Co-skipper Mark Fischer announced he would step off the boat for now, leaving open the possibility of returning later in the race. Rumours around the dock were that Fischer, a demanding and exacting skipper, had rubbed his crew the wrong way. Fischer brushed the criticism aside. "On any boat during the heat of competition you get some normal friction between a skipper and crew," he said. "Some crewmembers will like a skipper, while others will think he's a pain in the neck. That's normal." Regardless, Fischer did not return to the race. The team's founder and benefactor, George Collins, would replace him on Leg 3.

While other crews struggled to explain their failures, those crews who set records on the leg were basking in the glow of accomplishment. Swedish Match was awarded the Volvo Trophy as winner of the leg. She also laid claim to the highest average speed sailed on any leg in The Whitbread's 25-year history, at 13 knots. Silk Cut's crew claimed the 24-hour world monohull speed record. She broke the previous record by a convincing 15 miles, sailing 449.1 miles in 24 hours, averaging 18.7 knots.

As the crews settled in for a three-week stay in port, Toshiba co-skipper Dennis Conner arrived in Fremantle. Conner voiced satisfaction with the team's third-place showing on the leg. He was clearly proud his team had justified his elevation of Paul Standbridge after Dickson's departure. Skipper Standbridge said the leg actually marked the beginning of a comeback for the boat and crew. "They are doing a really good job and placed well this leg. Of course, they would have preferred to be first or second, but then everyone would." Conner denied rumours that he would skipper from Sydney, Australia, to Auckland, New Zealand, on Leg 4.

Leg 3: Fremantle, Australia, to Sydney, Australia

"The boat rises and climbs over the swells, only to fall banging and crashing into the trough and then shudder and slam to shake herself free."

Ken Venn, Toshiba

On Saturday, 13 December 1997, the fleet left Fremantle, heading for Sydney. It was summer Down Under and the day was perfect. Referring to the area's legendary prevailing winds, Cayard reported, "The Fremantle Doctor is in, so we will have a good wind from 210 degrees, at 20-plus knots."

Cayard and EF Language took good advantage of the running start. He arrived at the first buoy before the rest of the fleet, then rounded Rottnest Island first as well, one-and-a-half hours after the start. By the beginning of the second day, the fleet was tacking upwind. Innovation Kvaerner, currently the overall points leader in the race, suddenly hove to. The crew had discovered alarming dents and buckles in the lower part of the mast just above the step. After examining the dents, they decided to cautiously sail on. However, it was clear the mast needed repair, so skipper Frostad radioed shore crew for assistance. A helicopter was sent to drop a repair kit; in order to intercept it, in accordance with Whitbread rules, the boat headed to within one mile of shore and dropped anchor. No sooner had the repair kit hit the deck than the crew hoisted anchor and resumed racing, bracing the lower mast while under sail. By midnight, Innovation Kvaerner had struggled back into the pack, a mere nine miles astern of leader EF Language.

As the fleet fanned out into the Great Australian Bight, the boats encountered fierce headwinds. W60s are not designed for upwind conditions. When forced into them, the boats pound mercilessly, taking a toll on both boat and crew. Upwind conditions mean tacking, tacking and tacking again. Each time a boat tacks, all hands, even those trying to sleep, are pressed into service. They furiously shift tons of sails to provide added weight on the high side.

"No way can you call the last 24 hours pleasant," wrote Dalton. "Yesterday was filled with constant tacking in fresh wind, no sleep for the boys and lots of water flying around."

As the headwinds hit the fleet like an invisible wall, Toshiba positioned herself in the middle of the pack, slipping ahead. Chessie Racing, with George Collins acting as skipper on his first leg, pulled into second place. EF Language fell back into sixth, behind Merit Cup.

Meanwhile, aboard Silk Cut, fresh water supplies were in jeopardy. It was hot and the Silk Cut crew reported their watermaker had broken down. The prospects were grim. The boat could either go in for repairs or try to get by using hand-powered emergency desalinators. Skipper Lawrie Smith decided to see if they could make do on this short leg using just the hand-operated watermakers. The results were not promising. "The amount of fresh water produced is about equivalent to the amount of sweat lost using them," Smith reported. "We are now searching for a model that turns sea water into beer!"

Humour aside, in the hot conditions, the situation was serious. Besides having to produce enough drinking water for the 12 men aboard, it would take two men six hours of pumping to produce enough water to cook a single dehydrated meal. The crew continued working on the broken desalinator. Happily, the next day they reported they had it running again.

In a bold move, Innovation Kvaerner and Brunel-Sunergy — with new skipper Roy Heiner — headed almost due south while the rest of the boats continued to bash their way to Bass Strait. For a while, it appeared the dramatic move would pay off. Though Toshiba held her lead, Innovation

Kvaerner gained over 11 nautical miles on her with more favourable wind angles in the south. Swedish Match skipper Gunnar Krantz watched the gambit with interest. He, too, was beginning to consider a southern course. "At the moment, it looks good for Kvaerner and Brunel and they are 45 miles south of us," wrote Krantz. "If we get a good wind direction we have not excluded the option to go even more to the south."

However, fate, rather than tactics, was about to make that decision for Krantz. The upwind conditions were beginning to take their toll on his boat. The pounding was compressing the boat's mast each time the bow bashed into an oncoming wave. Finally, on Day 7, the stress took physical form. "Swedish Match has damage to the mast," Krantz reported to shore. "The damage is at the deck, just above the mast step, the mast has buckled in on both sides due to compression load." The problem was similar to the mast problem experienced earlier in the leg by Innovation Kvaerner.

Krantz was faced with a tough decision. He could request that a repair kit be flown to him as Innovation Kvaerner had done, or he could sail on, risking a total mast failure if these upwind conditions did not change soon. The choice of repairing the mast did not appear very attractive. The boats were farther offshore now than they had been when Innovation Kvaerner decided to make repairs. A decision to repair Swedish Match's mast would prove costly, as they would have to sail to shore and drop anchor in order to receive the repair kit. The skipper decided to sail on. As the boats headed into Bass Strait, Krantz turned south, seeking winds more favourable to his needs and weakened mast.

By 22 December, the fleet was packed in close formation by Whitbread standards, with only 28 miles separating the leader Toshiba from the last boat, BrunelSunergy. Within the pack the boats were in four groups. Toshiba, Silk Cut, and Chessie Racing were grouped in the north, with EF Education and Merit Cup sailing the middle course just below them. Positioned to the south were Swedish Match, EF Language, Innovation Kvaerner and BrunelSunergy.

Swedish Match's southern strategy paid off. The yacht slipped under the headwinds and found good reaching conditions. Swedish Match, damaged mast and all, slipped into second place, just behind EF Language. Then, during the early morning hours of December 22, Swedish Match nosed into first place. Cayard was not amused. "It is Monday morning, three days before Christmas, and we have got bogies all over the place," Cayard reported that morning. "There's going to be a big dogfight to the finish."

Swedish Match was in the lead, but with a weakened mast, she still had to sail conservatively — not so EF Language. Cayard smelled blood and hoisted sail. With just five hours to the finish line, Cayard passed Swedish Match to regain the front position.

The final hours of Leg 3 saw high drama when an Innovation Kvaerner crewman, Alby Pratt, was tossed overboard during an early morning sail change. He was not tethered at the time and the crew had to turn around and go looking for him. Fortunately, he was wearing his strobe light, and was scooped out of the water quickly.

With Sydney Harbour looming just ahead of the fleet, the leg became a sprint to the finish. Never had there been such a close Whitbread leg as this third one, which turned into a 2,250-nautical-mile drag race. "Now in sight of half the fleet and going like hell," reported BrunelSunergy's navigator, Stuart Quarrie.

By ocean-racing standards, it was a photo finish. Six of the competitors arrived within 11 minutes of one another; inside two hours, all nine of the W60s had finished in Australia's first settlement. The sailors glided into Sydney Harbour under the cover of darkness. At the finish line off the Sydney Opera House, EF Language's crew lit red flares to illuminate the darkness and announce their arrival.

Cayard and his crew were ahead of wounded Swedish Match, which finished in second place only five minutes and eight seconds behind. A bare 53 seconds later was third-placed Chessie Racing, skippered by her owner, George Collins. Chessie Racing arrived two minutes and 16 seconds ahead of fourth-placed Merit Cup, which came in one minute and 41 seconds ahead of Innovation Kvaerner. Just 46 seconds after Innovation Kvaerner crossed, Toshiba finished.

When Cayard stepped ashore after nine days, nine hours and nine minutes of sailing to receive the Volvo Trophy for Leg 3, he was visibly excited. "It was the tightest ocean race I have ever been in," Cayard said. "Everything balanced out perfectly and we had one hell of a boat race."

Cayard had reason to gush. He now had two leg victories in the bag and was the overall leader with 302 points. The Cayard-doubters fell silent once again.

On Chessie Racing, George Collins also had reason to be pleased. Having been written off early in the race by the odds-makers, Collins took his third place showing as proof that his boat and crew were competitive.

It was another disappointing leg for Toshiba, with a sixth-place finish. In seventh was Silk Cut, another team that so far had failed to live up to pre-race expectations. The change of skippers on BrunelSunergy had yet to pay off, as that team came in eighth.

The last boat to arrive was EF Education, after nine days, ten hours and 47 minutes at sea, just one hour and 38 minutes behind the first boat. She had been doing well and held off advances by Merit Cup until two days before the finish, when her runner and topmast terminals came completely unscrewed. "It was only gear failure that hindered us," said EF Education crewmember Keryn McMaster. Many of the other teams shared the feeling.

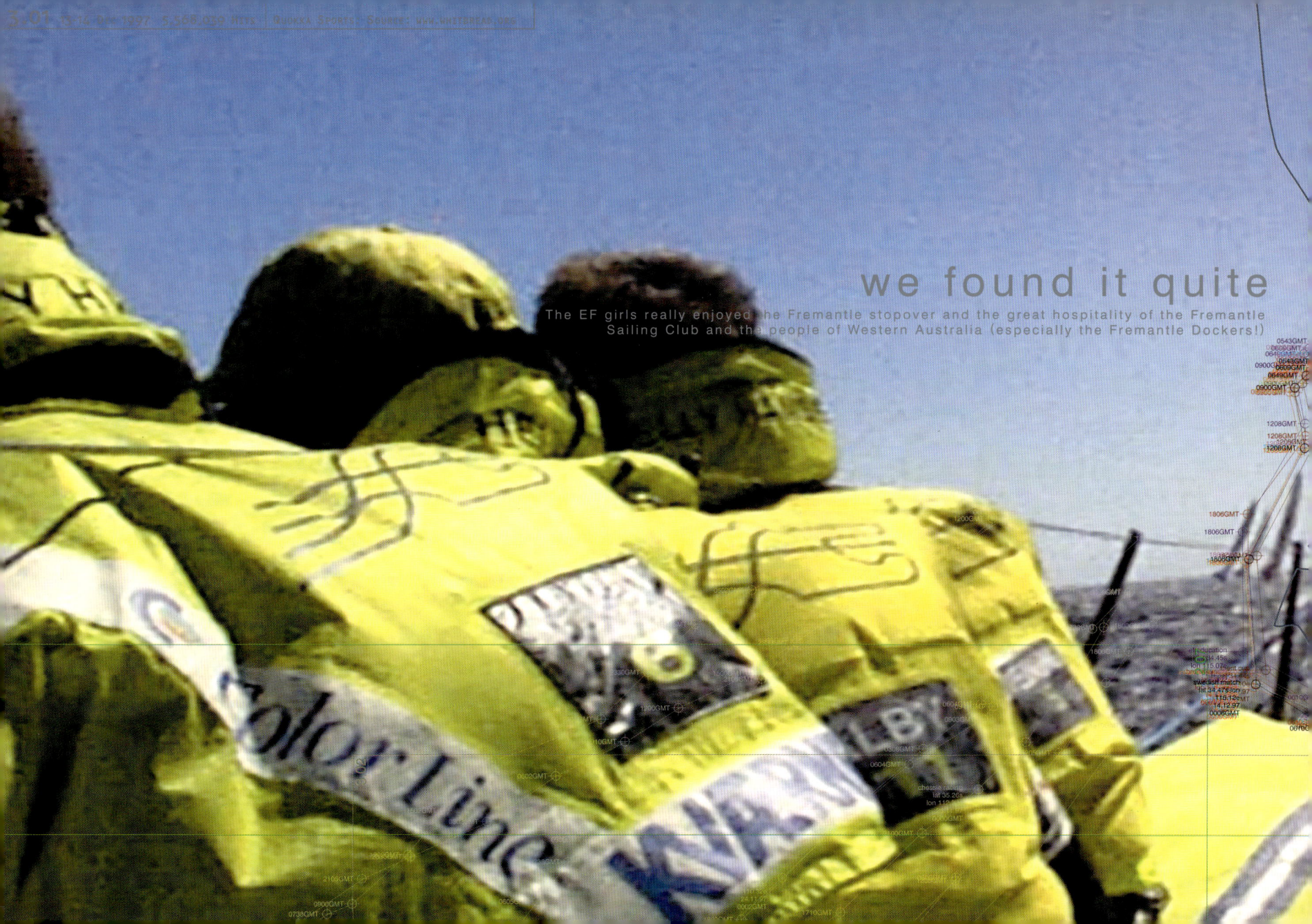

we found it quite

The EF girls really enjoyed the Fremantle stopover and the great hospitality of the Fremantle Sailing Club and the people of Western Australia (especially the Fremantle Dockers!)

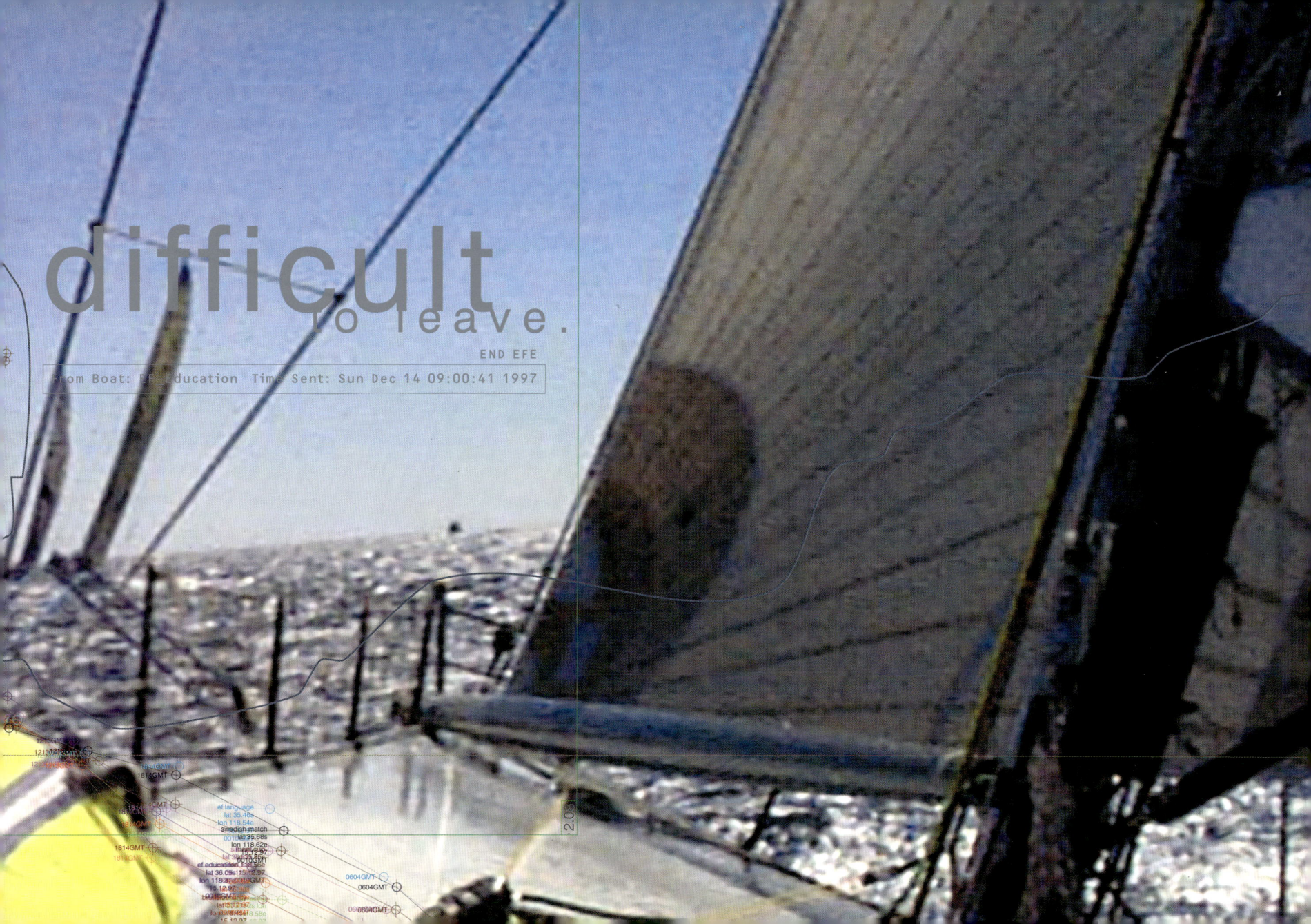

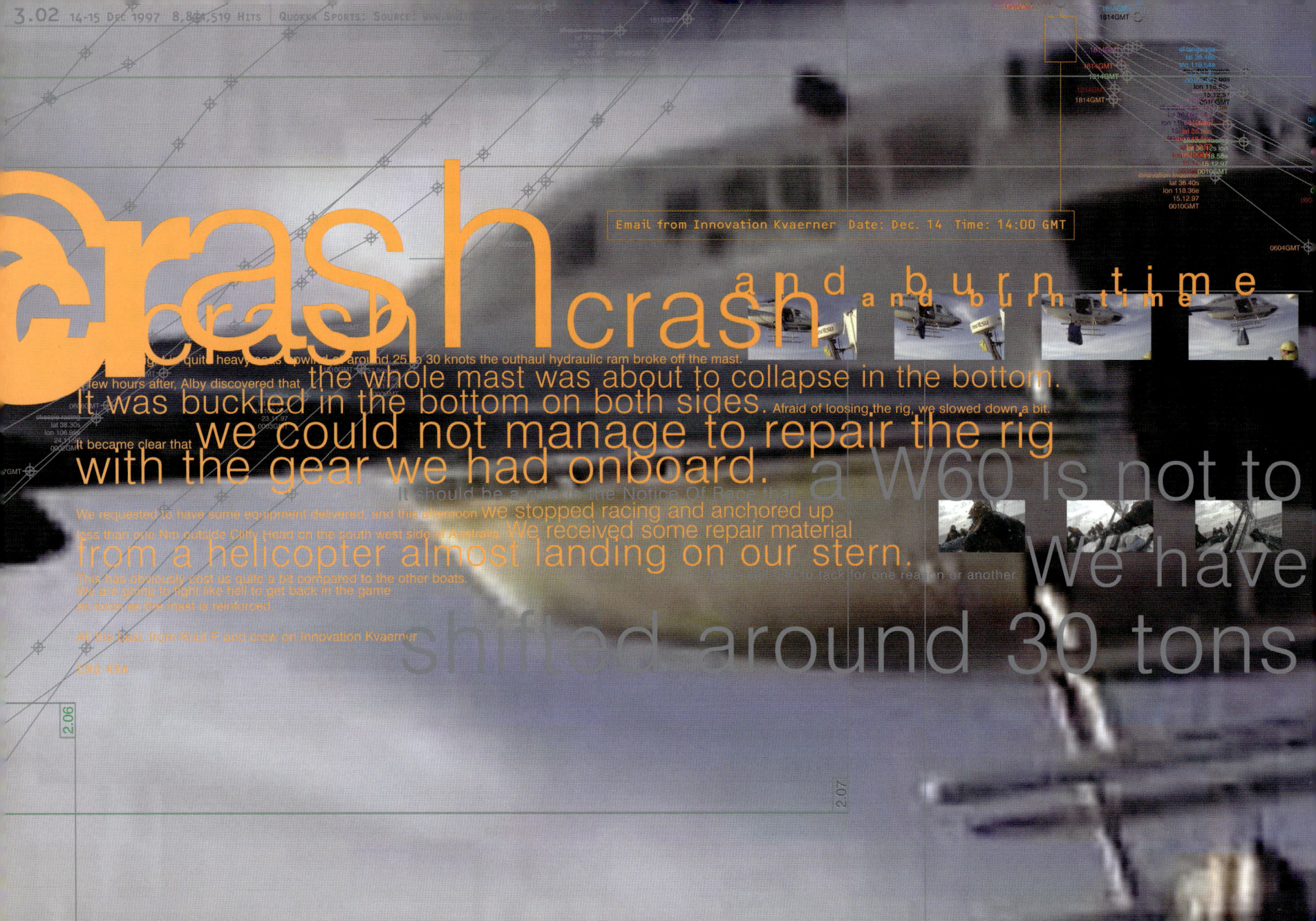

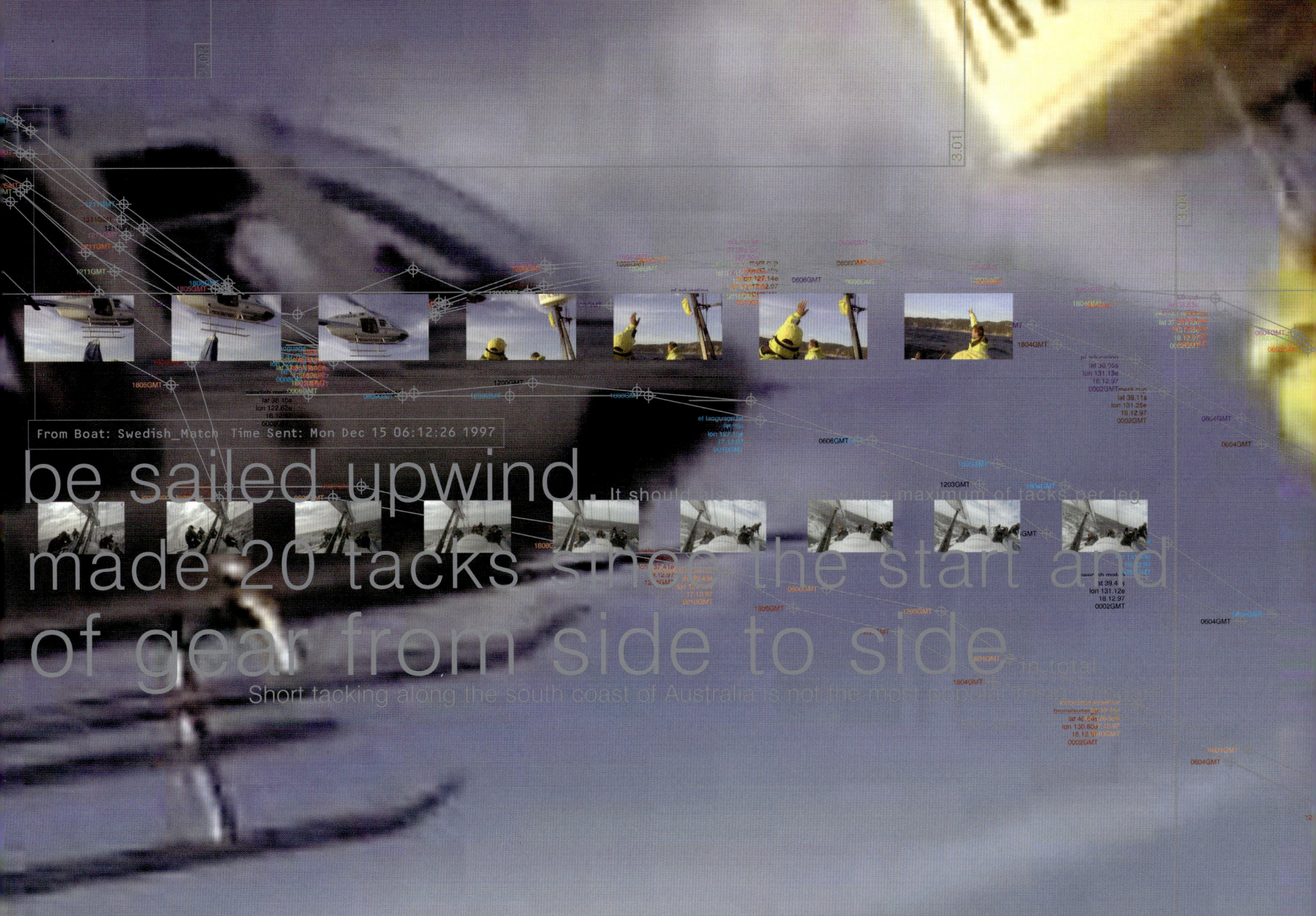

From Boat: Swedish_Match Time Sent: Mon Dec 15 06:12:26 1997

be sailed upwind. It should... ...with a maximum of tacks per leg... made 20 tacks since the start and ...of gear from side to side... in total. Short tacking along the south coast of Australia is not the most...

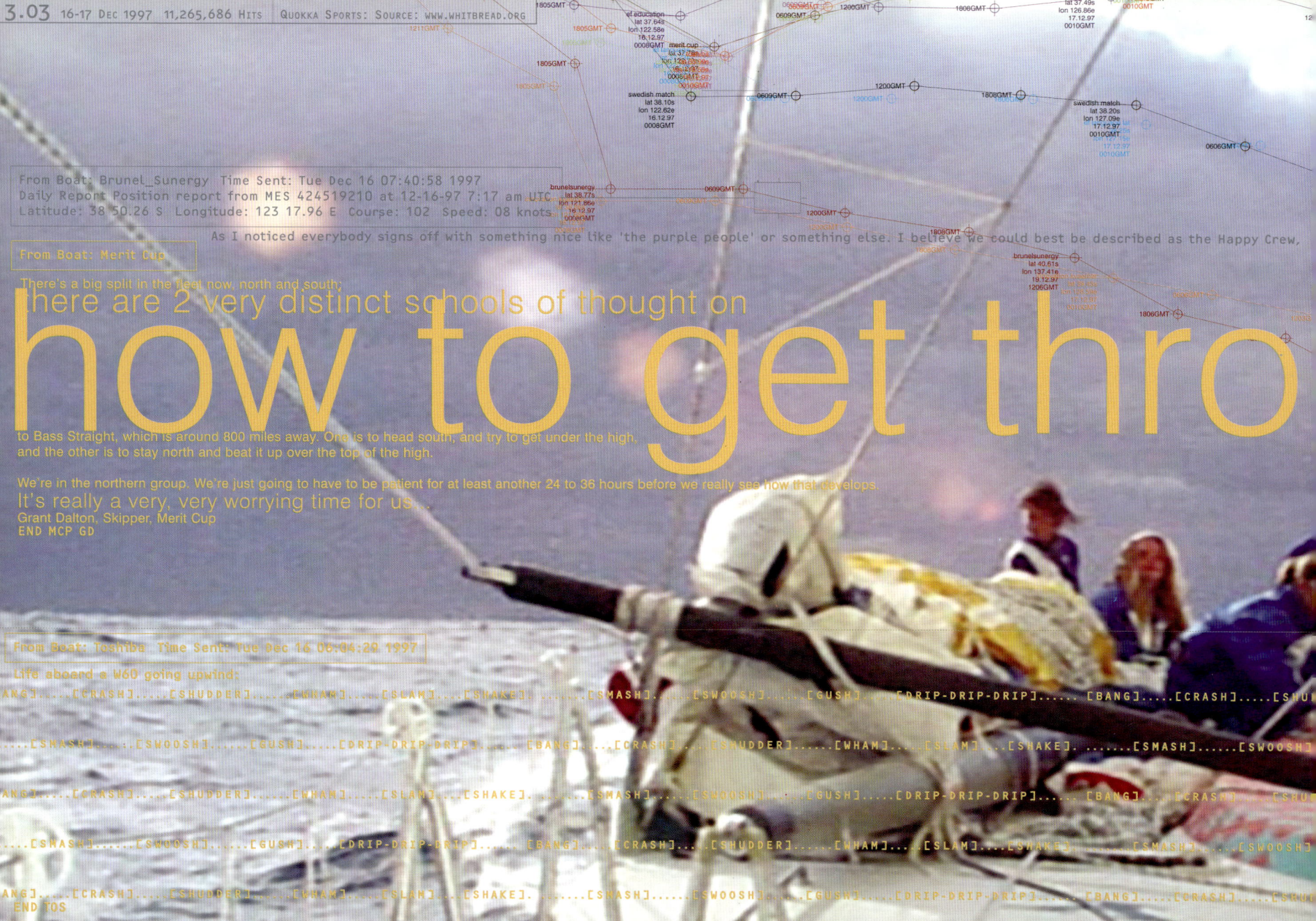

how to get thro

3.03 16–17 Dec 1997 11,265,686 Hits Quokka Sports: Source: www.whitbread.org

From Boat: Brunel_Sunergy Time Sent: Tue Dec 16 07:40:58 1997
Daily Report Position report from MES 424519210 at 12-16-97 7:17 am UTC
Latitude: 38 50.26 S Longitude: 123 17.96 E Course: 102 Speed: 08 knots

As I noticed everybody signs off with something nice like 'the purple people' or something else, I believe we could best be described as the Happy Crew.

From Boat: Merit Cup

There's a big split in the fleet now, north and south; there are 2 very distinct schools of thought on how to get through to Bass Straight, which is around 800 miles away. One is to head south, and try to get under the high, and the other is to stay north and beat it up over the top of the high.

We're in the northern group. We're just going to have to be patient for at least another 24 to 36 hours before we really see how that develops.
It's really a very, very worrying time for us...
Grant Dalton, Skipper, Merit Cup
END MCP GD

From Boat: Toshiba Time Sent: Tue Dec 16 06:04:28 1997
Life aboard a W60 going upwind:
[BANG]....[CRASH]....[SHUDDER]....[WHAM]....[SLAM]...[SHAKE]....[SMASH]....[SWOOSH]....[GUSH]....[DRIP-DRIP-DRIP]....[BANG]....[CRASH]....[SHU
....[SMASH]....[SWOOSH]....[GUSH]....[DRIP-DRIP-DRIP]....[BANG]....[CRASH]....[SHUDDER]....[WHAM]....[SLAM]...[SHAKE]....[SMASH]....[SWOOSH]
....[CRASH]....[SHUDDER]....[WHAM]....[SLAM]...[SHAKE]....[SMASH]....[SWOOSH]....[GUSH]....[DRIP-DRIP-DRIP]....[BANG]....[CRASH]
....[SMASH]....[SWOOSH]....[GUSH]....[DRIP-DRIP-DRIP]....[BANG]....[CRASH]....[SHUDDER]....[WHAM]....[SLAM]...[SHAKE]....[SMASH]....[SWOOSH]
[BANG]....[CRASH]....[SHUDDER]....[WHAM]....[SLAM]...[SHAKE]....[SMASH]....[SWOOSH]....[GUSH]....[DRIP-DRIP-DRIP]....[BANG]....[CRASH]....[SHU
END TOS

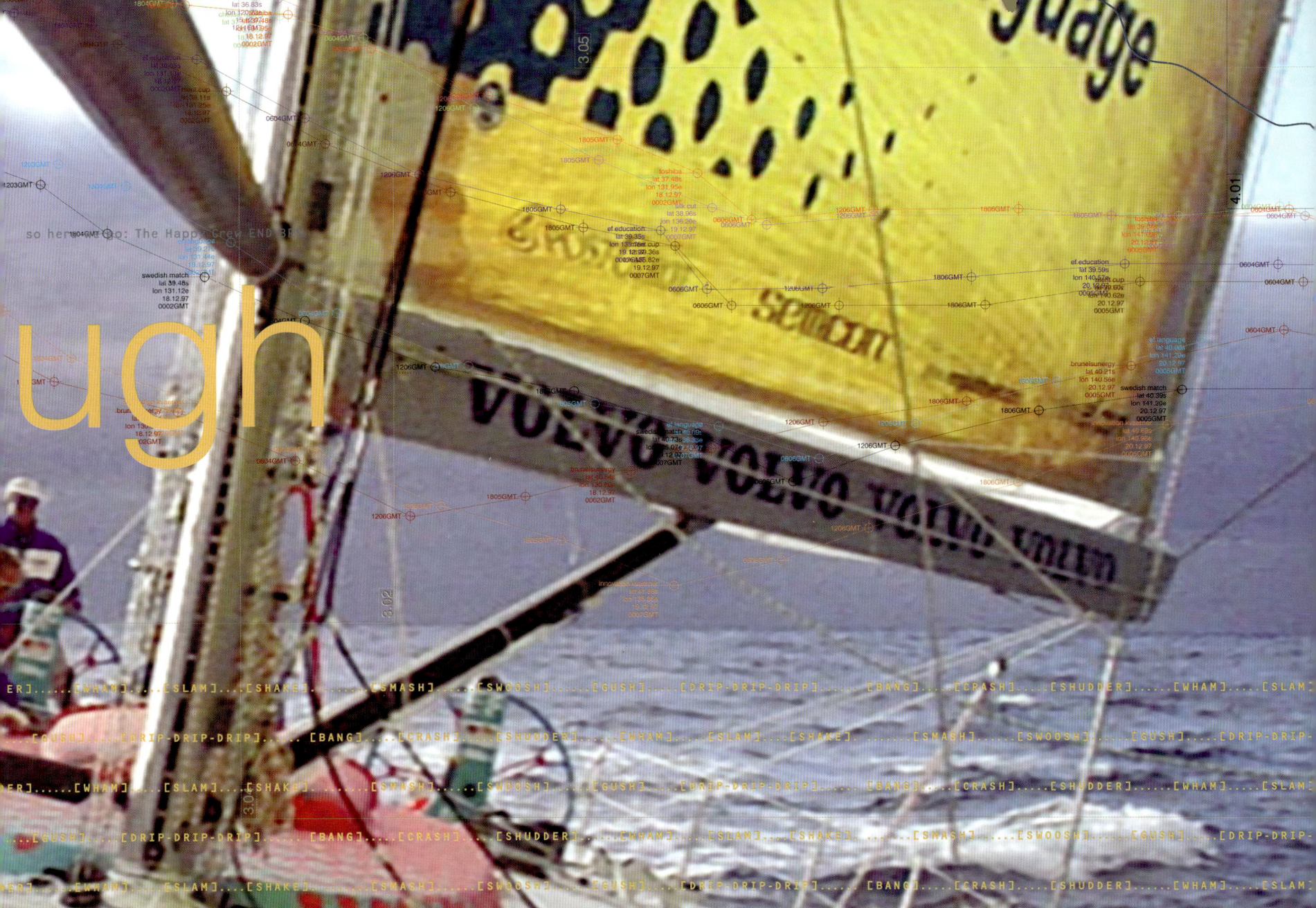

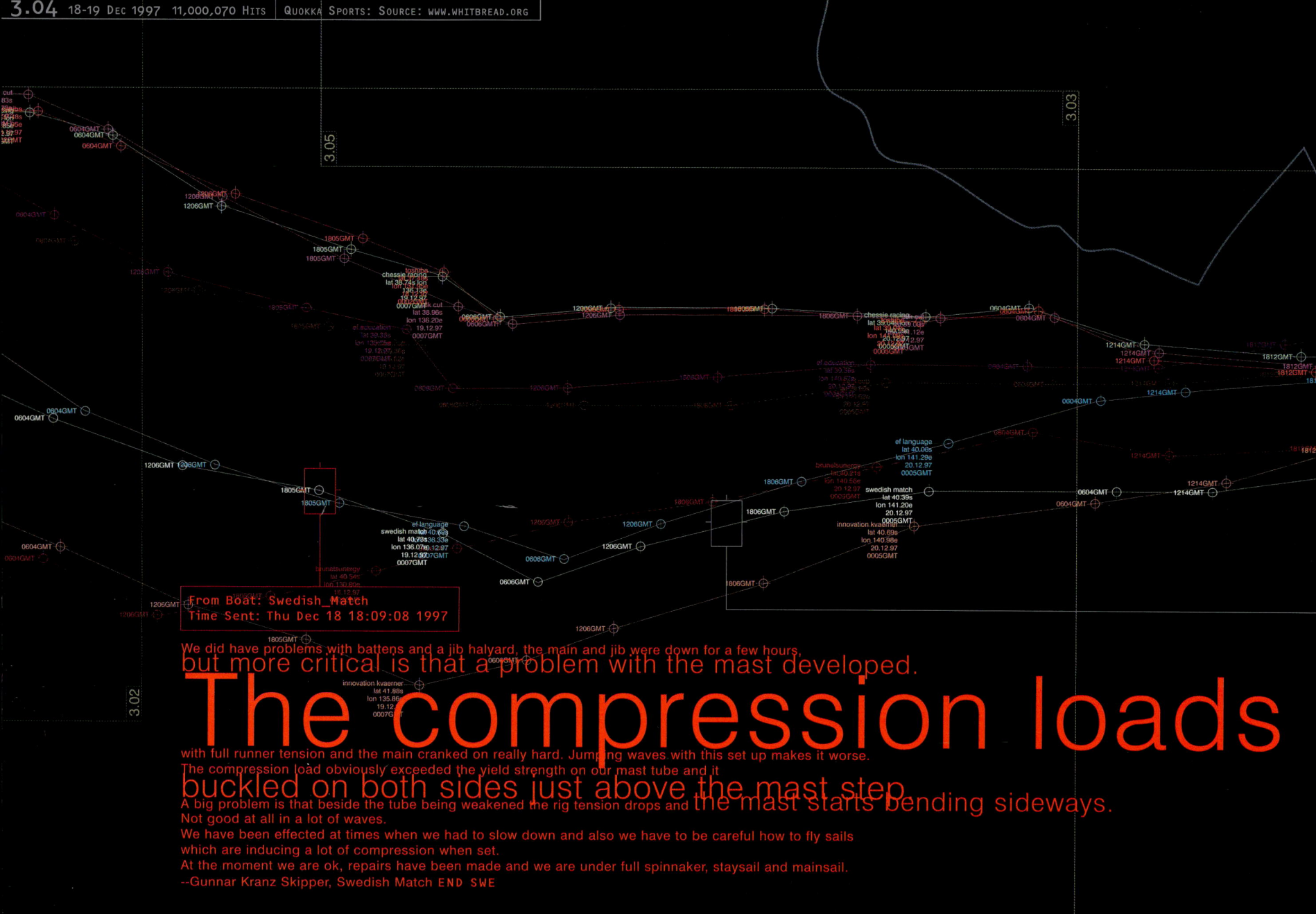

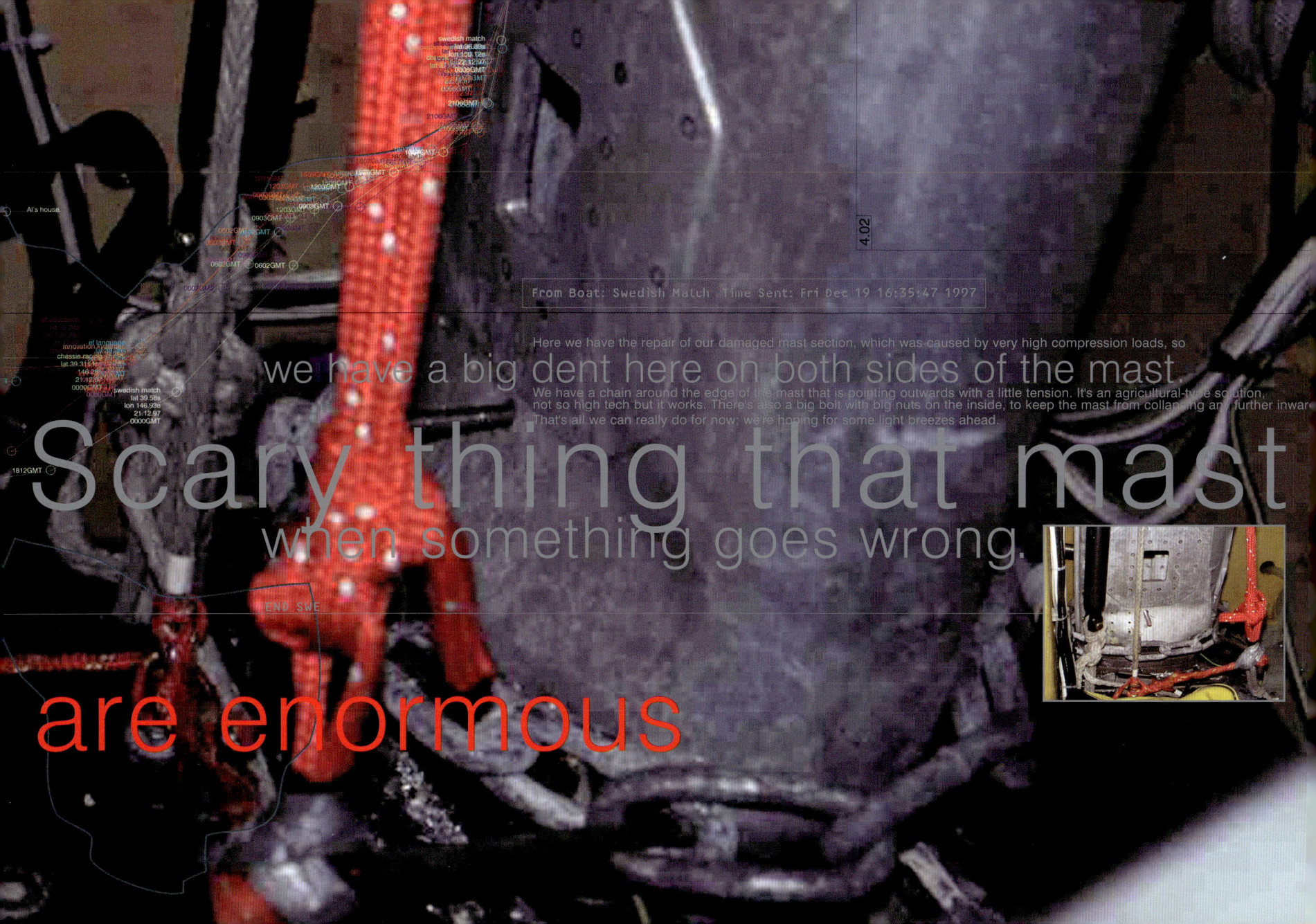

From Boat: Swedish Match Time Sent: Fri Dec 19 16:35:47 1997

Here we have the repair of our damaged mast section, which was caused by very high compression loads, so we have a big dent here on both sides of the mast. We have a chain around the edge of the mast that is pointing outwards with a little tension. It's an agricultural-type solution, not so high tech but it works. There's also a big bolt with big nuts on the inside, to keep the mast from collapsing any further inward. That's all we can really do for now; we're hoping for some light breezes ahead.

Scary thing that mast when something goes wrong.

are enormous

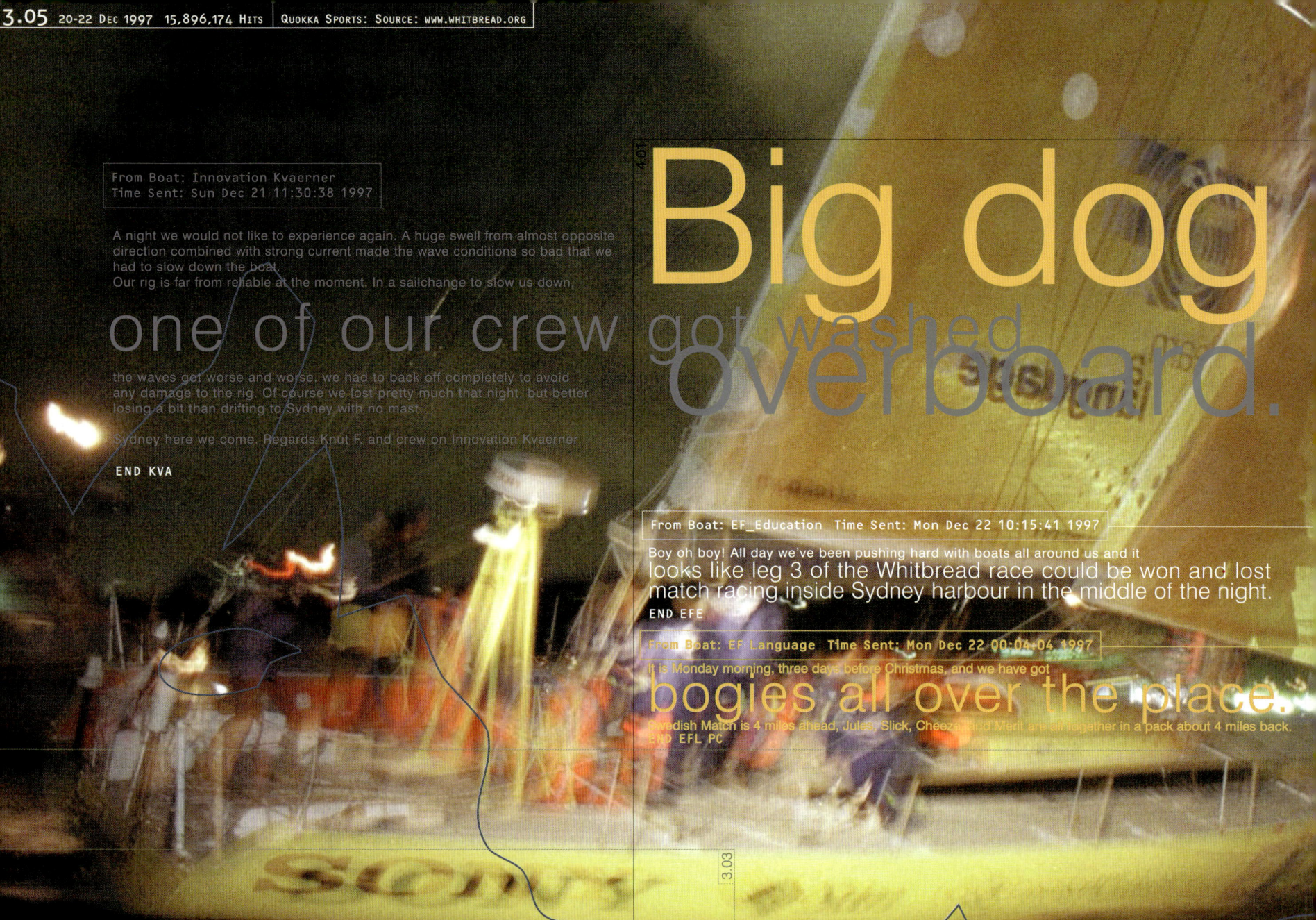

3.05 20-22 Dec 1997 15,896,174 Hits Quokka Sports: Source: www.whitbread.org

Big dog got washed overboard.

From Boat: Innovation Kvaerner
Time Sent: Sun Dec 21 11:30:38 1997

A night we would not like to experience again. A huge swell from almost opposite direction combined with strong current made the wave conditions so bad that we had to slow down the boat.
Our rig is far from reliable at the moment. In a sailchange to slow us down, one of our crew got washed overboard. the waves got worse and worse. we had to back off completely to avoid any damage to the rig. Of course we lost pretty much that night, but better losing a bit than drifting to Sydney with no mast.
Sydney here we come. Regards Knut F. and crew on Innovation Kvaerner

END KVA

From Boat: EF_Education Time Sent: Mon Dec 22 10:15:41 1997

Boy oh boy! All day we've been pushing hard with boats all around us and it looks like leg 3 of the Whitbread race could be won and lost match racing inside Sydney harbour in the middle of the night.
END EFE

From Boat: EF Language Time Sent: Mon Dec 22 00:04:04 1997

It is Monday morning, three days before Christmas, and we have got bogies all over the place. Swedish Match is 4 miles ahead, Jules, Slick, Cheeza and Merit are all together in a pack about 4 miles back.
END EFL PC

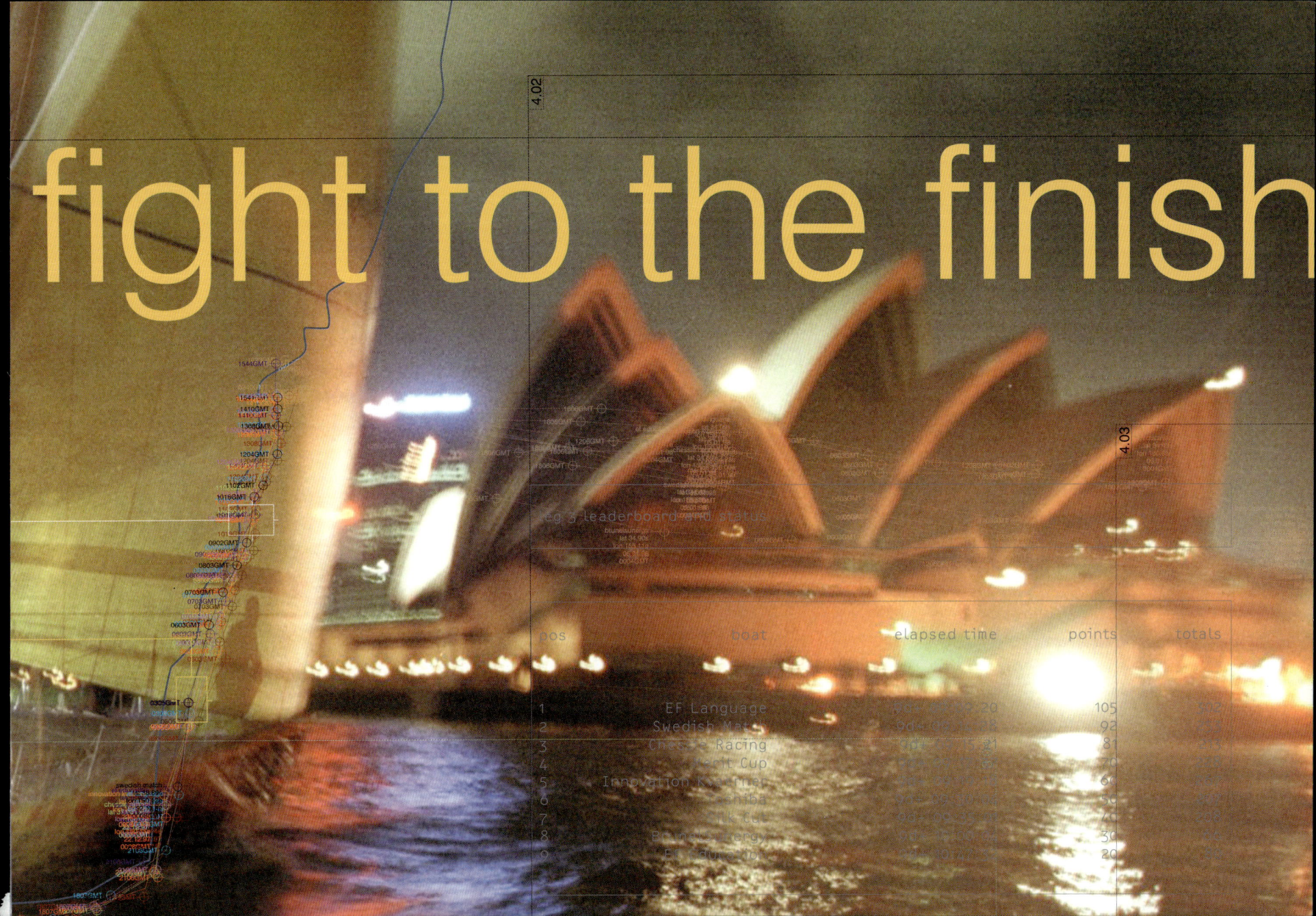

4.0.0 04 Jan – 09 Jan 1998 37,814,474 Hits | Quokka Sports: Source: www.whitbread.org

Leg 4

Distance:

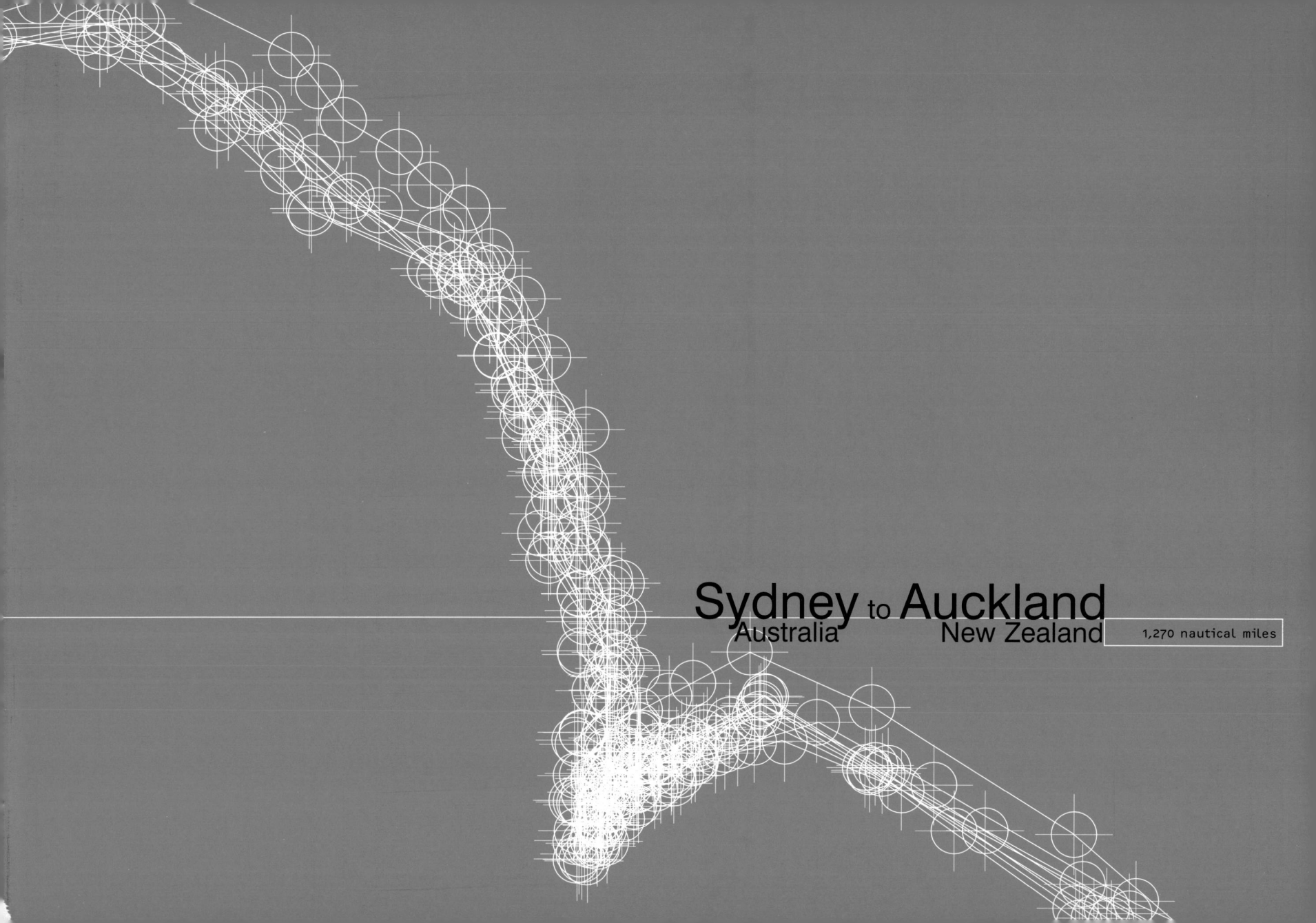

Leg 4: Prelude

After a couple of days off to celebrate Christmas in Sydney, the crews were soon back at work on their boats, preparing for the 4 January 1998 start of Leg 4. The first order of business was to deal with the rash of mast problems that had struck the fleet. During the last leg, three W60s had suffered mast problems. Norway's Innovation Kvaerner was the first, reporting buckling at the mast step on their first night out. Five days later, Swedish Match experienced the same problem. Again, the mast had buckled under the deck around the mast step. Skipper Krantz reported the unnerving experience of sitting on the toilet watching the mast flexing. He said it was the wrong place to be if the mast gave way.

Next, Chessie Racing reported mast difficulties, although Chessie's problem was not as serious as the others. Her mast had cracks where the spreaders met the mast. To get their wounded boats ready for Leg 4, Swedish Match and Innovation Kvaerner amputated the compressed sections of their masts, a piece about 300 millimetres (12 inches) in length. The damaged sections were then encased in a reinforcing sleeve which had a second inner sleeve that fit inside the original mast. The pieces were both glued and riveted together.

The fix would, it was hoped, take Swedish Match the 1,270 miles to Auckland, but Krantz did not want to take his repaired mast around Cape Horn on Leg 5 — he applied to the Whitbread Race Office to replace the mast during the stopover in New Zealand. The request was granted.

As start day approached, it was learned that Dennis Conner had experienced a change of heart. In Fremantle, he had categorically denied he would skipper Leg 4. After the boat's dismal showing on the last leg, however, it should not have surprised anyone to see the 'take charge' Conner decide he needed to get aboard to see why his team couldn't break into the top three. For the record, Conner simply said he wanted to get out from behind a desk. "I've been part of this programme for two years," said Conner, "and I don't think anyone would begrudge me a few days at sea."

This would not be Conner's first taste of The Whitbread. In the 1993-94 Whitbread, Conner sailed the yacht Winston from Fremantle to Auckland. During that leg, Conner took the team on a huge flyer south, leading the fleet for many days before being caught by a weather system and overtaken. This would be a shorter leg, and Conner said he was not planning any big surprises. "I don't think there will be any flyers," he said. "I think the boats will be closer together than they were on the first two legs. In a six-day race, you're not going to see anyone get too far ahead."

Conner's announcement sent a stir through the Race Village. Few people in sailing evoke stronger feelings, pro or con, than Dennis Conner. Fans either accept his brash, take-no-prisoners style as honest and refreshing, or reject it as arrogant and abrasive. He is such a powerful presence in an event that fans inevitably line up on either the 'love him' or 'hate him' sides, leaving no one but race officials in the middle.

Conner's decision to take the helm now also set the stage for a confrontation with EF Language's skipper, Paul Cayard. He was the man many saw as the most likely contender for the America's Cup mantle worn so long by Conner. In a reference to Cayard's lengthy emails during the past three legs, Conner took a jab at his rival for fan attention. "I keep up to date by reading Paul Michener's accounts of the race," Conner said with a wry smile. "He's working toward a Pulitzer."

George Collins, still upbeat after his third-place Leg 3 finish, announced that he would skipper Chessie Racing on Leg 4 as well. "We said we had a long learning curve to go on," said Collins. "Clearly, I've ratcheted it up."

As the crews boarded their boats for the start, Merit Cup skipper Grant Dalton, who had spent the stopover suffering from a serious throat infection, was seen stepping aboard carrying a plastic bag full of antibiotics and painkillers. The story amongst the crew was that Dalton had the same infection prior to the 1993-94 race, and he won that one.

Leg 4: Sydney, Australia, to Auckland, New Zealand

"It's a yachtsman's worst nightmare — when you are leading to fall into a [wind] hole and to know that the others are coming at you."
Swedish Match co-skipper, Erle Williams

It was under leaden skies on 4 January 1998 that the fleet lined up in Sydney Harbour for the start of Leg 4. Aboard Toshiba, as the seconds ticked down, Dennis Conner was clearly visible at the helm as he jockeyed for position. While the rest of the fleet sailed well away from the line, Conner suddenly tacked and made a dash toward the line. Clearly, he was cutting it close — in fact, Toshiba crossed three seconds early. Instead of one, two shots from the starting cannon sounded — as the rest of the fleet crossed the line and raced on, Conner had to return and re-cross the line.

"I just could not wait for the chance to put Toshiba across the starting line first," Conner said later. "Well, I got my wish as we crossed a half-boatlength ahead at the favoured end, only to hear another gun, meaning we started prematurely and had to return to the line and restart, which of course meant we went from first to last. Talk about dreams turning to ashes."

The Leg 4 start out of Sydney Harbour was one of the quickest starts of the race and gave the fleet a chance to display their controversial 'Code 0' sails. Half an hour after the start, the crews were outside Sydney Heads and on their way to New Zealand.

Three-and-a-half hours later, EF Language was in the lead with Silk Cut 1.5 miles astern. Once out to sea, EF Language's Cayard reported to race headquarters that the wind had suddenly lightened and swung from 155 degrees to 120, then back to 135 degrees. The shifting conditions were forecasted to continue, sending navigators to their charts looking for the most favoured route from the Australian east coast to the northern tip of New Zealand. The question was whether to point north or head south. "If anything, we would like to stay south of the Great Circle as the wind should fill in from the south in a couple of days," wrote Swedish Match skipper Krantz. "But, this area seems to be capable of very quick shifts in weather patterns and currents. I believe that getting through the fickle wind areas on the east side of New Zealand will be the deciding factors in this leg." They would be prophetic words.

At the end of 24 hours of sailing, the three boats in front were EF Language, Silk Cut and Toshiba. As the next day progressed, the fleet began to spread out on a north/south axis 51 miles wide as each boat made its choice. Cayard headed north. At the end of the second day the lead had shifted to Toshiba, with Swedish Match just a mile behind her. Both boats had headed south. Conner was clearly enjoying himself and felt redeemed from his bad start back in Sydney, noting that had he not led the boat to the front of the pack, "I am sure my name would be mud with the crew."

The southern route was paying off handsomely for Toshiba and Swedish Match, with both boats reporting good sailing in a fresh 26-knot breeze. Behind them in third place was Merit Cup, carrying her crew of Kiwis determined to make a good showing before the hometown crowd in Auckland. These were familiar waters to skipper Dalton, so he pushed his boat hard, reporting that they were sailing under spinnaker and averaging around 16 knots. During the night, the wind shifted a full 45 degrees on the Merit Cup crew, which rolled the boat into a broach at about 20 knots. "We ended up having to cut the halyard," Dalton reported. "After laying on our side for five to ten minutes, we dragged the spinnaker back over the stern. We were really lucky not to do any real damage."

In fourth place, Chessie Racing had overtaken Silk Cut, now in fifth. Cayard and his navigator Mark Rudiger had decided the northerly route offered more promise in the long term. This decision cost EF Language 24 miles to Toshiba in just six hours of sailing. "Looks like the south is paying," Cayard wrote the next morning. "This could be bad for us northerners as the advantage to the south could last for quite some time of sailing."

Knut Frostad on Innovation Kvaerner also had time to bemoan the northerly course he'd chosen. He was now over 77 miles behind Swedish Match, having dropped a staggering 40 of those miles in just 24 hours.

Aboard EF Education, the women were having another bit of bad luck. Trailing 100 miles behind the leader, the boat suffered damage to her bow when the fitting holding the headsail to the deck gave way, taking a piece of the bow along with it. "This exposed a large hole," reported navigator Lynnath Beckley, "with daylight and water pouring in." The team had to drop the headsail and sail under the main only while emergency repairs were made. "Never a dull moment on EF Education," Beckley quipped.

On the third day, with just two full days of sailing remaining in this short leg, Swedish Match was maintaining a six-mile lead over second-placed Toshiba. The fleet was now heading north toward Cape Reinga, on the northern tip of New Zealand. It was clear that Swedish Match, just 180 miles from the cape, would be the first boat to pass it. "We are all trying to reach Cape Reinga on a starboard fetch or close-hauled," Krantz wrote. Before the leg started, Krantz had noted that coming down the New Zealand coast from the cape would be a dangerous moment, because of the unpredictable winds that swirl off the mountains that line the shore.

On EF Language, Cayard saw the error of his ways. He deserted the northerly route and took the yacht south. Regrettably, the decision cost him even more miles, and he fell to eighth place. "When it goes bad, I guess it really goes bad," said Cayard. "We can't seem to get anything right today." However, the south began to slowly repay Cayard; he gained 20 miles the next day, overtaking BrunelSunergy and Innovation Kvaerner.

In an interview before the leg, Cayard reflected on his shortcomings. He noted one of them was his inability to relax at all during a race. "I find that I can't go off duty," Cayard said. "No matter how many days or weeks it may be, I simply can't disengage. Even in my bunk when I am supposed to be getting some sleep, I can't. One ear is always tuned into what is happening up on deck. It's exhausting, and I know it is not good from a competitive standpoint for me to let myself get so exhausted."

It was that sleep-deprived Paul Cayard who, on this leg's last full day of sailing, was still clawing his way back. "I did not sleep much in the last 24 hours," Cayard emailed. "My anxiety built with our demise. There is no way for me to drop it from my mind."

One by one, the boats rounded Cape Reinga and began a sprint down the coast. Swedish Match, as expected, was the first around. To her crew's horror, she didn't get far. After sailing around the cape, near North Island the wind suddenly disappeared. Swedish Match's sails fell limp and the boat glided to a stop. Krantz had fallen into one of the shore-effect wind holes he had been concerned about before the leg started.

One by one, the sight that confronted them — the leader dead in the water — flabbergasted the boats behind Swedish Match. Dennis Conner recalled the moment: "Someone said it looked like there was an America's Cup boat meeting us, and I told them they must be nuts," said Conner. "Then we realised it was a Whitbread boat and when it turned out to be Gunnar Krantz and Swedish Match we were all laughing."

From being the odds-on favourite to win the leg, the Swedish Match crew had been reduced to the job of warning buoy. They marked the wind hole for the rest of the fleet as one by one they sailed past in procession. "It's a yachtsman's worst nightmare," said Swedish Match co-skipper Erle Williams. "When you are leading to fall into a hole and to know that the others are coming at you."

After four boats passed them, a puffy breeze freed the hapless crew, and Swedish Match rejoined the procession along the coast. It was too late: The largely Kiwi crew aboard Merit Cup, with the smell of their homeland in their nostrils, were not to be denied. Merit Cup pulled into the lead with Toshiba right on her stern.

If a Hollywood studio had choreographed the Leg 4 finish it could not have created a more spectacular finale. As the hometown crew aboard Merit Cup match-raced the famed Dennis Conner to the finish line, everything was just the way it should be for such a moment. After two weeks of light breezes in the area, the wind suddenly kicked up to an impressive 45 knots for the finish. Thousands of Kiwis lined the shore to cheer their countrymen on.

In lumpy seas and surrounded by an enormous fleet of spectator boats, Merit Cup crossed the finish line to capture the leg victory. Two minutes and 36 seconds later, Toshiba crossed in second place — close enough, but it could have been a lot closer. No sooner had Merit Cup crossed the line than her mainsail disintegrated in a gust of wind. The drama of it all was almost more than the normally stoic Dalton could take.

"I was telling my crew on the way in of the two greatest days in my life," Dalton said in a dockside interview. "The first was four years ago when we beat Tokio into here, and the second was today."

Ten minutes behind Toshiba, Chessie Racing crossed to claim her second third-place slot in as many legs. EF Language crossed in fourth place, a finish that gave the team enough points to retain the overall lead in the race.

Salvaging what he could of his doomed lead, Gunnar Krantz steered Swedish Match to a fifth-place finish, 17 minutes behind EF Language. Over two hours would pass before the sixth boat crossed — another disappointing performance for the once highly rated Silk Cut team. Innovation Kvaerner, which had plotted a too-northerly course early in the leg, came in 41 minutes behind Silk Cut.

The last two boats to finish were BrunelSunergy and EF Education. BrunelSunergy's skipper, Roy Heiner, said he believed improvements needed to be made to his Judel/Vrolijk-designed yacht. Since the Alan Andrews-designed entry, America's Challenge, had dropped out of the race after Leg 1, the only boat in the fleet that was not designed by Bruce Farr was the Dutch boat. "Our boat is designed by a person who has designed for the first time," said Heiner. "We can still see improvements and by the end of the race we might be happy we have our boat than another boat."

Even though they were the last to arrive, the EF Education crew was clearly becoming a sentimental favourite amongst the fans. A beaming barefooted skipper, Christine Guillou, brought the boat in to a rapturous welcome by thousands of fans, who had waited two additional hours just to cheer the women into port.

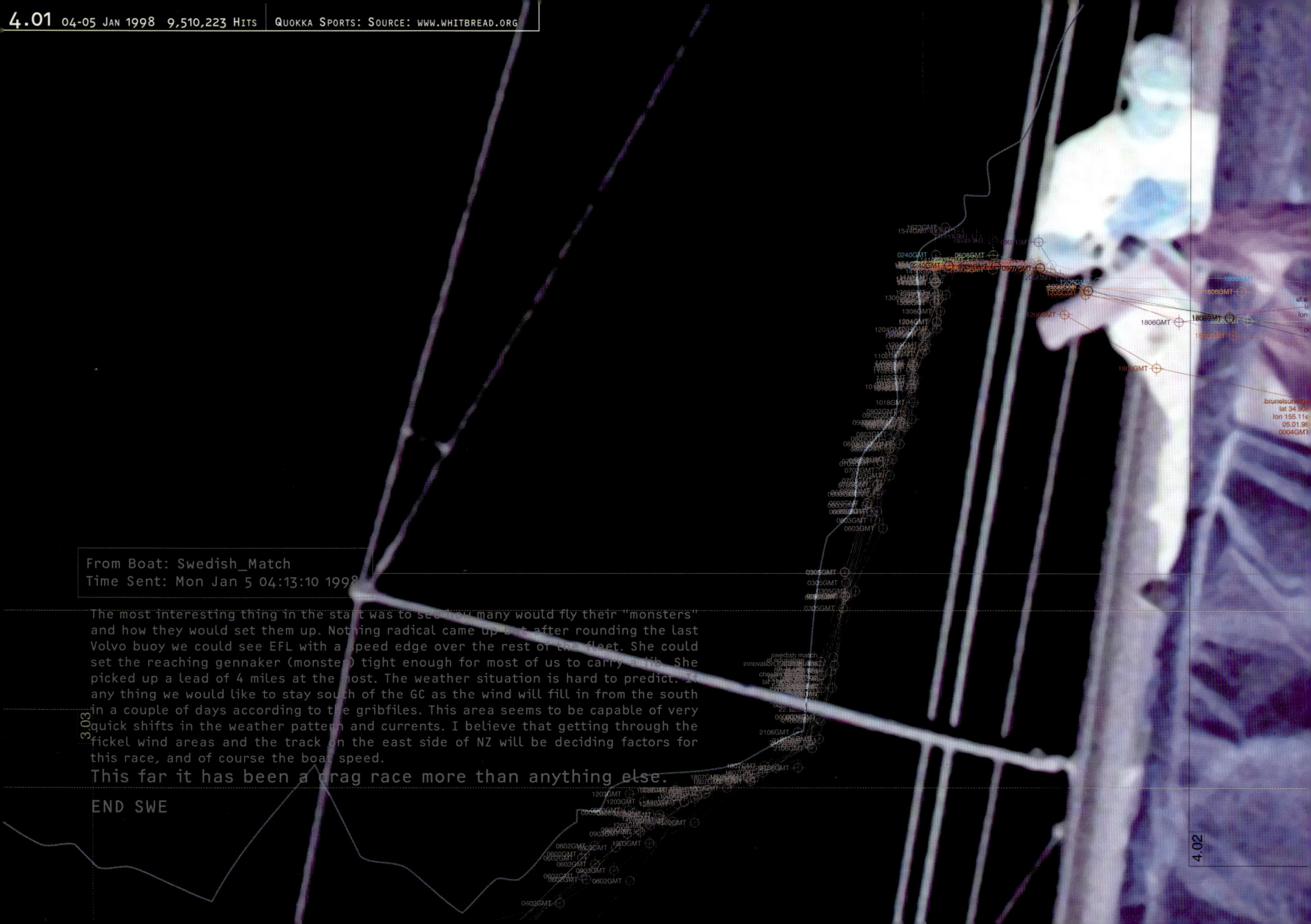

4.01 04-05 JAN 1998 9,510,223 HITS QUOKKA SPORTS: SOURCE: WWW.WHITBREAD.ORG

From Boat: Swedish_Match
Time Sent: Mon Jan 5 04:13:10 1998

The most interesting thing in the start was to see how many would fly their "monsters" and how they would set them up. Nothing radical came up but after rounding the last Volvo buoy we could see EFL with a speed edge over the rest of the fleet. She could set the reaching gennaker (monster) tight enough for most of us to carry a jib. She picked up a lead of 4 miles at the most. The weather situation is hard to predict. If any thing we would like to stay south of the GC as the wind will fill in from the south in a couple of days according to the gribfiles. This area seems to be capable of very quick shifts in the weather pattern and currents. I believe that getting through the fickel wind areas and the track on the east side of NZ will be deciding factors for this race, and of course the boat speed.
This far it has been a drag race more than anything else.

END SWE

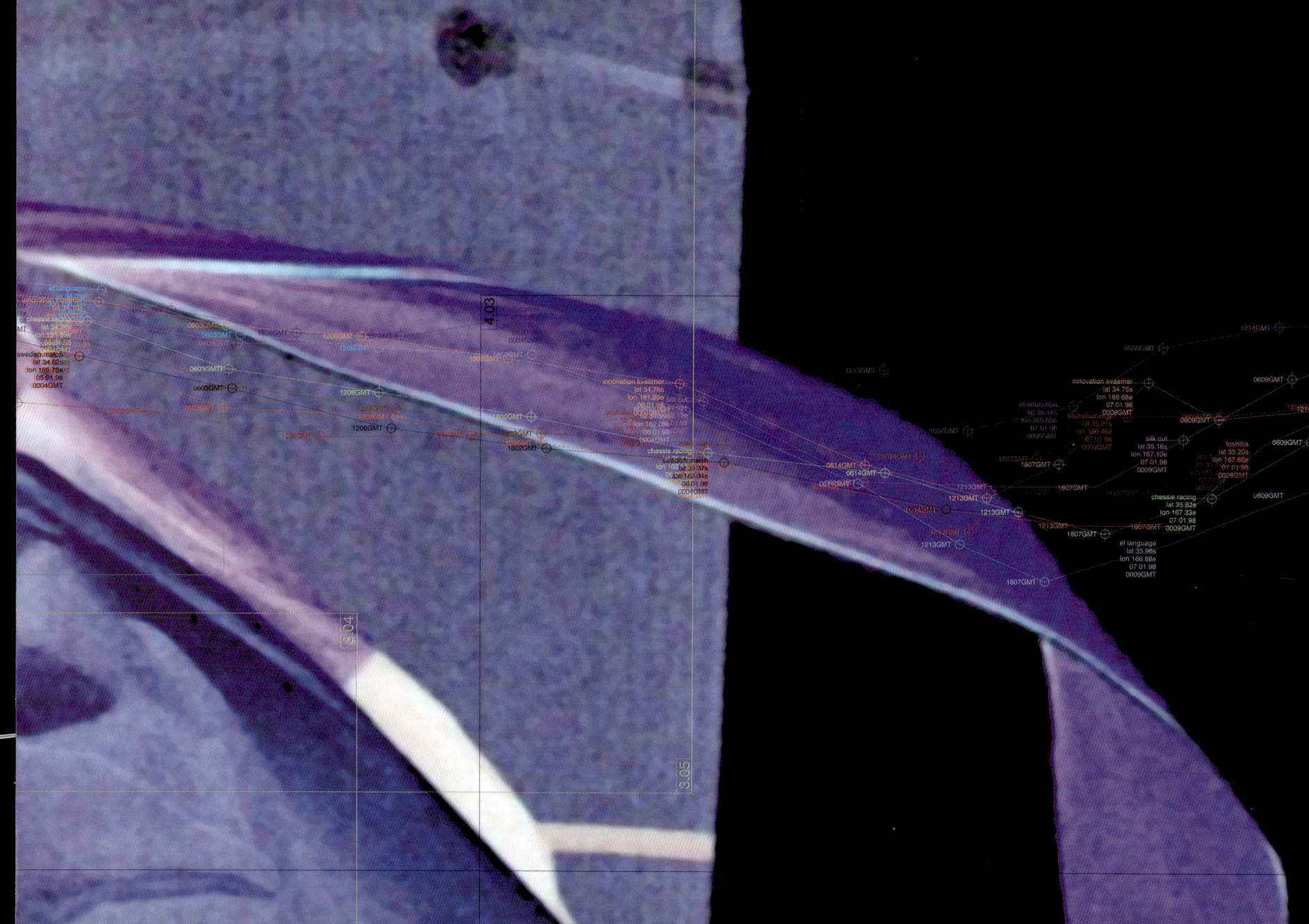

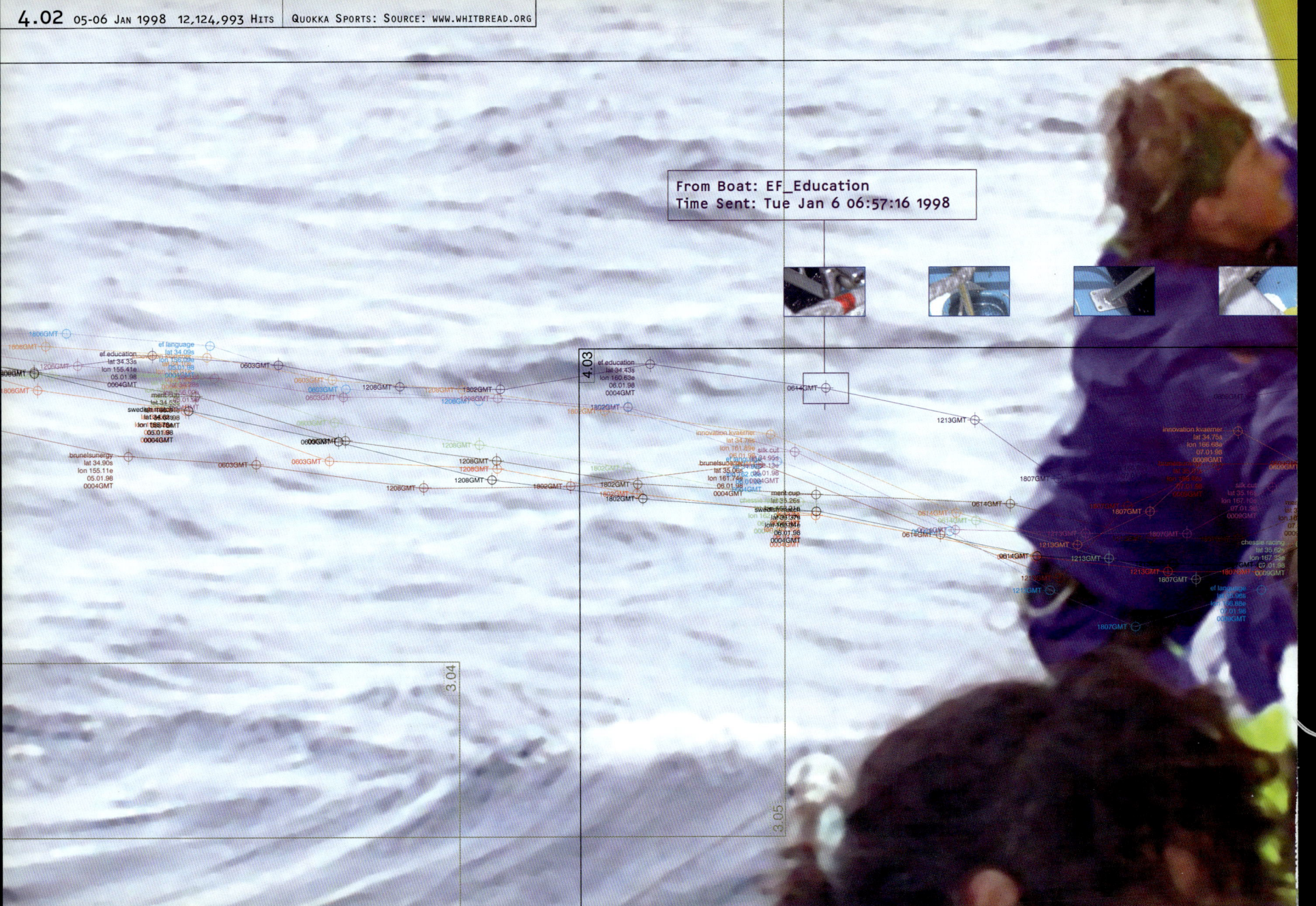

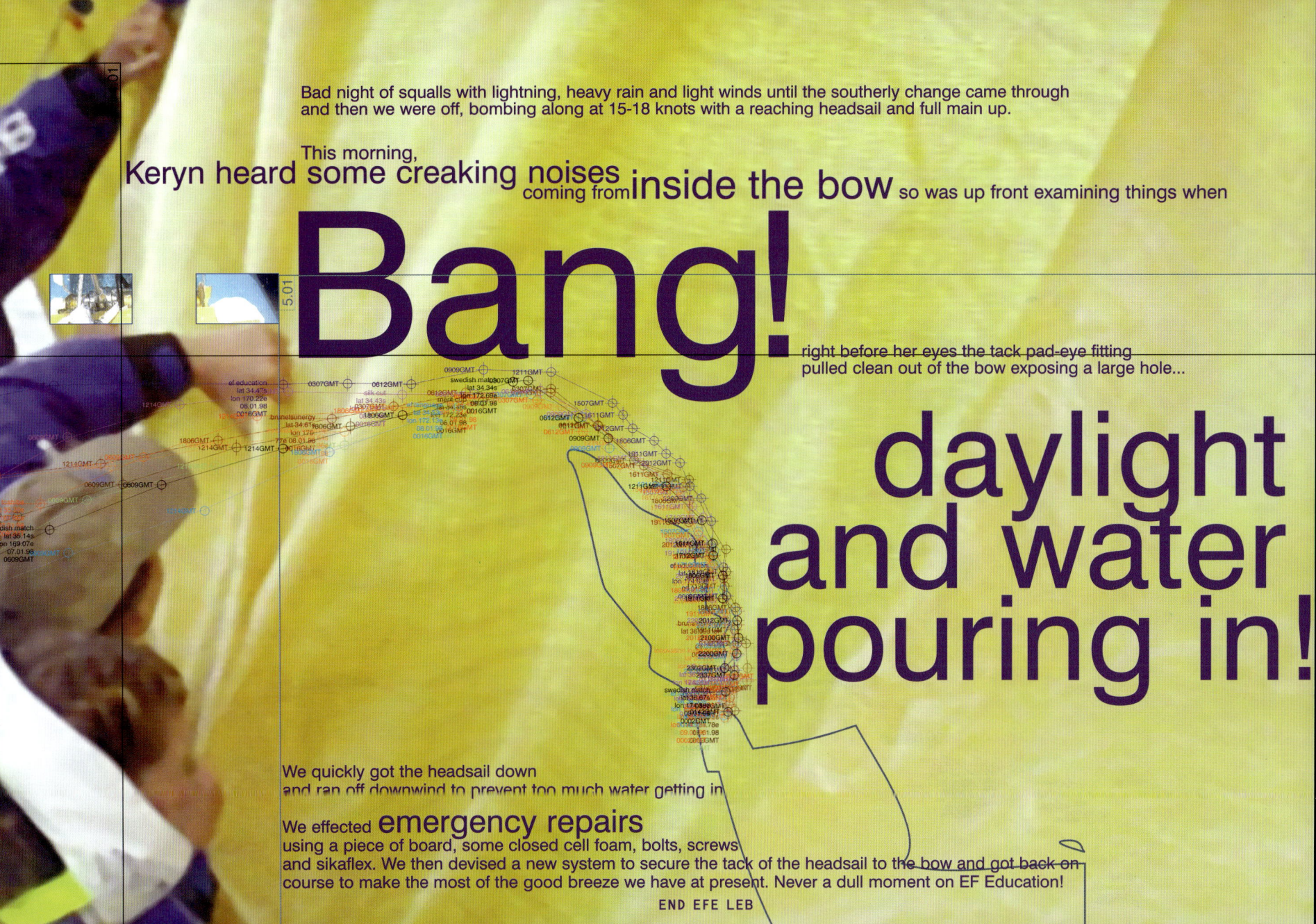

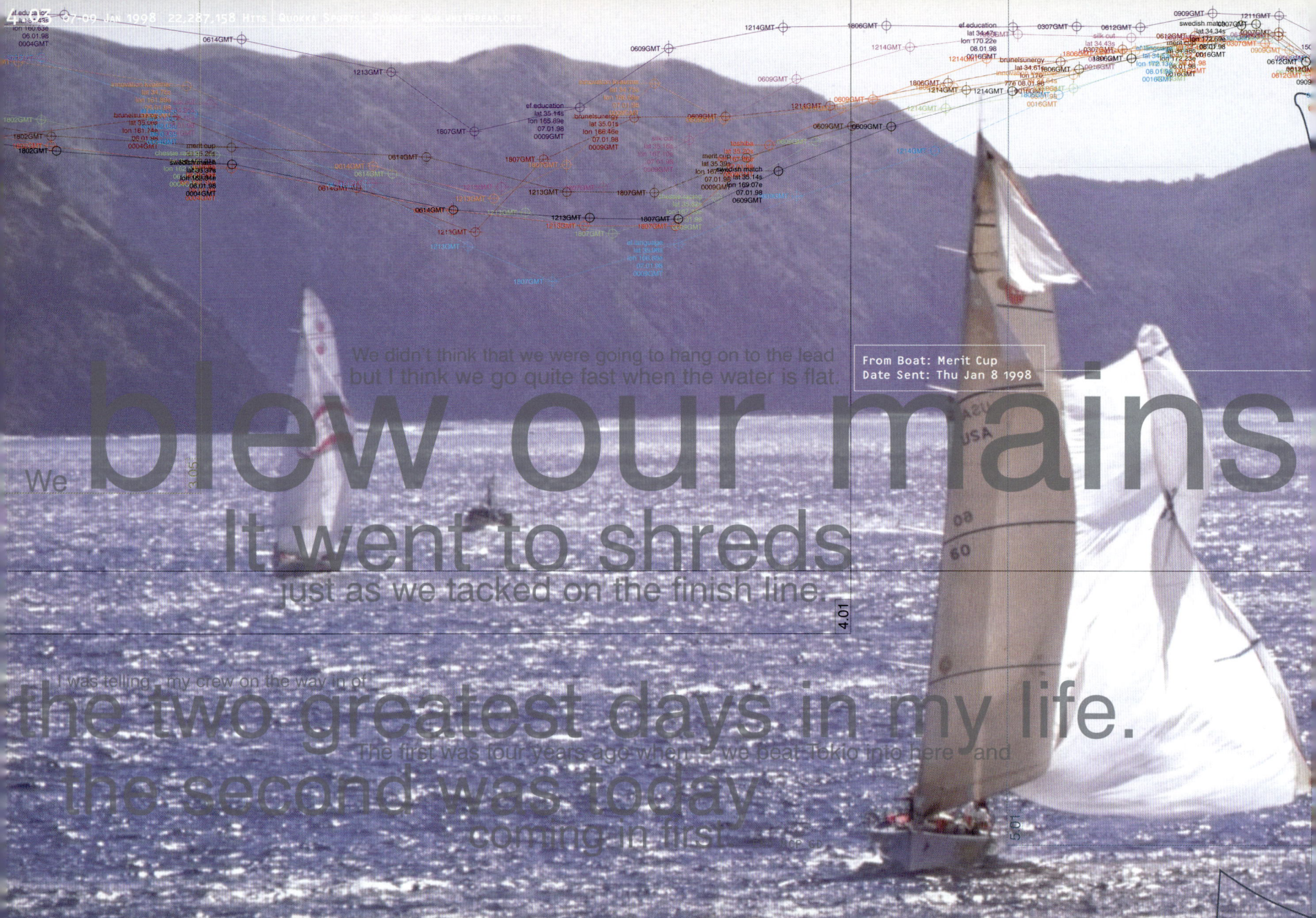

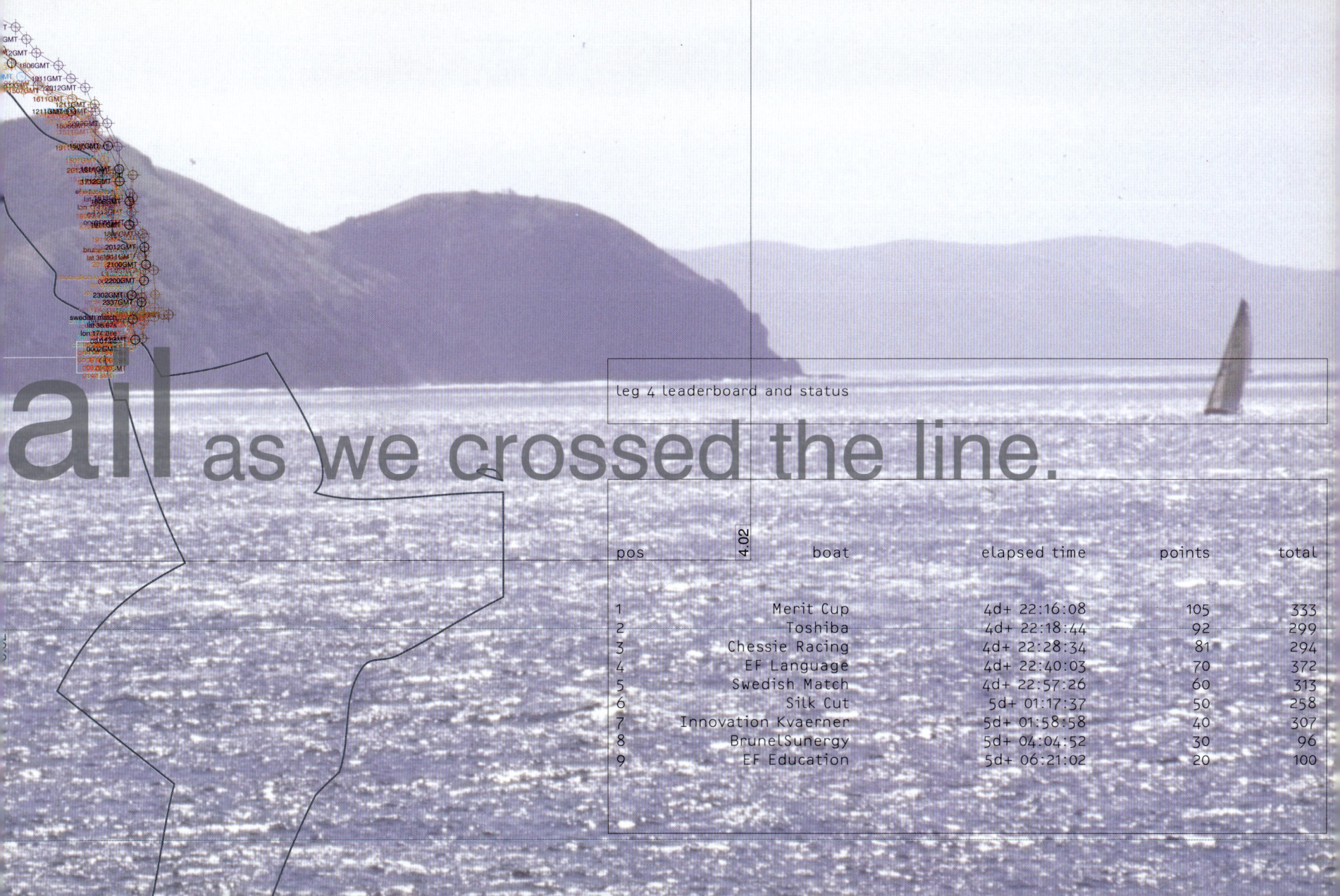

all as we crossed the line.

leg 4 leaderboard and status

4.02

pos	boat	elapsed time	points	total
1	Merit Cup	4d+ 22:16:08	105	333
2	Toshiba	4d+ 22:18:44	92	299
3	Chessie Racing	4d+ 22:28:34	81	294
4	EF Language	4d+ 22:40:03	70	372
5	Swedish Match	4d+ 22:57:26	60	313
6	Silk Cut	5d+ 01:17:37	50	258
7	Innovation Kvaerner	5d+ 01:58:58	40	307
8	BrunelSunergy	5d+ 04:04:52	30	96
9	EF Education	5d+ 06:21:02	20	100

5.0.0 01 Feb – 28 Feb 1998   140,495,087 Hits | Quokka Sports: Source: www.whitbread.org

Leg 5

Distance:

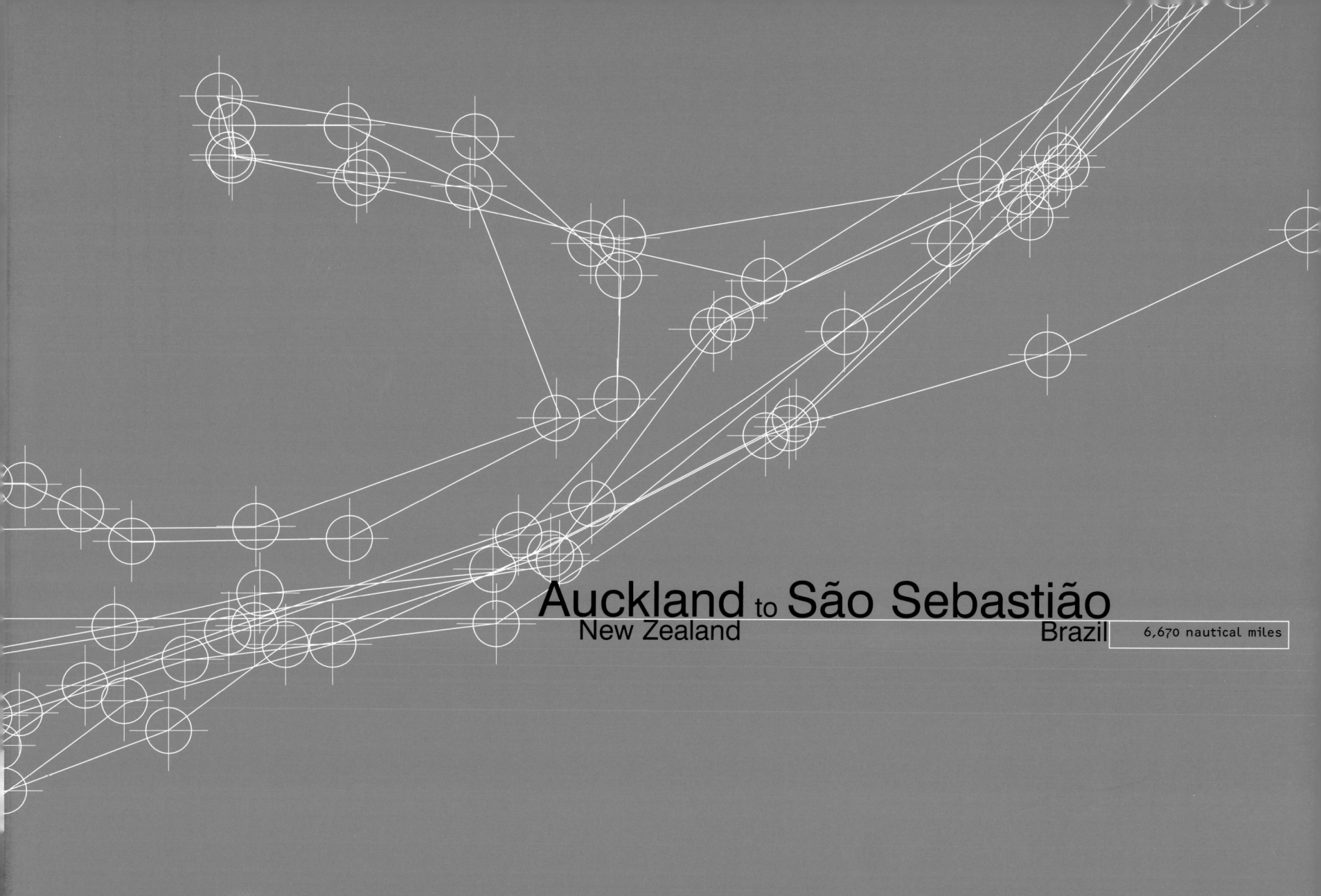

Leg 5: Prelude

A day after arriving in Auckland at the finish of Leg 4, the Toshiba team filed a formal protest against EF Language. Conner alleged that the boat had failed to display navigation lights after sunset on 8 January, in violation of race rules. The team also claimed EF Language had failed to turn her lights on even after being notified by Toshiba of the violation. At the time, the boats were in a tight tactical race, so Conner said EF Language's failure to turn on her lights put Toshiba at a disadvantage, "by not being able to keep visual contact with our close competition."

It was the first protest of the race, and fans flooded the Whitbread Web site with mail either berating Conner for injecting litigious 'America's Cup' tactics into The Whitbread, or praising him for insisting that race rules be respected.

The protest meant members of the International Jury had to be flown in from around the world to hear the case. On 13 January, the jury convened at the Royal New Zealand Yacht Squadron headquarters and listened to Toshiba's complaint. Conner alleged that, as the rules required, he had sent a message to EF Language regarding her running lights violation.

Though the message was received by the Whitbread Race Office, no record existed that EF Language ever received Toshiba's protest. The team claimed they had not. After brief deliberations, noting that "no verbal communication was made at the time or subsequently by Toshiba to advise EF Language that Toshiba was protesting," the jury ruled Toshiba's protest invalid.

With the protest out of the way, attention shifted to preparations for the race's most dramatic and potentially dangerous leg. It would be a 6,670-nautical-mile trek from Auckland, through the Southern Ocean, around Cape Horn, and up the eastern coast of South America to São Sebastião, Brazil.

The fleet had now covered over 15,000 nautical miles, just less than half of the total 31,600 miles. For most, Leg 5 meant more than simply crossing the halfway point. The Southern Ocean leg is the one that most Whitbread competitors feel embodies the race's essence, exposing sailors and yachts to every extreme condition Poseidon can produce. From the warm waters of New Zealand, the boats nose-dive south, into the Screaming Sixties. There, gale-force winds whip up giant seas, and hull-puncturing chunks of ice sailors call 'growlers' lurk just below the surface. As the boats head toward Cape Horn, they are over 2,000 miles from the nearest land or help if disaster should strike.

For EF Language skipper Paul Cayard, this Southern Ocean leg held an additional challenge. His first taste of Southern Ocean conditions had been neither pleasant nor successful, earning him and his team their worst standing of the race so far. "We will see how much I learned when we go back down into that danger zone," Cayard said, reflecting on the leg ahead. "My learning curve is a lot steeper than most people's. We have talked a lot about what happened on the second leg and we feel ready to go."

It was also make-or-break time for Silk Cut. Rumours surrounded the team's poor showing, focusing on the lack of trust between skipper Lawrie Smith and his young navigator, Steve Hayles. Hayles eventually resigned, replaced by a Smith campaign veteran, Vincent Geake.

Chessie Racing skipper George Collins had taken the helm on the last two legs, and had put the team on the podium both times with two third-place finishes. The 57-year-old retired businessman knew that the Southern Ocean was no place for him. Before the race began, he promised he would not impose himself on the crew in conditions better suited to younger men. "When conditions get tough, it takes a full crew of twelve to sail one of these boats," Collins noted. "When I am on board in those conditions, I am like half a crewmember. I will step off when appropriate and get out of the way."

On Leg 5, Collins did so, relinquishing the skipper's cap to an experienced offshore sailor, Dee Smith.

On Toshiba, Paul Standbridge, 39, returned as skipper, as Dennis Conner, 56, also stepped aside to let a younger man sail this punishing leg.

Leg 5: Auckland, New Zealand, to São Sebastião, Brazil

"What we are doing down here is indescribable. It is on the brink of being madness."

Swedish Match skipper, Gunnar Krantz

The fleet of nine boats left Auckland harbour as they arrived, listening to the cheers of tens of thousands of fans and surrounded by an enormous spectator fleet. The boats crossed the line in stately order under spinnakers in a light breeze. It would soon prove a frustrating start for the geared-up crews. After rounding the first turning mark 4.5 nautical miles from the starting line, the breeze died and sails went limp. It took another 45 minutes for the fleet to inch its way 2.5 miles to the second mark. A brief blast of wind got all the boats around the mark in just seven minutes — then the wind died again.

The fleet, still surrounded by thousands of pleasure craft, wallowed in the Hauraki Gulf. Five hours after the start, the WRO issued the first official position report, showing Chessie Racing in the lead, 2.1 miles ahead of Merit Cup. Essentially, the report was meaningless, as the boats were making no appreciable headway. Just over five miles separated the boats as they inched their way out to sea.

The first week proved slow and frustrating. Once offshore, the fleet spread out across a 48-mile east/west axis, with EF Language the most westerly of the boats. The yachts were still running downwind as they pointed south in light northwesterly breezes. By the fifth day at sea, Paul Standbridge had had enough of the light conditions — that night, under cover of darkness, Toshiba broke away. She gybed, pointing her bow farther south. The next morning, Toshiba was in the lead, followed by Merit Cup and EF Language.

As the boats crawled south, the weather finally began to change. Lynnath Beckley aboard EF Education reported chilly conditions and fog. Nevertheless, though the area was known for fierce winds, none materialised. "Definitely slower than you expect for this part of the world," Merit Cup skipper Grant Dalton reported.

By the end of the first week, conditions had changed for the leaders. They finally tasted wind, though not the kind they wanted. The leading six boats — Toshiba, EF Language, Swedish Match, Silk Cut, Chessie Racing and Merit Cup — suddenly found themselves beating in a stiffening 30-knot easterly breeze. Well behind them, the last three boats, Innovation Kvaerner, BrunelSunergy and EF Education, were running downwind in 45 knots of westerly breeze. It was a classic example of being on the correct side of a low-pressure system. The leaders were on the wrong side.

"We are now on the south side of the low [pressure system], hard on the wind with very confused seas (and crew!)," emailed Swedish Match skipper Gunnar Krantz. Aboard EF Language, Paul Cayard reported, "It has been a tough 24 hours. A low-pressure system has come and wreaked havoc with the race course." Cayard added that he was forced to rewrite half his email report because he found he could not hold on and write at the same time.

By Day 8, Silk Cut had snatched the lead briefly from EF Language. By the end of the day, however, she was back in third position behind Swedish Match. The real action was at the tail end of the fleet, where the EF Education crew were having gear problems again. A turnbuckle on the starboard rod had ripped out of the stud atop the first spreader. The crew immediately dropped the main and gybed to avoid a catastrophic mast failure. In the dark, with the wind howling, Bridget Suckling and Lisa Charles climbed the rig to see if they could reconnect the rod, but were unable to do so. The next morning the crew reinforced the mast by winching lines tight around it. Even with this repair, clearly the boat was in no condition to race. Plans were laid for a cautious sail around Cape Horn to the small town of Ushuaia, Argentina, for additional repairs. It seemed the only break the sailors on EF Education were going to get in this race was broken gear.

Wind and sea conditions continued to build as the Southern Ocean began to live up to its billing.

Aboard Innovation Kvaerner, holding on in seventh place, skipper Knut Frostad reported conditions had reached the limit. "I have just experienced some of the toughest days ever on the sea," Frostad wrote. "Winds gusting up to 68 knots. Suddenly you are not in the race anymore, but rather just focused on survival."

The question facing the crews was just how far south they dared go. The farther south, the shorter the distance to the finish; simultaneously, the greater the danger. The Antarctic ice and frigid conditions would only add to the already fierce wind and seas. "How far south?" Krantz asked, noting that the choice of a southerly route also determined a boat's approach to Cape Horn, "one of the most important decisions of the leg."

The first boat to report ice was leader EF Language, who sighted a one-mile-long iceberg just off her lee side. The weather continued to deteriorate. Grant Dalton reported that the only remaining dry spot aboard Merit Cup was the navigation station. He went on to report that conditions had become so rough that it was literally impossible to stand on deck without getting washed off your feet in seconds. EF Language navigator Mark Rudiger complained that he did not even dare leave the nav station to go 10 feet forward to fetch a much-needed cup of coffee. The reason wasn't his fear of falling, but rather a desperate need to keep as much weight in the boat's stern as possible so the bow would not bury itself in the fierce oncoming waves.

Dawn on the tenth day brought the second boat casualty of the leg. The sole UK entry in the race, Silk Cut, radioed race headquarters and reported a problem. While running hard in 30 knots of wind with a masthead kite up, the crew suddenly heard a loud bang. All eyes instinctively turned upward, to discover that the mast had snapped off just above the second set of spreaders. The wounded Silk Cut yacht now joined EF Education, over 2,000 miles from land, limping along with a jury-rigged mast. After assessing their options — all grim — skipper Smith reported that they too would head for Ushuaia for repairs.

The tenth day also saw a dangerous battle over third place, between Toshiba and Merit Cup. In raging winds and seas, the two boats were sailing nearly side by side, both hoisting sail despite the ugly conditions and recent reports of ice. "As I look out the hatch, not more than 200 metres away there is Toshiba absolutely flying," reported Dalton. "This is not safe at all, the way we are sailing now, but what choice do you have?"

Two hours later, Dalton said he had had enough. "With the wind getting to over 40 knots and the boat absolutely out of control, I pulled the plug and left Toshiba to it." Dalton wrote the next day that the violent match race had left his crew mending torn sails, a spinnaker pole snapped in two places, and three broken battens in the mainsail. Still, discretion seemed to triumph over valour. At the end of the day, Merit Cup had regained third place, passing Toshiba and gaining nearly 20 miles on leaders EF Language and Swedish Match.

It was now time for the front of the fleet to begin lining up for an approach to Cape Horn. Swedish Match was trailing the leader, EF Language, by about 50 miles — skipper Gunnar Krantz was determined to close the gap. He was pushing his boat and crew to the breaking point. "What we are going through is indescribable," Krantz wrote in his daily dispatch. "It is on the brink of being madness. Pushing the boat as hard at night as in the day. It is very, very scary, but you just do it."

Aboard Chessie Racing, which had been holding in sixth position, trouble struck belowdecks. A small but critical part on the boat's main generator gave out. Without the generator, the boat did not have enough electrical power to produce fresh water or to shift water ballast when the boat tacked. "My mind didn't focus on The Whitbread race any longer," reported watch captain Grant Spanhake, "but on how we could survive."

Though less spectacular than a mast failure, Chessie's broken generator was no less serious a problem. With most of the food aboard requiring rehydration, no fresh water meant no food. In the brutal cold of the Southern Ocean, crews burnt between 3,500 and 4,000 calories a day. (Typically, humans burn roughly 2,000 calories a day.)

Meanwhile, on deck the wind was howling at over 45 knots. If the boat had to tack, there was no way to shift the water ballast to maintain trim and stability. Plans were immediately put in motion to get a replacement part flown from Baltimore, Md., US, to Rio de Janeiro, Brazil. From there the part would be flown by private plane to a point on the coast near Cape Horn, where a launch would deliver it to the yacht. This made three wounded yachts heading for the desolate southern tip of South America for repairs.

At the head of the fleet, EF Language was having a flawless race. She had extended her lead to nearly 130 miles by 15 February 1998, Day 15. Cayard rounded Cape Horn before the end of the day. To add insult to injury, as well as frustration for those chasing him, the good winds lasted just long enough for his boat, then dropped to nothing.

For Swedish Match's skipper, it was like reliving the Cape Reinga nightmare. "It seems like the word Cape is the same as wind hole for the blue boat," wrote a dejected Krantz. "We are rocking from side to side in the waves. Toshiba is suddenly even with us. Frustrating!"

Aboard Merit Cup, having slipped again to fourth behind Toshiba, the lull was infuriating. "I am indignant," Dalton wrote. "After eight days of gale-force winds, it has now deserted us at such a critical time." He said conditions were so tame at the normally dreaded spot that "if we had a dinghy we could almost row ashore to Cape Horn."

Almost 1,500 miles back in the fleet, conditions were much different for EF Education. While her crew was trying to nurse her severely weakened rig, a 35-knot easterly battered the yacht — the mast snapped just above the first set of spreaders. "Everyone on deck at the moment," navigator Lynnath Beckley reported in a terse message to the Whitbread Race Office. "Rig broken at first and second spreader...all OK. Now trying to disconnect remains of rig before it damages boat."

Back up front, Day 17 saw frustration build for the four boats chasing EF Language. Cayard continued to sail away, now 350 miles ahead of the nearest boat. Swedish Match, Toshiba, Merit Cup and Innovation Kvaerner inched slowly north in the unusually windless seas between South America and the Falkland Islands. Besides the lack of wind, the boats were also bedevilled by thick kelp that kept wrapping itself around their keels and props. Several boats reported having to stop, back their jibs and sail in reverse to free the tangled mess.

The next day brought no relief. The 'Gang of Four' spent the day trading places as they tacked back and forth looking for a breeze. As a measure of how bad the situation was, Innovation Kvaerner reported the fastest average speed for the previous 24 hours: 4.3 knots. The WRO reported that the crew aboard Toshiba had become so frustrated by the conditions that their most recent report — one line only — was "unprintable."

Over 200 miles behind, the Dutch boat, BrunelSunergy, had just rounded Cape Horn. Skipper Roy Heiner was aware of the pileup ahead. Twenty miles behind her, Chessie Racing was back on the race course after an Indy 500-style pit stop near shore. She picked up parts for her broken generator, plus additional food, water and fuel. Chessie, in seventh place, was breathing down BrunelSunergy's neck. Heiner decided he did not want to become boat No. 5 in the parking lot ahead and suddenly bore east.

The course he set took him on a risky eastern passage around the Falkland Islands. The favoured route, leaving the Falklands well to starboard, was proving a disappointment for the four boats ahead of him. Heiner knew that high pressure and fluky winds normally dominated the area east of the Falklands. He was betting the high-pressure system normally east of the Falklands was the one sitting on top of the Gang of Four. If he could get around the Falklands before the high moved back east, he could flank the four boats ahead of him, jumping into second place before they got moving again. It was a high-stakes play.

Dee Smith, skipper of Chessie Racing, saw Heiner's move, but decided it was too risky. Chessie had already beaten the odds once on this leg, and he was in no mood to press his luck. Smith was betting that by the time he caught up with the four boats parked ahead, the winds would have increased enough for him to plot a course just to the east and around them. If Heiner's guess was right, Smith calculated he would not do as well as BrunelSunergy, but would still benefit from the winds farther east. If, on the other hand, Heiner was wrong, then Chessie's skipper figured he would at least not end up stuck east of the Falklands.

One day later, Heiner's gambit had paid off, big time. While Swedish Match, Toshiba, Merit Cup and Innovation Kvaerner floated helplessly in light and shifty conditions to the west, BrunelSunergy found steady winds 25 miles east of the Falklands. Heiner, who had taken other, less successful flyers in this race, crowed. "I always knew we would get it right some day," Heiner said when BrunelSunergy moved into second place. "It is difficult to imagine that we thought to have lost it all as we lay becalmed before the Horn."

Dee Smith's calculations seemed to have panned out as well. Chessie Racing moved steadily up through the fleet. By sunset on Day 20, the order of the fleet had changed remarkably. EF Language remained in the lead by 530 miles. Next, however, was BrunelSunergy, after her successful eastward rounding of the Falklands. Chessie Racing had cut in behind Innovation Kvaerner to take fourth position.

As predicted, the winds did return for the four boats stuck west of the Falklands, but it didn't help. Grant Dalton bemoaned the fact that although they were sailing "at least as fast as the boats to the east of us, the current was hitting us so hard that we took some heavy losses to Chessie and Brunel." The current also "kicked up a nasty sea way," he reported. It was even worse for Innovation Kvaerner. The Norwegian team had elected to hug the coastline, ending up, in skipper Frostad's words, "completely hammered." The team dropped back to seventh position.

The dawn of Day 22 saw EF Language blasting along just 570 miles from the finish line. A fierce battle was under way between Chessie Racing, Swedish Match and Merit Cup — all within single-digit miles of one another — for third place. Chessie stubbornly held off each challenge.

Suddenly, Leg 5 was over. After 23 days and one hour at sea EF Language crossed the finish line in São Sebastião to capture Southern Ocean honours. It was Cayard's third victory of the race, and he was at the wheel when the boat crossed the line over 500 miles ahead of second-place BrunelSunergy. Amid the din of samba drummers and dancers, a beaming Cayard yelled answers to reporters' questions quayside. "For us to be first to Cape Horn and to finish first shows that we learned from our mistakes on Leg 2," he said. "And that is very satisfying." Cayard's navigator and friend, Mark Rudiger, agreed. "Paul definitely learned his lesson, and this time he listened to the guys who had been in the Southern Ocean before."

The second-place finish for BrunelSunergy three days later was particularly sweet for the Dutch team. For once in this race, the self-proclaimed "Happy Crew" had something to be happy about. Not only was it their best showing of the race so far, but the way they had pulled it off made it all the more satisfying. Heiner was asked about the Falklands manoeuvre that catapulted BrunelSunergy from the back of the fleet to the front. "We thought about it half a day before we got to Cape Horn," he said. "We saw it as a possibility then. And I was surprised that none of the others did it. We expected them to. But they all just followed each other. We were in the right position."

The Chessie team sailed into São Sebastião less than six hours behind BrunelSunergy, capturing another third-place win — three in three legs. No one was giving the Chessie team short shrift any longer. The crew had proven Chessie Racing could leave far more experienced Whitbread teams in her wake.

Swedish Match came in fourth. Toshiba crossed the line in fifth, followed three miles behind by Merit Cup. Shockingly, the order would not stand after allegations surfaced that shook the Toshiba team to its core.

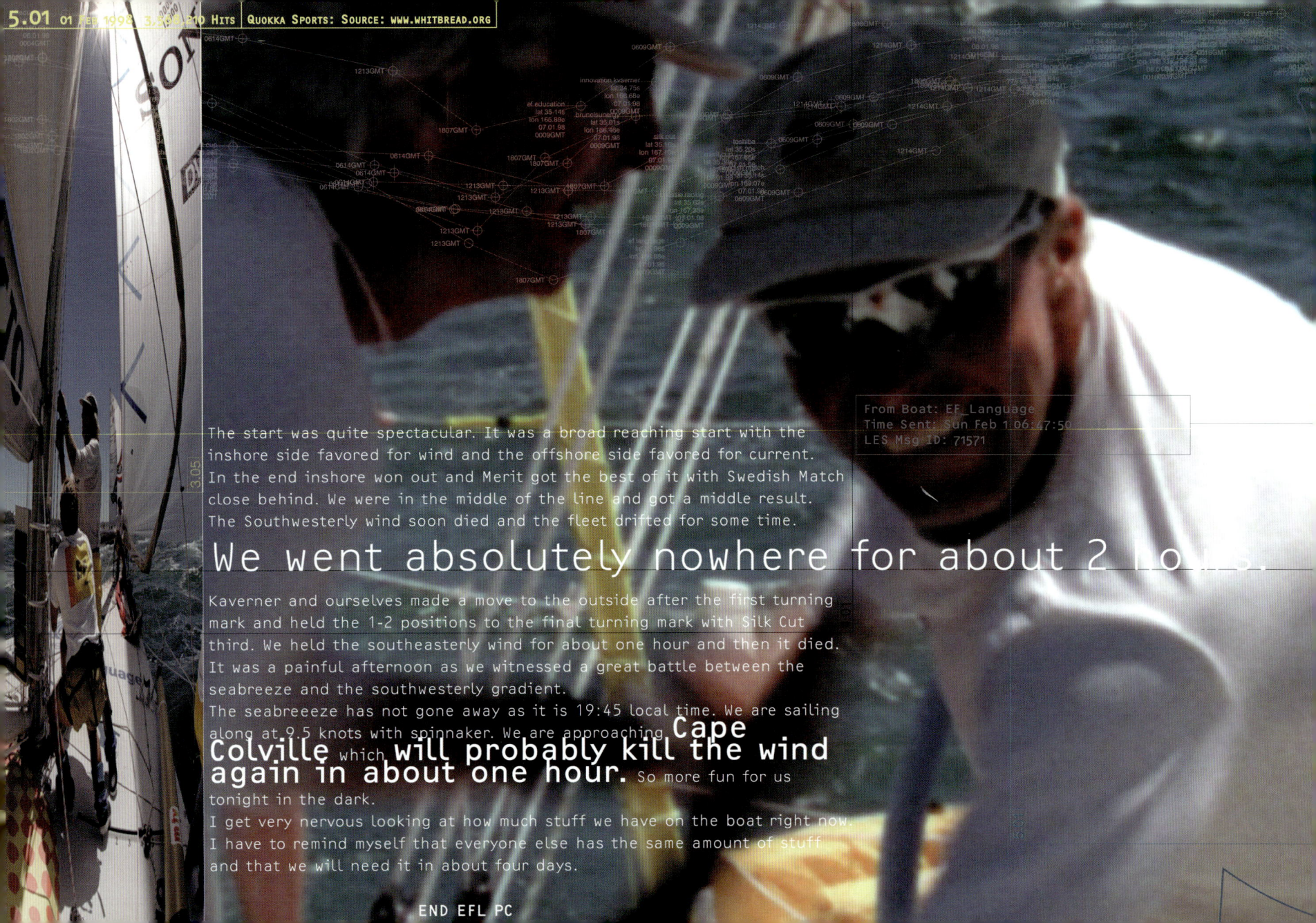

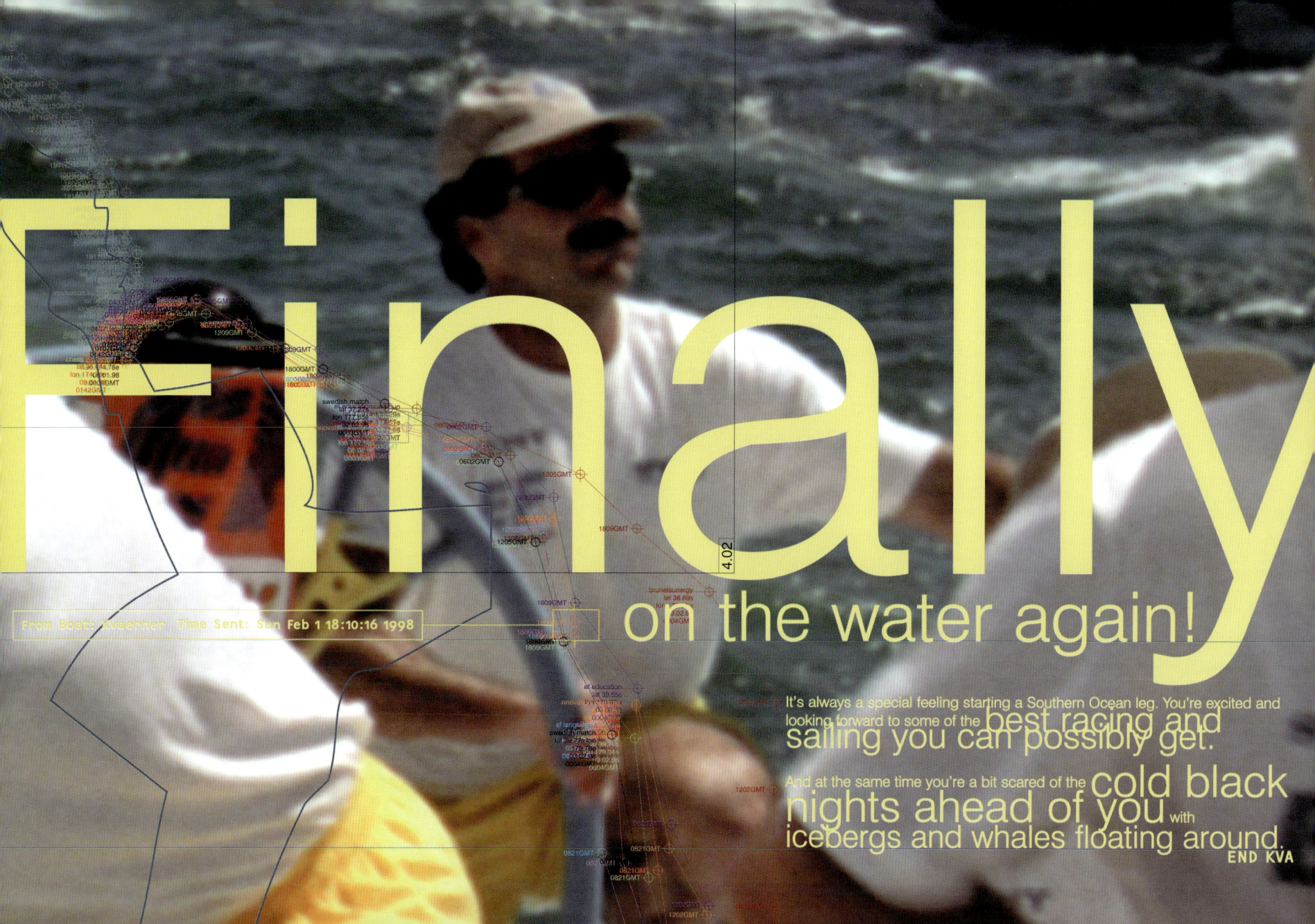

Finally
on the water again!

From Boat: Kvaerner Time Sent: Sun Feb 1 18:10:16 1998

It's always a special feeling starting a Southern Ocean leg. You're excited and looking forward to some of the best racing and sailing you can possibly get. And at the same time you're a bit scared of the cold black nights ahead of you with icebergs and whales floating around.
END KVA

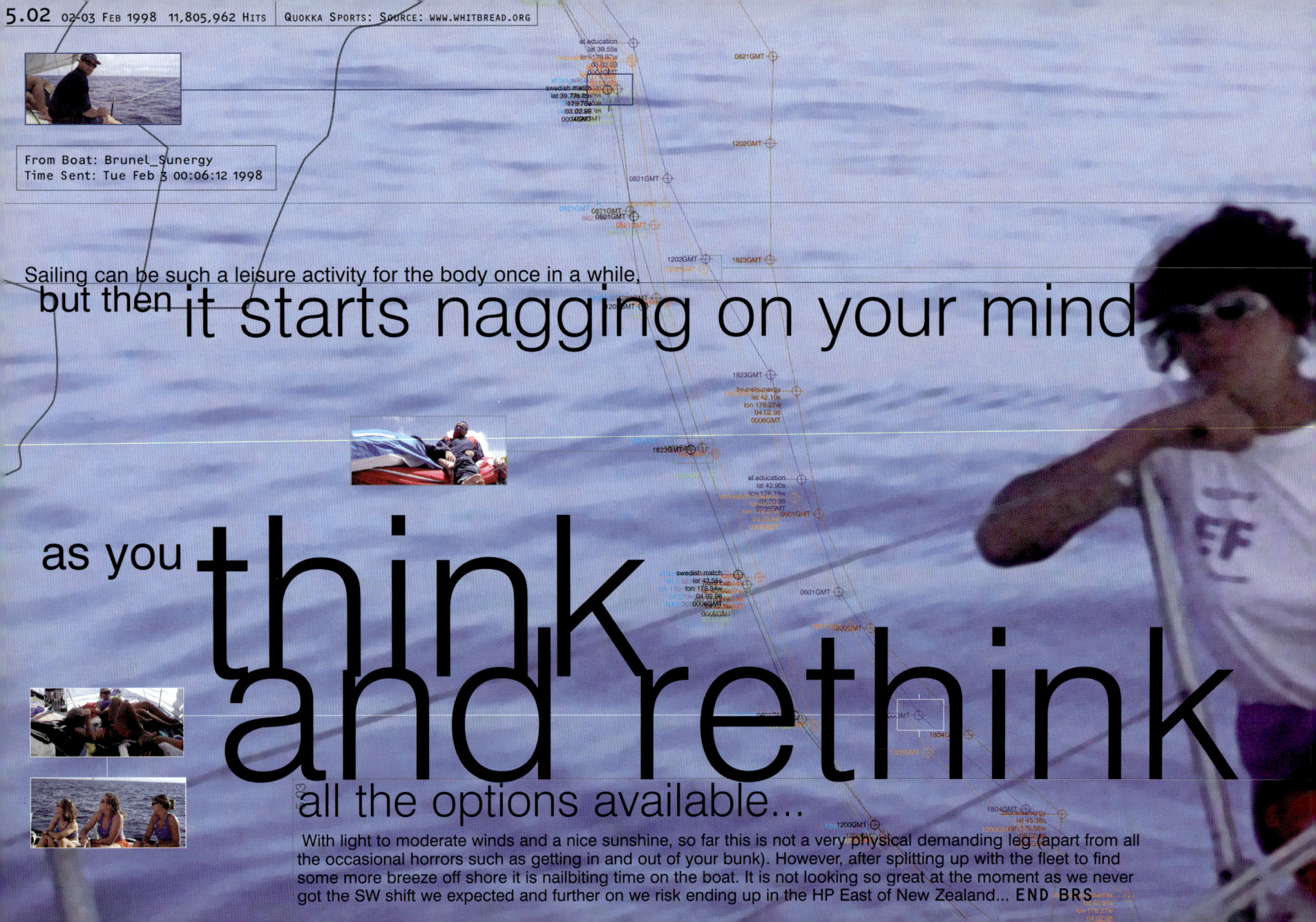

From Boat: Kvaerner
Time Sent: Tue Feb 3 12:09:00 1998

What a close race. Not that we don't like being chased by girls, but EF Education has really been giving us a hard time out here. **We have been fighting for every inch,** but at least it seems like we have positioned ourselves on the right side so far. It's still going to be light winds for some time, and I believe it's still too early to position yourself for the strong westerlies.
The next 24 hour will again be very important. It will be critical to get south of the fleet to be positioned well for the strong west and north west winds arriving from the west. Passed the date line today, so tomorrow should be Tuesday as well. Nick just missed out on having his birhday twice, as he had his day yesterday.

Getting colder at night now—
I guess it's sign of what to expect.   END KVA

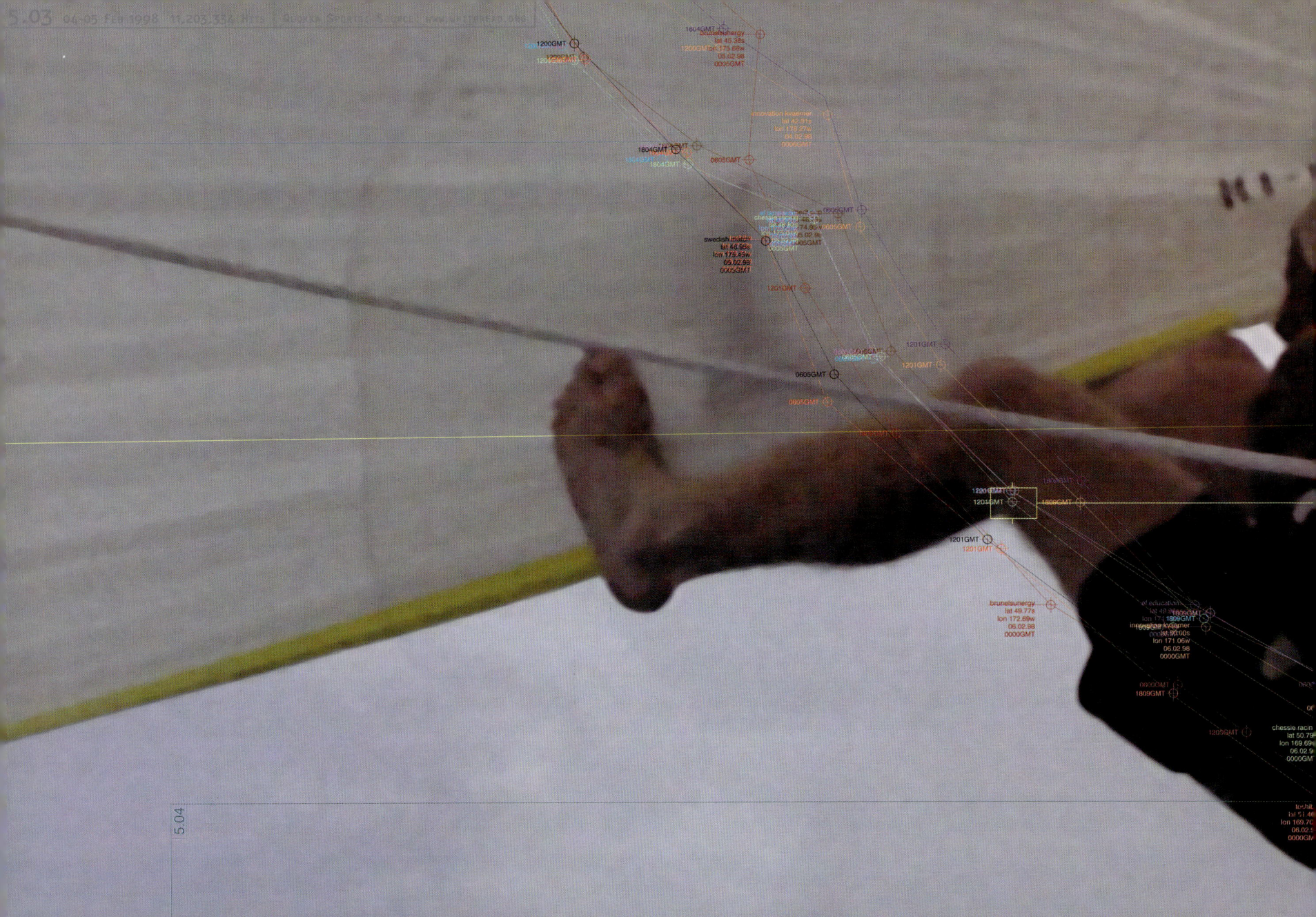

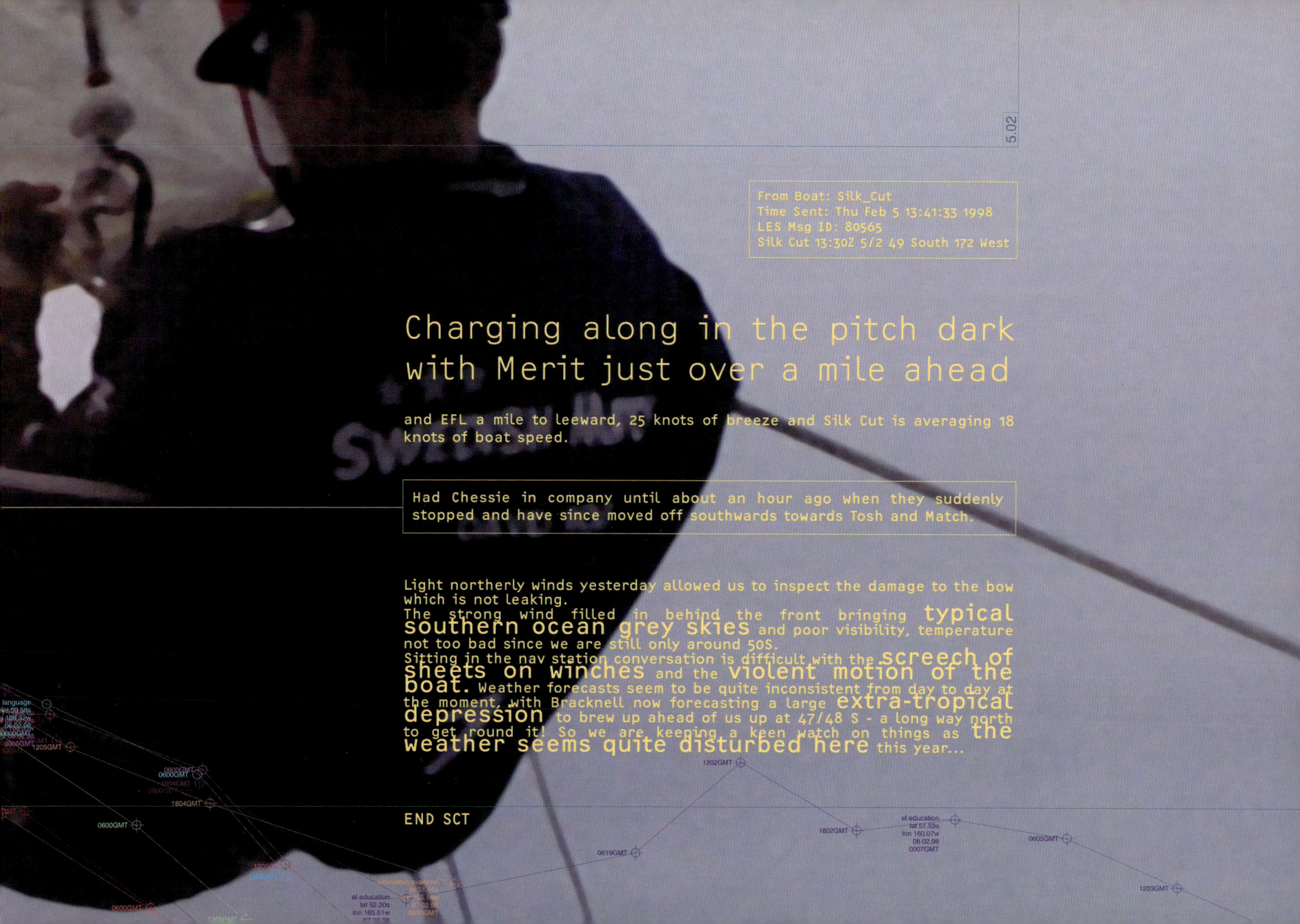

From Boat: Silk_Cut
Time Sent: Thu Feb 5 13:41:33 1998
LES Msg ID: 80565
Silk Cut 13:30Z 5/2 49 South 172 West

Charging along in the pitch dark with Merit just over a mile ahead

and EFL a mile to leeward, 25 knots of breeze and Silk Cut is averaging 18 knots of boat speed.

Had Chessie in company until about an hour ago when they suddenly stopped and have since moved off southwards towards Tosh and Match.

Light northerly winds yesterday allowed us to inspect the damage to the bow which is not leaking.
The strong wind filled in behind the front bringing **typical southern ocean grey skies** and poor visibility, temperature not too bad since we are still only around 50S.
Sitting in the nav station conversation is difficult with the **screech of sheets on winches** and the **violent motion of the boat.** Weather forecasts seem to be quite inconsistent from day to day at the moment, with Bracknell now forecasting a large **extra-tropical depression** to brew up ahead of us up at 47/48 S - a long way north to get round it! So we are keeping a keen watch on things as **the weather seems quite disturbed here** this year...

END SCT

5.04 06-07 Feb 1998 8,234,121 Hits Quokka Sports: Source: www.whitbread.org

From Boat: Swedish Match Time Sent: Fri Feb 6 05:47:44 1998

Weather is always hard to understand. It seems to have the right to change, be wrong, unpredictable, developing faster or slower than predicted etc. All the rights in the world at any point of time. Nobody is responsible and in charge, nobody to complain to and most of all, it just is what it is. It is funny that the single factor that influences this race most is untouchable.
This leg in particular is very hard to read right at all stages.

Our wind is now dropping

and we must choose the right course not to stop completely. We are already timeless on the boat after six days. Days are rolling on without us taking any notice, just race, eat and sleep.
Regards Gurra END SWE

From Boat: Swedish_Match Time Sent: Sat Feb 7 06:36:50 1998

I did talk about low pressure system in my last report and

I should probably have kept my m

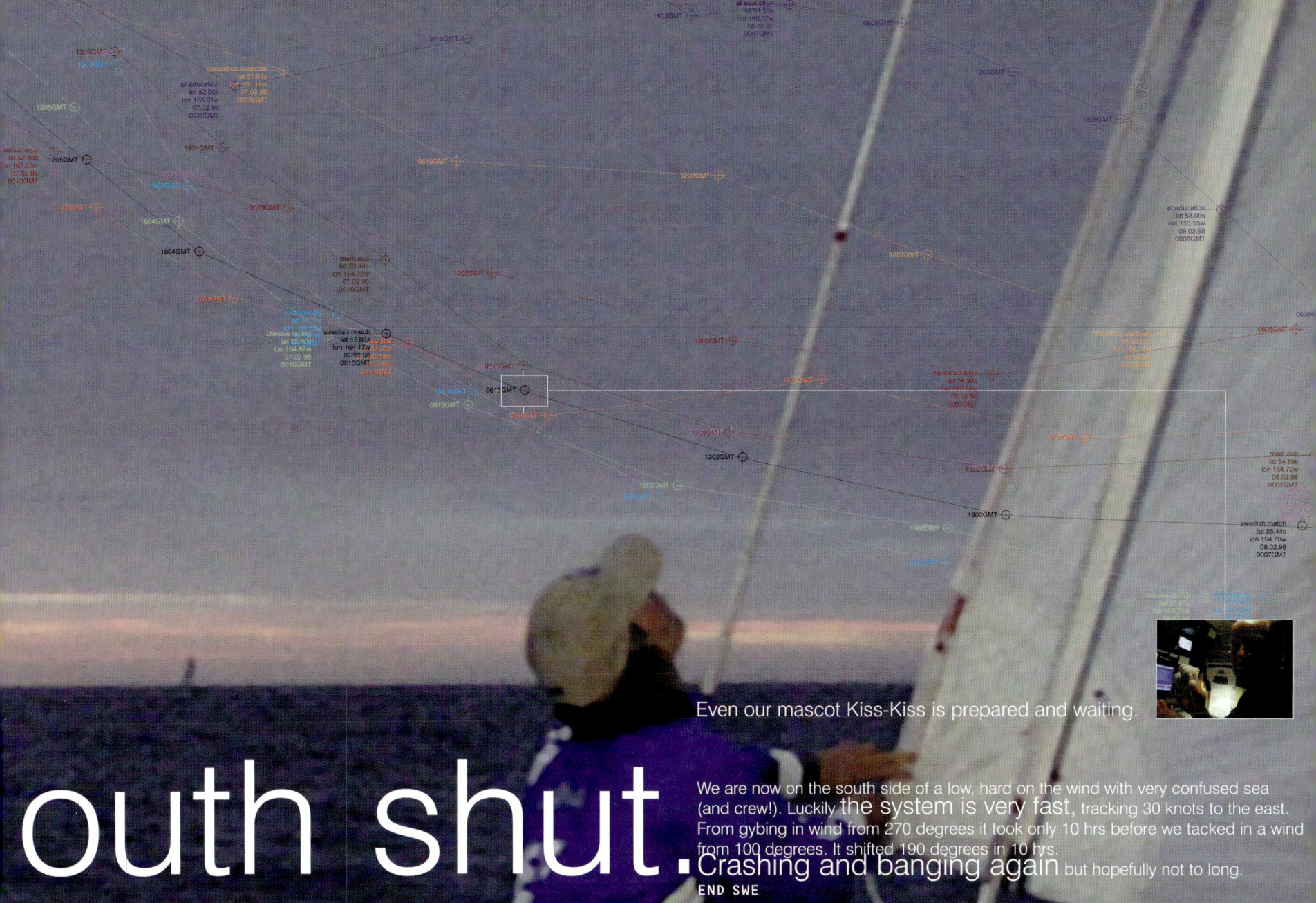

outh shut.

Even our mascot Kiss-Kiss is prepared and waiting.

We are now on the south side of a low, hard on the wind with very confused sea (and crew!). Luckily the system is very fast, tracking 30 knots to the east. From gybing in wind from 270 degrees it took only 10 hrs before we tacked in a wind from 100 degrees. It shifted 190 degrees in 10 hrs. Crashing and banging again but hopefully not to long.

END SWE

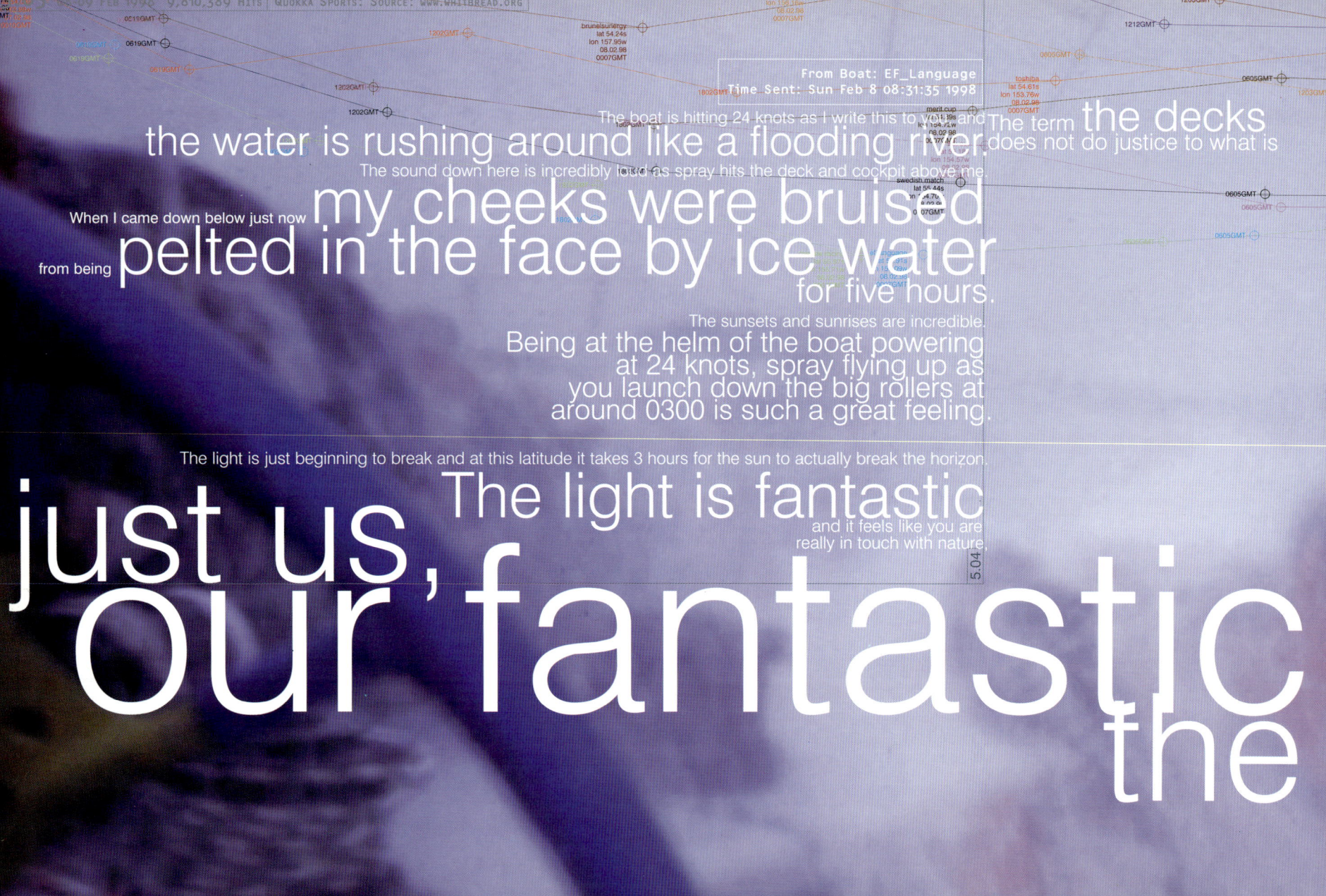

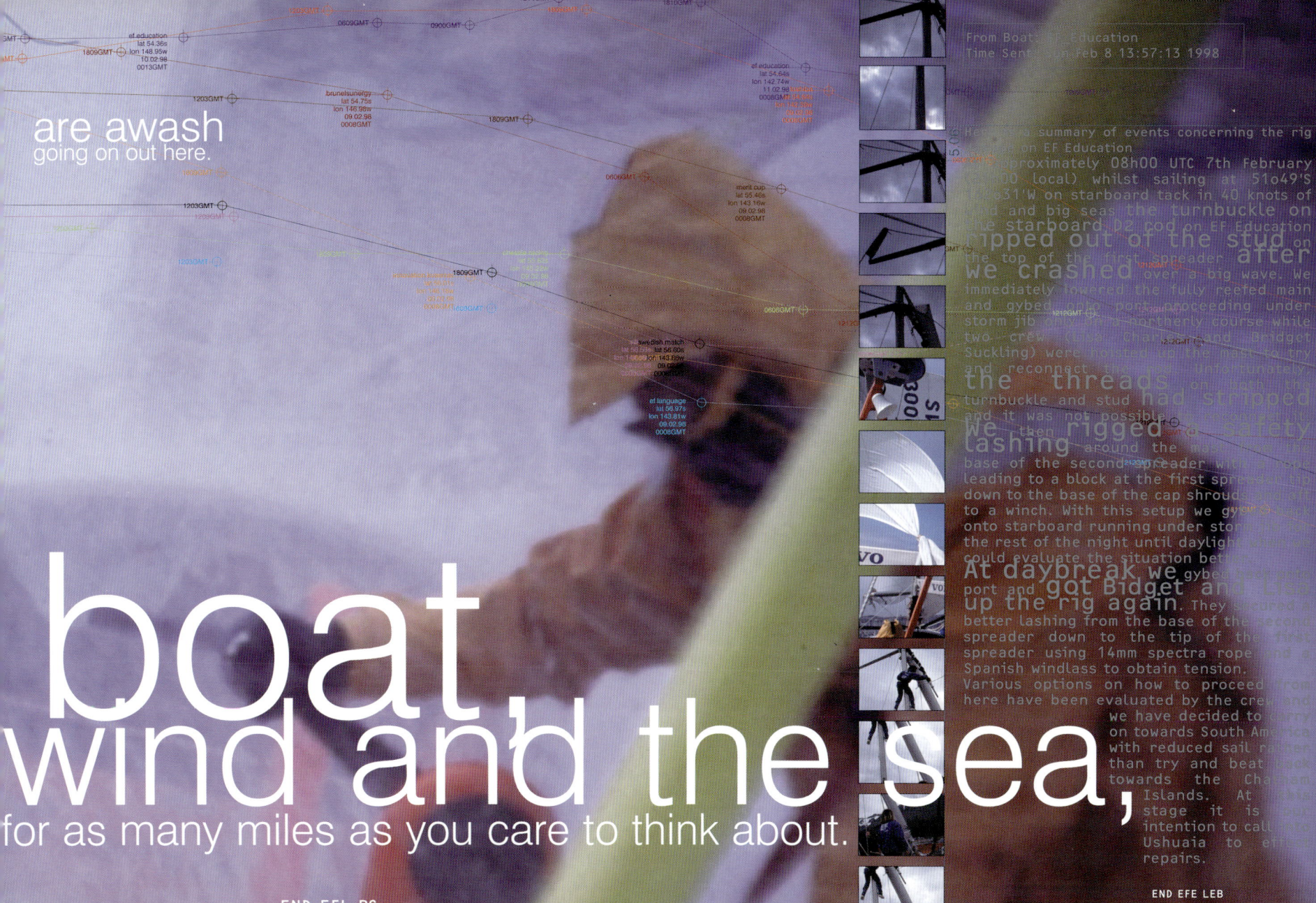

are awash
going on out here.

boat
wind and the sea,
for as many miles as you care to think about.

END EFL PC

From Boat: EF Education
Time Sent: Sun Feb 8 13:57:13 1998

Here is a summary of events concerning the rig failure on EF Education.

At approximately 08h00 UTC 7th February (05h00 local) whilst sailing at 51o49'S 64o31'W on starboard tack in 40 knots of wind and big seas the turnbuckle on the starboard D2 rod on EF Education ripped out of the stud on the top of the first spreader after we crashed over a big wave. We immediately lowered the fully reefed main and gybed onto port, proceeding under storm jib on a northerly course while two crew (Paul Champ and Bridget Suckling) were hoisted up the mast to try and reconnect the turnbuckle. Unfortunately the threads on both the turnbuckle and stud had stripped and it was not possible. We then rigged a safety lashing around the base of the second spreader with a line leading to a block at the first spreader and down to the base of the cap shroud and to a winch. With this setup we gybed onto starboard running under storm jib the rest of the night until daylight so we could evaluate the situation better.

At daybreak we gybed back to port and got Bridget and Paul up the rig again. They secured a better lashing from the base of the second spreader down to the tip of the first spreader using 14mm spectra rope and a Spanish windlass to obtain tension. Various options on how to proceed from here have been evaluated by the crew and we have decided to continue on towards South America with reduced sail rather than try and beat back towards the Chatham Islands. At this stage it is our intention to call in at Ushuaia to effect repairs.

END EFE LEB

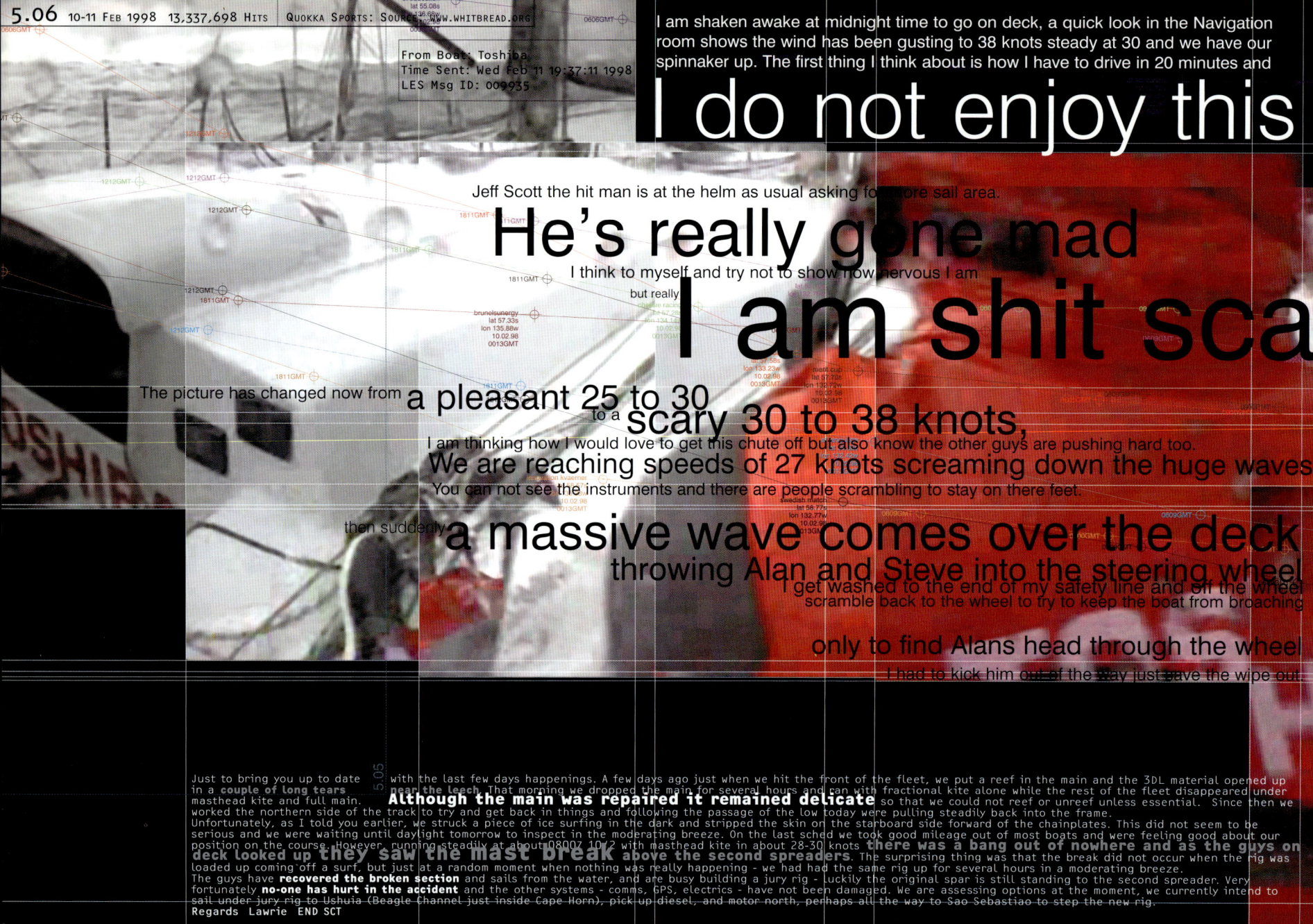

stuff.

red.

A quick cup of coffee and put some wet wet weather gear on.
Safety harnesses are a must in these conditions as

there are 2 tons of water rushing over the deck at 25 knots,

you get washed off your feet all the time.

This is not safe at all, the way we are sailing now, but what choice do you have?

The heater has now broken and Capey reckons he has an
ice berg on the bow
which he has spotted on the radar,
thankfully it's Merit Cup.

With Ross at the Helm the next day we sail past.
It was

a spectacular sight; two w60s screaming along at 25 knots only 4 boat lengths apart.

Well every one is very tired and cold but know we have only a few more days in this hell hole.
Someone get a gun and threaten me with death if you hear me talking about doing this race again.
Kelvin END TOS

From Boat: Merit_Cup
Time Sent: Tue Feb 10 17:59:41 1998

As I look out the hatch, not more than 200 metres away there is Tos absolutely flying. It is one of the most dramatic sailing scenes you could imagine. These two yachts at a point on the globe which is as far away from land as anywhere else on earth, going as hard as they can. We are averaging around 20 knots in up to 40 knots of breeze. As Tos starts to surf often their hull will come clear right back to the keel. At the same time a huge plume of water rises above the topsides and the boat is hurled into the trough. I have never scene a boat look like that before.
Prior to being caught up by Tos, last night, we had been sailing under storm spinnaker in control but still on edge. We got absolutely smacked by the rest of the fleet sailing that way and changed up to the bigger size spinnaker, the same as Tos.

Come last or hammer it with the chance of crashing like Silk Cut just has...2 hours later— with the wind getting to over 40 knots and the boat absolutely out of control I pulled the plug and left Tos to it. But 10 minutes after we had set our storm spin again there was Tos trying to pull what was left of their spin down. Now just in front of us they to are on a storm spin. I heard one of the guys mention last night that if you made your dog live in conditions like we are at present you would be had up by the SPCA, he's probably right. But the boys are self motivated and push on regardless. For me its a matter of balancing the need to push hard but not over the top. I think my sheer fear of what could happen to us stops that. We are all very sorry today for Lawrie and the team of Silk Cut. That is a rotten blow and no one deserves that.
END MCP

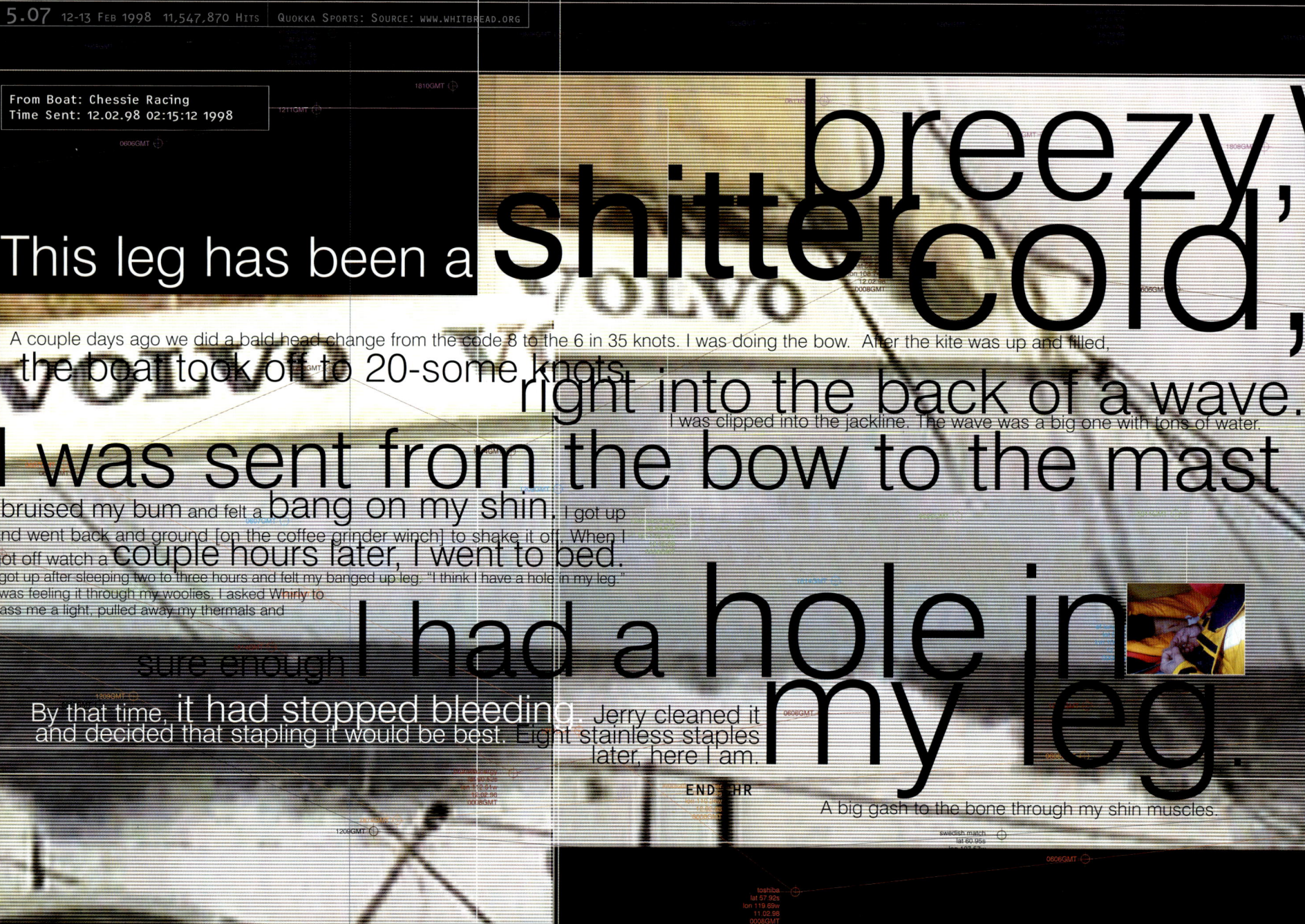

5.07 12-13 Feb 1998 11,547,870 Hits Quokka Sports: Source: www.whitbread.org

From Boat: Chessie Racing
Time Sent: 12.02.98 02:15:12 1998

This leg has been a **shitter, breezy, cold,**

A couple days ago we did a bald head change from the code 8 to the 6 in 35 knots. I was doing the bow. After the kite was up and filled, the boat took off to 20-some knots, right into the back of a wave. I was clipped into the jackline. The wave was a big one with tons of water. I was sent from the bow to the mast, bruised my bum and felt a bang on my shin. I got up and went back and ground [on the coffee grinder winch] to shake it off. When I got off watch a couple hours later, I went to bed. I got up after sleeping two to three hours and felt my banged up leg. "I think I have a hole in my leg." I was feeling it through my woolies. I asked Whirly to pass me a light, pulled away my thermals and sure enough I had a hole in my leg. By that time, it had stopped bleeding. Jerry cleaned it and decided that stapling it would be best. Eight stainless staples later, here I am. A big gash to the bone through my shin muscles.

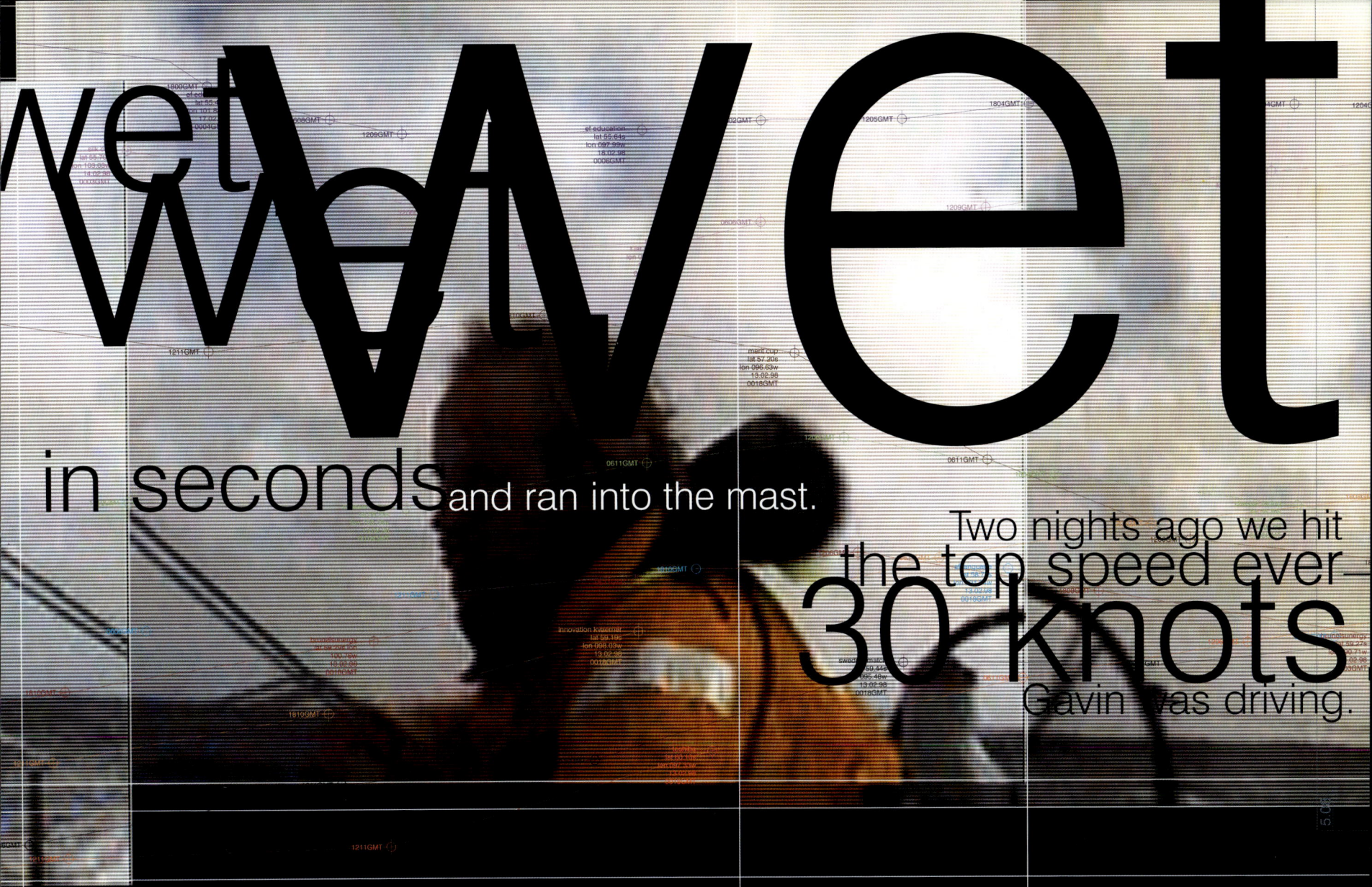

EF Language rounded

From Boat: EF_Education
Time Sent: Sat Feb 14 08:42:26 1998
LES Msg ID: 397885

Valentine's Day
and all the men are so far away...

In fact, unless there's an Antarctic research ship floating around the area, the nearest are probably in the Whitbread fleet. So the EF girls sent them, by kind favour of the Whitbread office, a fleet message to wish them a happy Valentine's day:

"Roses are red, violets are blue, Can't be with you, 'cos we broke our D2!"

Although not in the running for this leg anymore we do still follow the progress of all the boats at every report. We're really pleased that the guys on EF Language are still out in front.

Hang in there boys!!

END EFE LEB

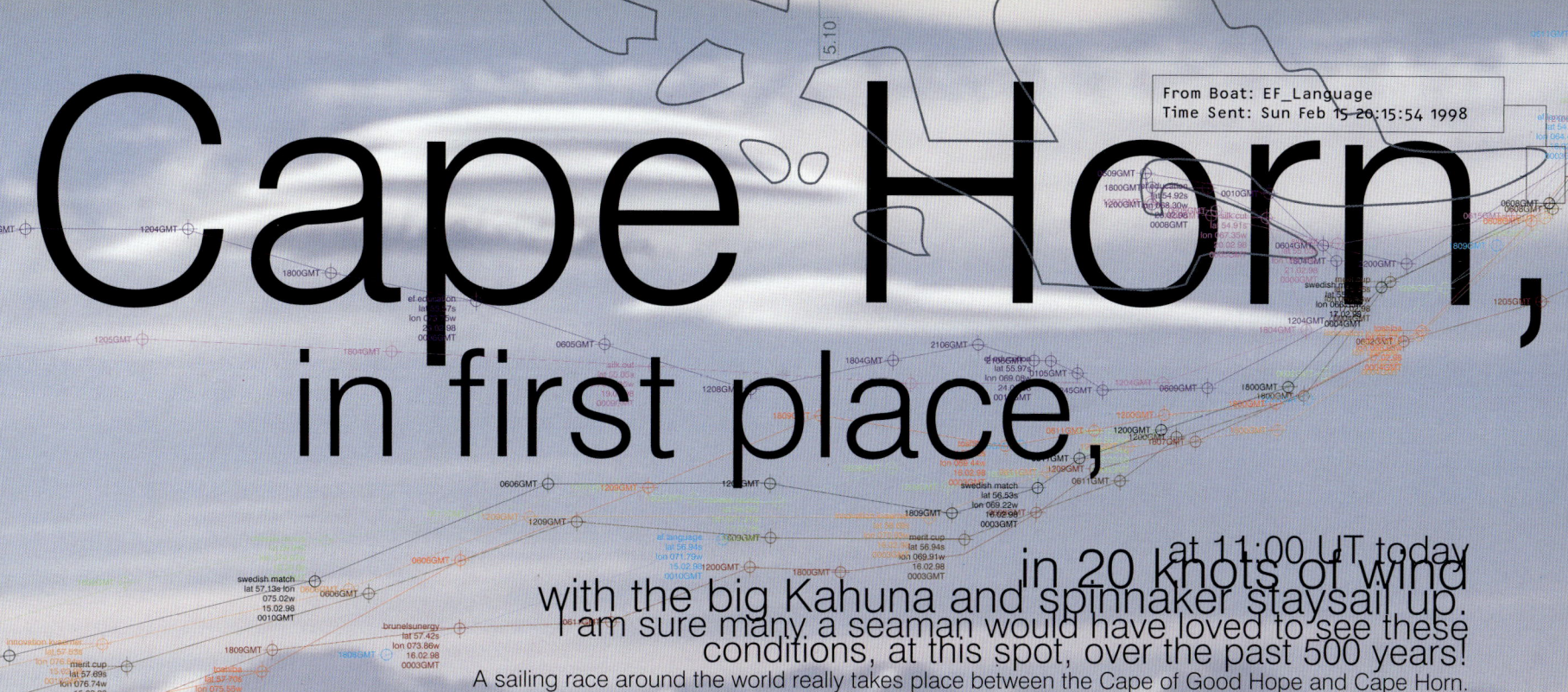

From Boat: EF_Language
Time Sent: Sun Feb 15 20:15:54 1998

Cape Horn,
in first place,
at 11:00 UT today in 20 knots of wind with the big Kahuna and spinnaker staysail up. I am sure many a seaman would have loved to see these conditions, at this spot, over the past 500 years! A sailing race around the world really takes place between the Cape of Good Hope and Cape Horn. This is where you go around. Before and after are just the delivery to where the circumnavigation is possible. There is tough racing before and after, that is for sure, but the Southern Ocean is one of the unique spots on this planet. Like Everest or the Sahara, **it is extreme** and not many go there. I am a bit nostalgic already as I know I may never come back. In some way, last week was the "good old days," already.

I will remember and talk about what I did during the last two weeks for the rest of my life.

END PC EFL

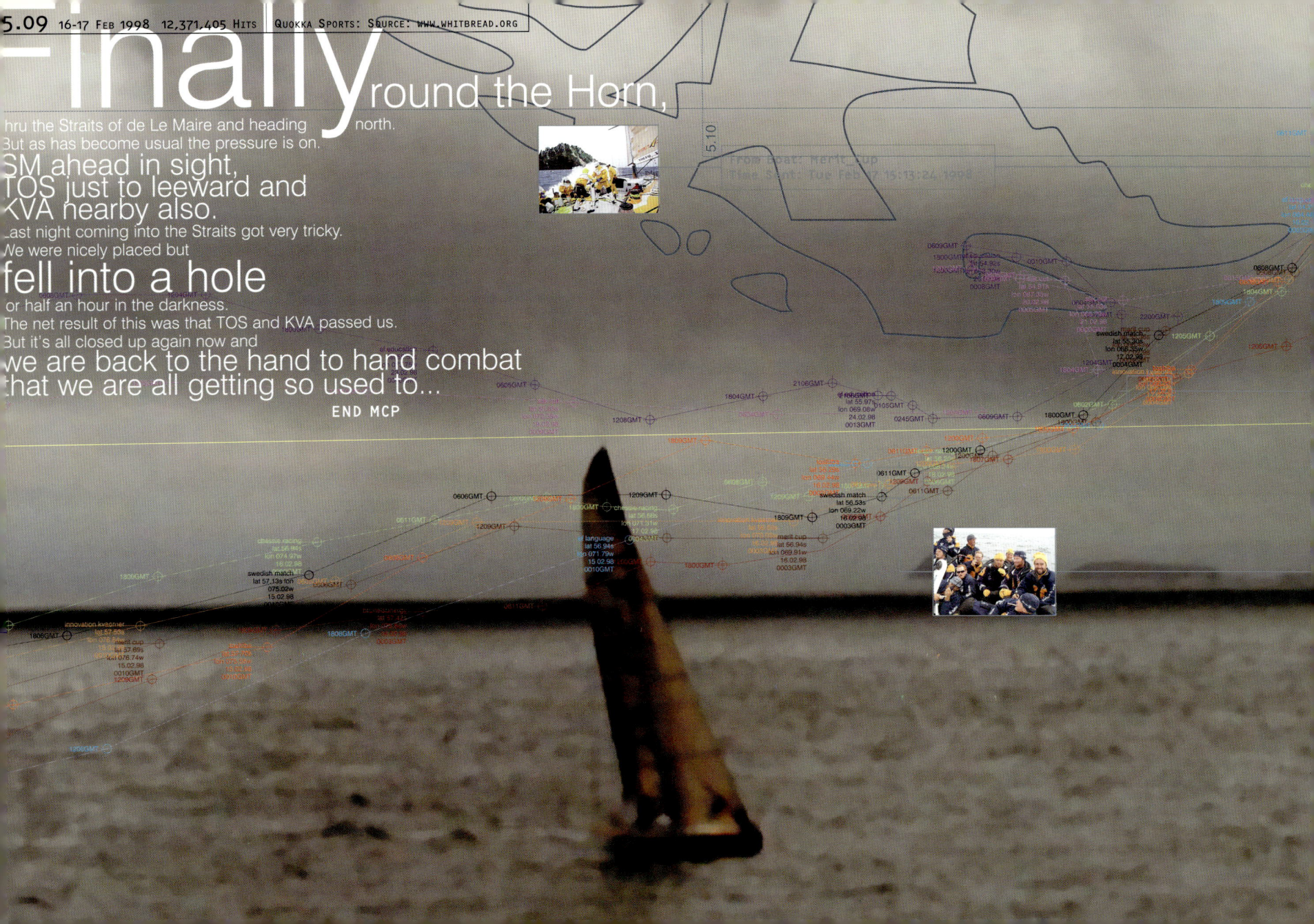

finally

We got round the maritime mile stone Cape Horn at noon today.

As we rounded, Nick did the honourable thing and had his ear pierced as per tradition with a sail needle and then inserted a fine gold earing.

END TOS

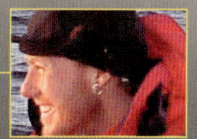

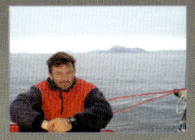

From Boat: Swedish Match
Time Sent: Mon Feb 16 02:53:55 1998

It seems like the word Cape is the same as wind hole for the blue boat. We are stuck at the furious and wellknown for it's violent weather Cape Horn, trying our best to stay over 2 knots of boatspeed in absolutely no wind. We are rocking from side to side in the waves and that creates some wind in the sails and we are moving forward. TOS is suddenly even with us and it was the blue boat alone that got stuck. Frustrating. We are still in a good race mode, just need a little wind so we can race!
Regards Gurra

END SWE

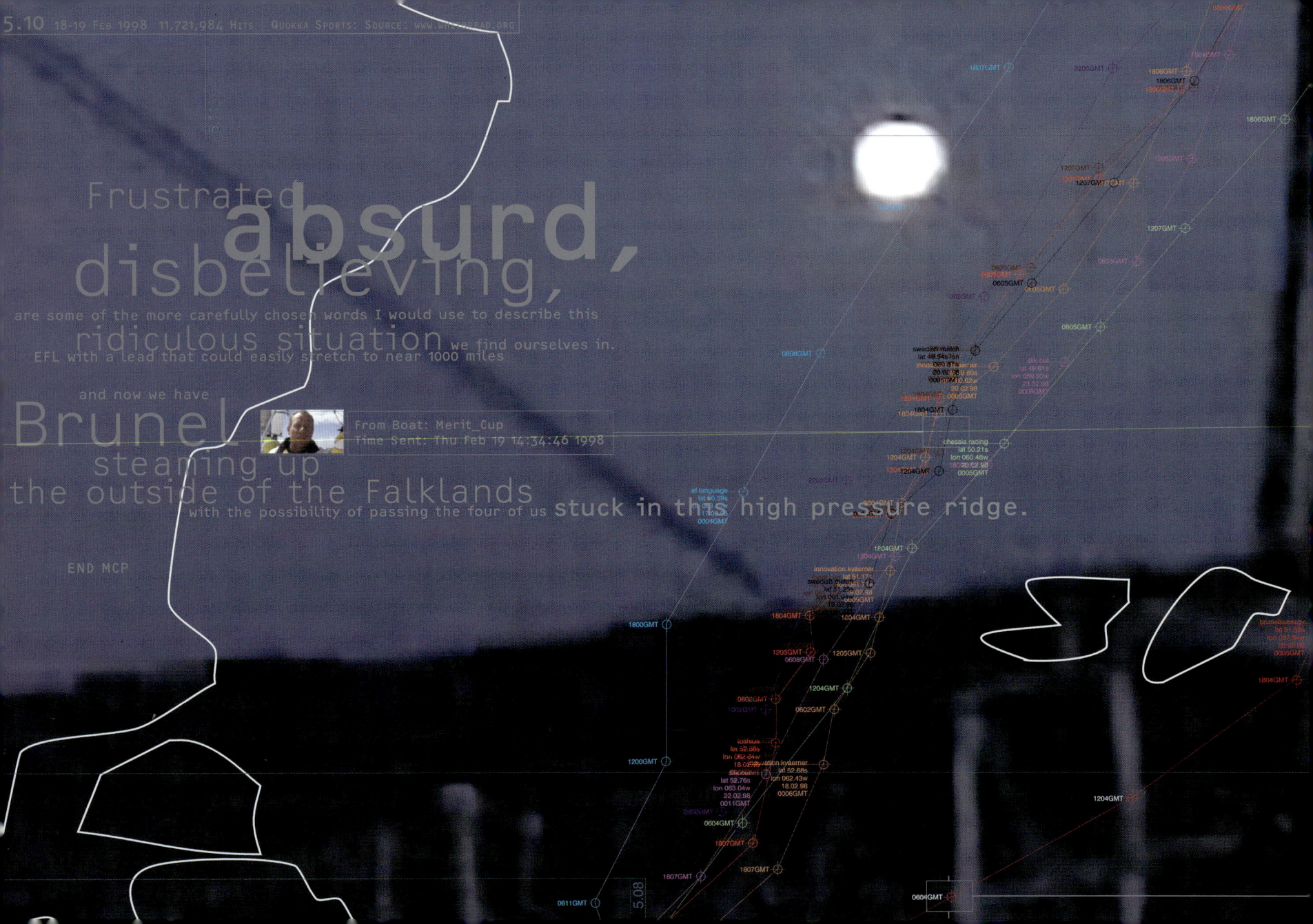

What a wonderfull thing happened some eight hours ago!

A thick fog was approaching as once again we lay becalmed.
As soon as we entered the fog the wind picked up to an unbelievable 20 knots

Quick shouts for foul weather gear came from deck

and ever since we have been reaching, now even with spinnaker, to keep within this breeze to the side of the High Pressure.
It sure feels good to be gaining on the boats in front. END BRS

From Boat: Brunel_Sunergy   Time Sent: Thu Feb 19 05:34:54 1998
MES 424519210 at 19-02-98 5:28 UTC   Lat: 53 45.89 S   Long: 061 15.50 W

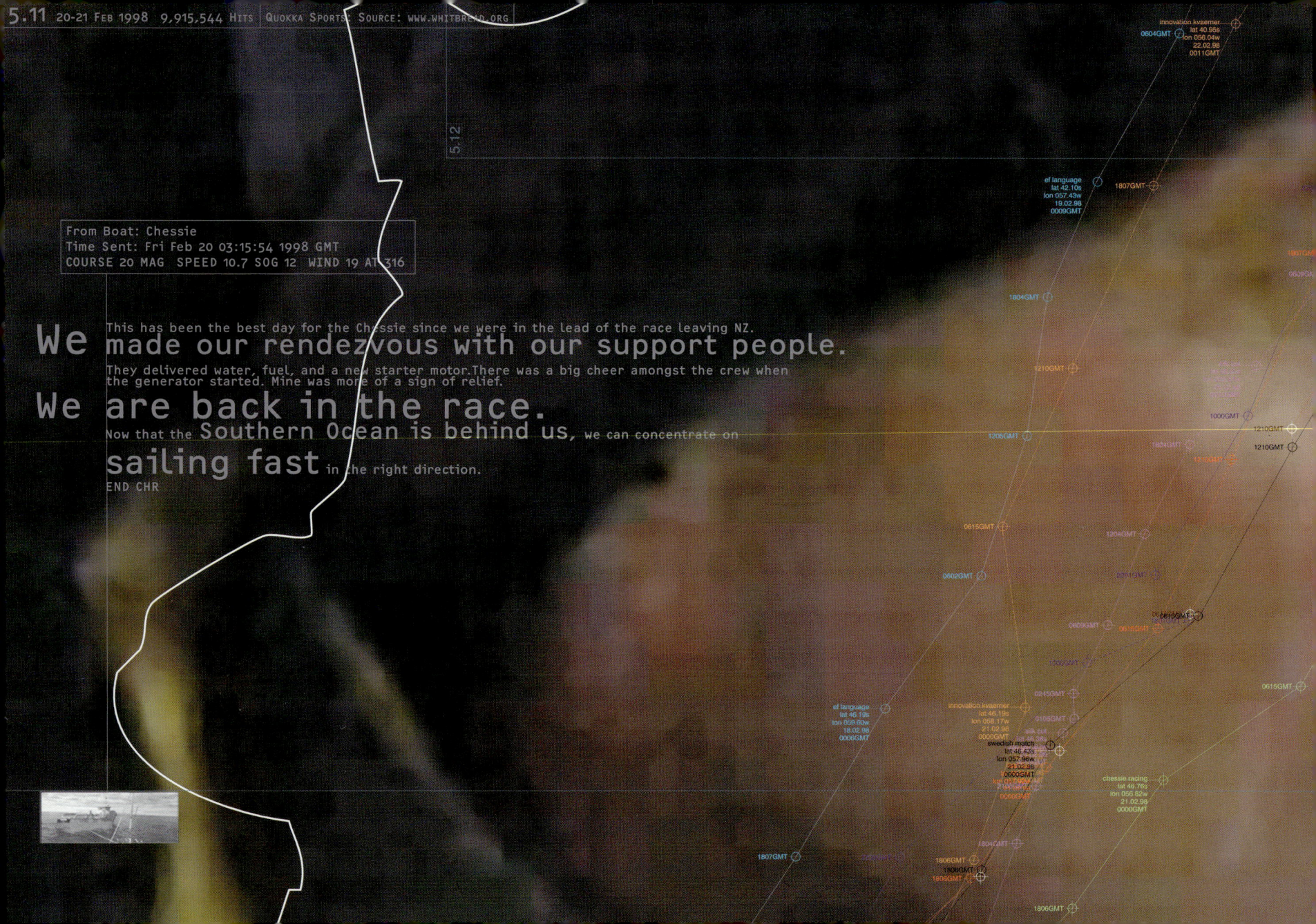

From Boat: Chessie
Time Sent: Fri Feb 20 03:15:54 1998 GMT
COURSE 20 MAG SPEED 10.7 SOG 12 WIND 19 AT 316

This has been the best day for the Chessie since we were in the lead of the race leaving NZ.
We made our rendezvous with our support people.
They delivered water, fuel, and a new starter motor. There was a big cheer amongst the crew when the generator started. Mine was more of a sign of relief.
We are back in the race.
Now that the Southern Ocean is behind us, we can concentrate on sailing fast in the right direction.
END CHR

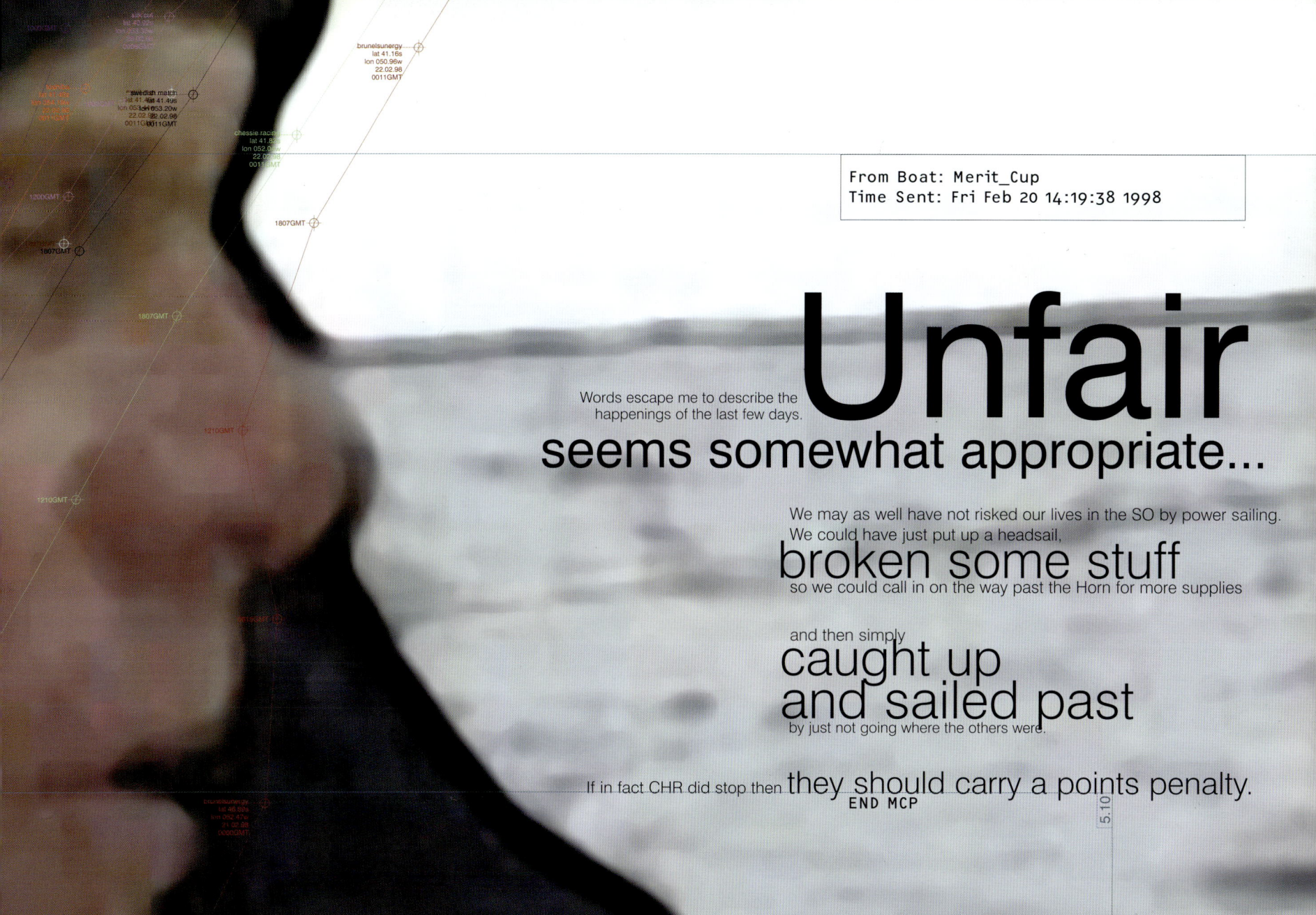

5.12 22-23 Feb 1998 10,036,728 Hits | Quokka Sports: Source: www.whitbread.org

Last night was a weird one as we survived some squalls up to 39 knots of windspeed with the masthead code 4 up.
No one ever thought about peeling to a smaller one, but it did get a bit scary now and then.
With the waves being very high and steep, there is not much surfing going on.
It is more like falling off the waves, a trick anybody could do. A lot of noise and a quick acceleration from 12 to 25 knots, followed by flapping sails as the apparent wind direction moves forward.
As daylight has returned you finally get to see the size of the waves, not a very reassuring sight.
But if any, this is the time to push hard and that is what we are doing.

Everybody is slowly getting tired, with most limbs hurting from grinding, driving and holding sheets.
Did two gybes with masthead spinnakers at 30-35 knots and not a problem.
A few broaches now and then, but nothing too alarming, seems like after the Southern Ocean we are not scared anymore.

END BRS

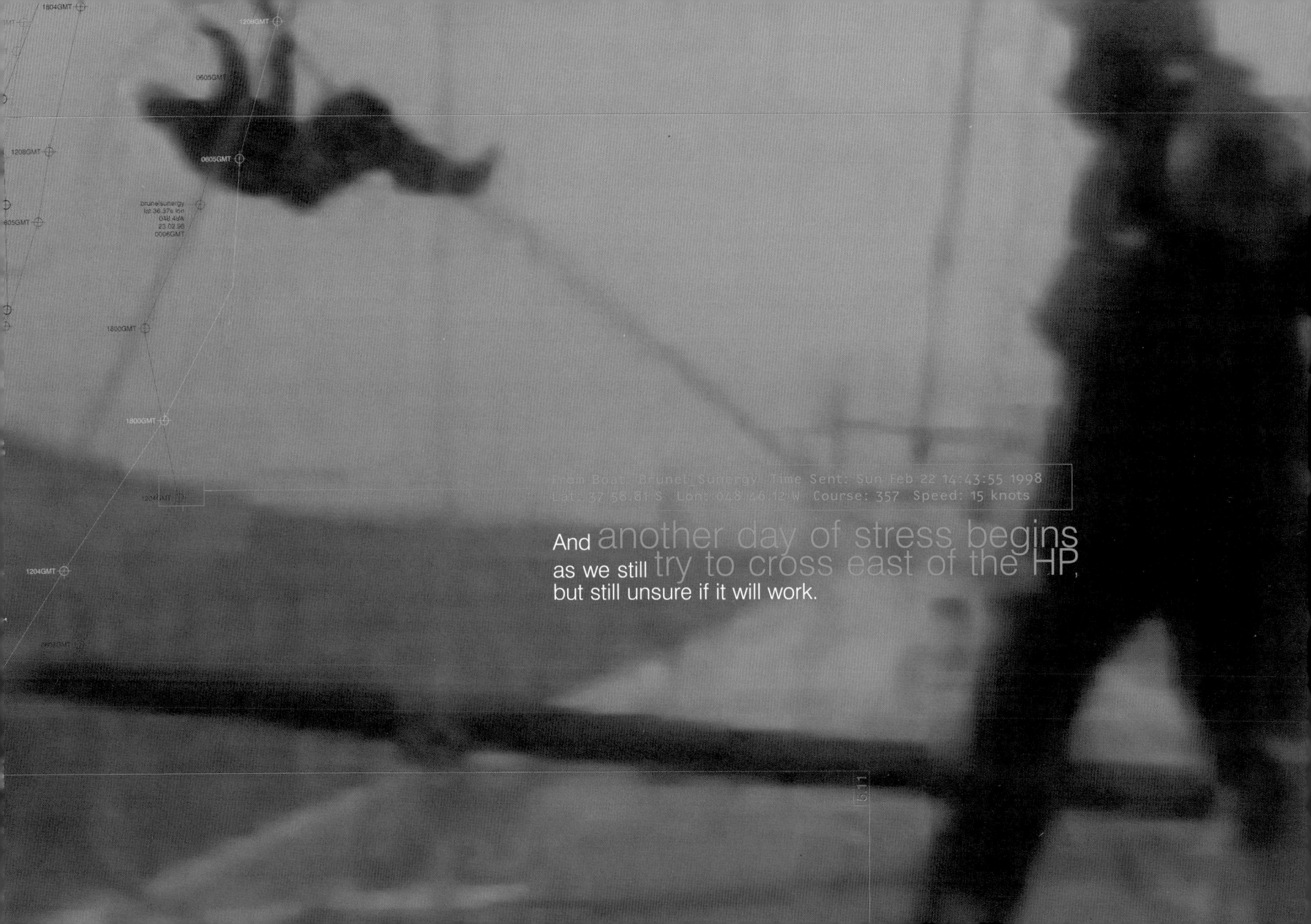

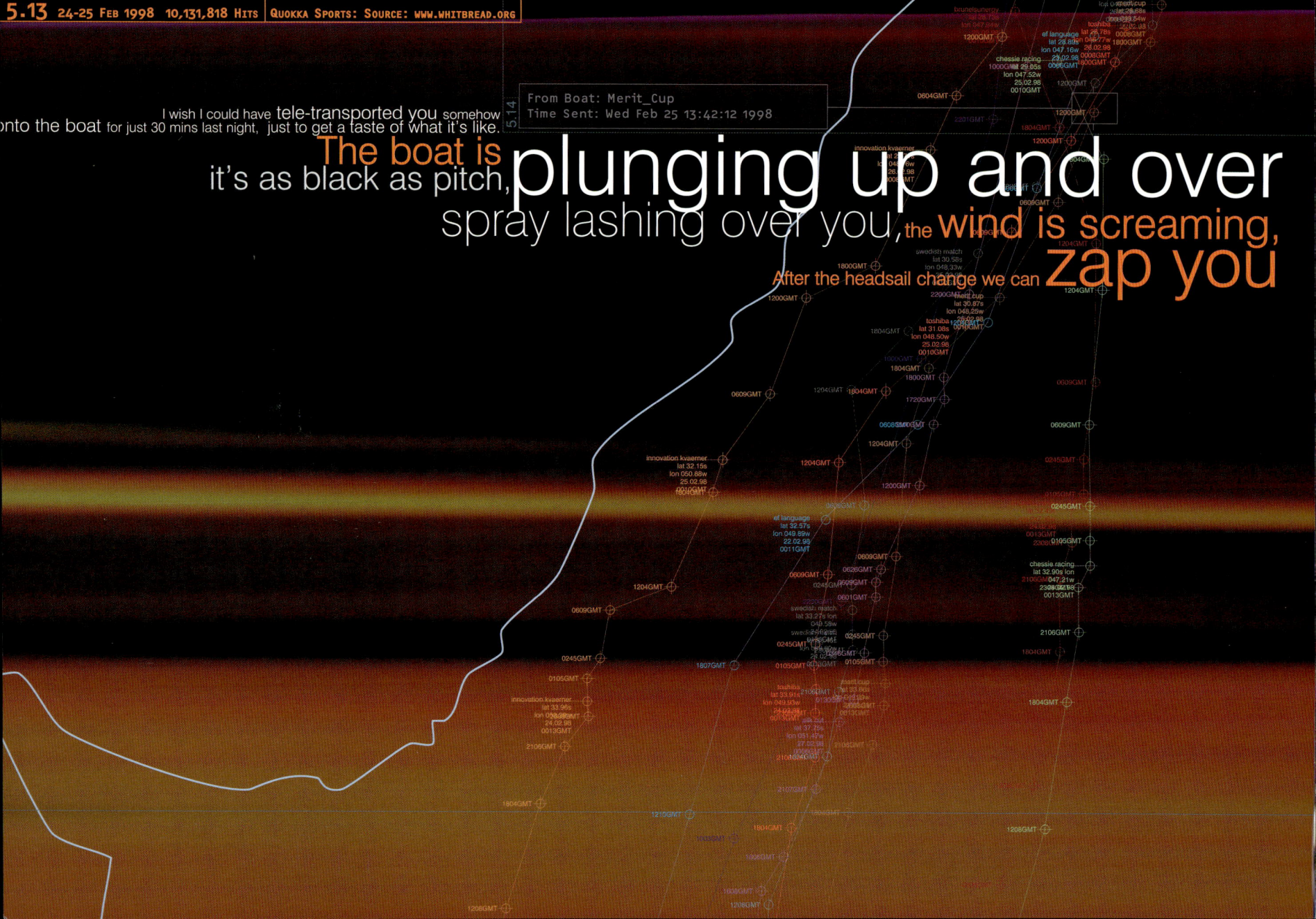

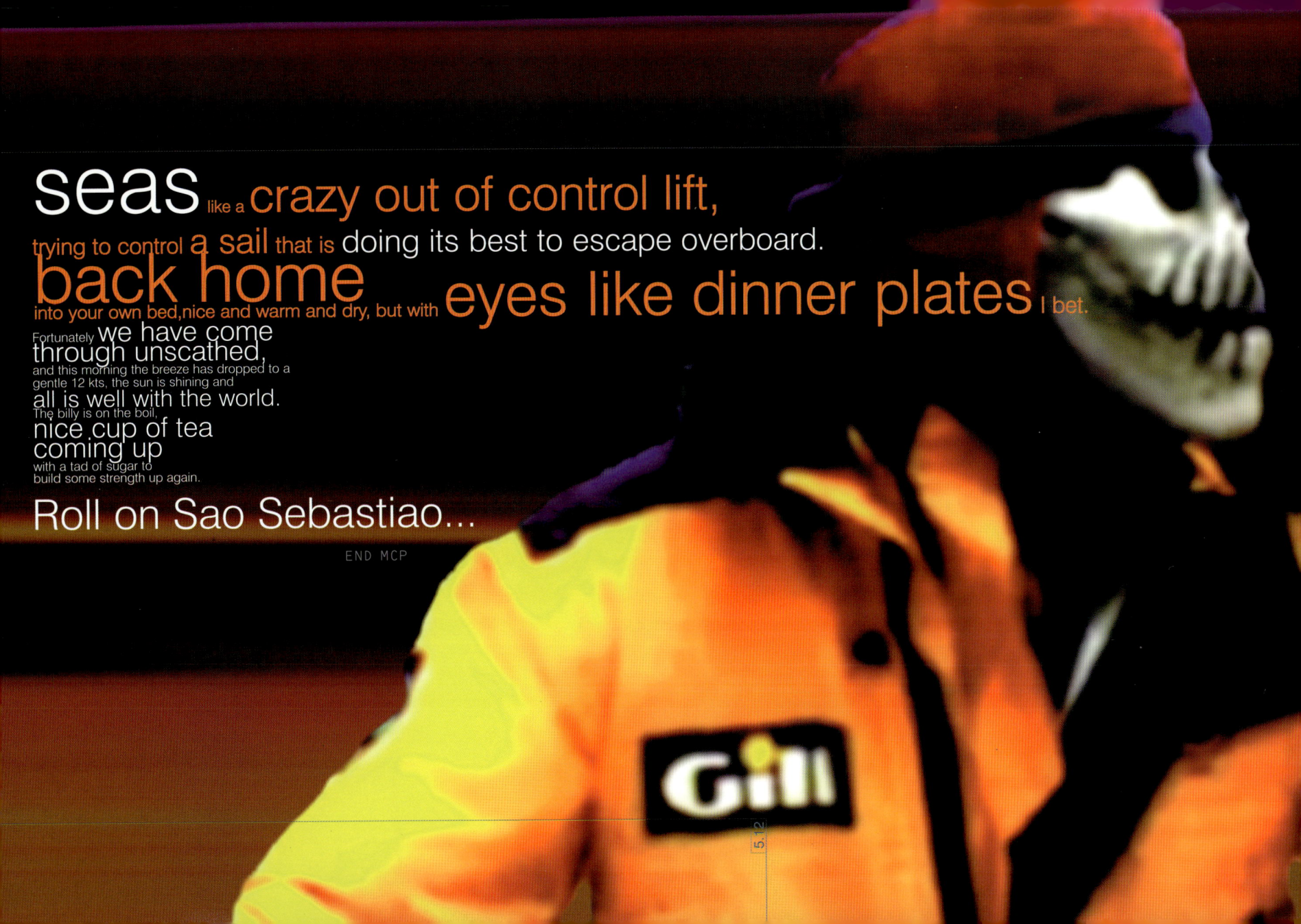

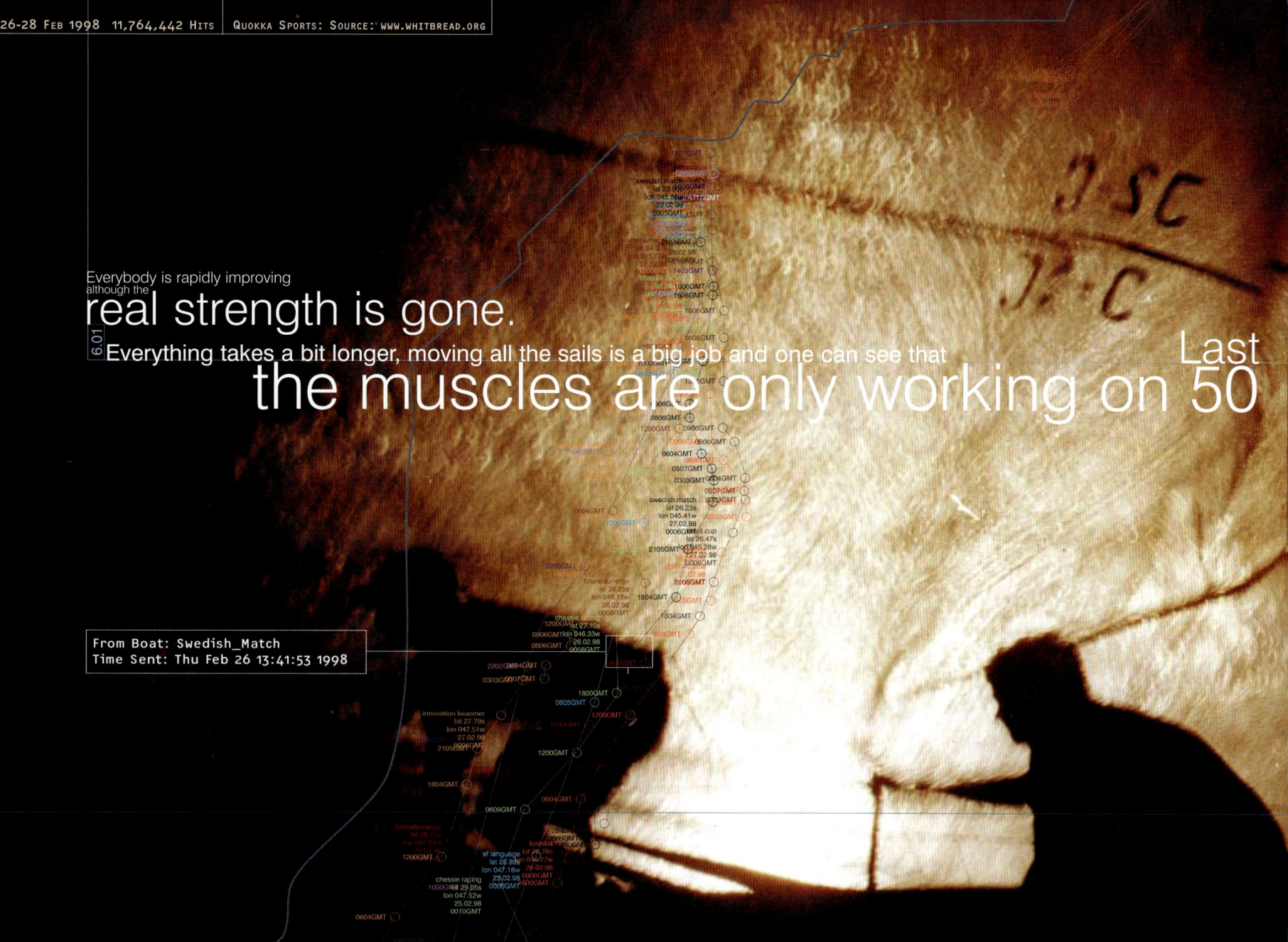

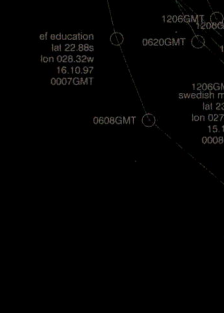

night's upwind was a nightmare.
percent. We had to slow down not to break the boat.

Lots of current and strong winds made it into the worst kind of sailing we can find on a W60. We are sailing together with TOS and MCP and it looks like we cannot live without each other. Same distance and same tracking all the time except for small variations.

Slowly we are getting closer to the finish.
If we look at how much sailing we get for each dollar we spend in this project we are looking very good. We would have liked to catch BRS and CHR but **the weather has not been on our side** and they have sailed well on their easterly track and protected their position.

Regards Gurra

END SWE

leg 5 leaderboard and status

pos	boat	elapsed time	points	totals
1	EF Language	23d+ 01:09:23	135	507
2	BrunelSunergy	26d+ 04:07:17	119	215
3	Chessie Racing	26d+ 10:33:48	105	399
4	Swedish Match	27d+ 01:19:09	91	404
5	Merit Cup	27d+ 01:50:27	78	411
6	Innovation Kvaerner	27d+ 16:12:15	65	372
-	EF Education	retired from leg	26	126
-	Silk Cut	retired from leg	26	284
-	Toshiba*	28d+ 02:19:32	0	299

*disqualified from leg

6.0.0 14 Mar – 31 Mar 1998   78,341,448 Hits | Quokka Sports: Source: www.whitbread.org

Distance:

Leg 6

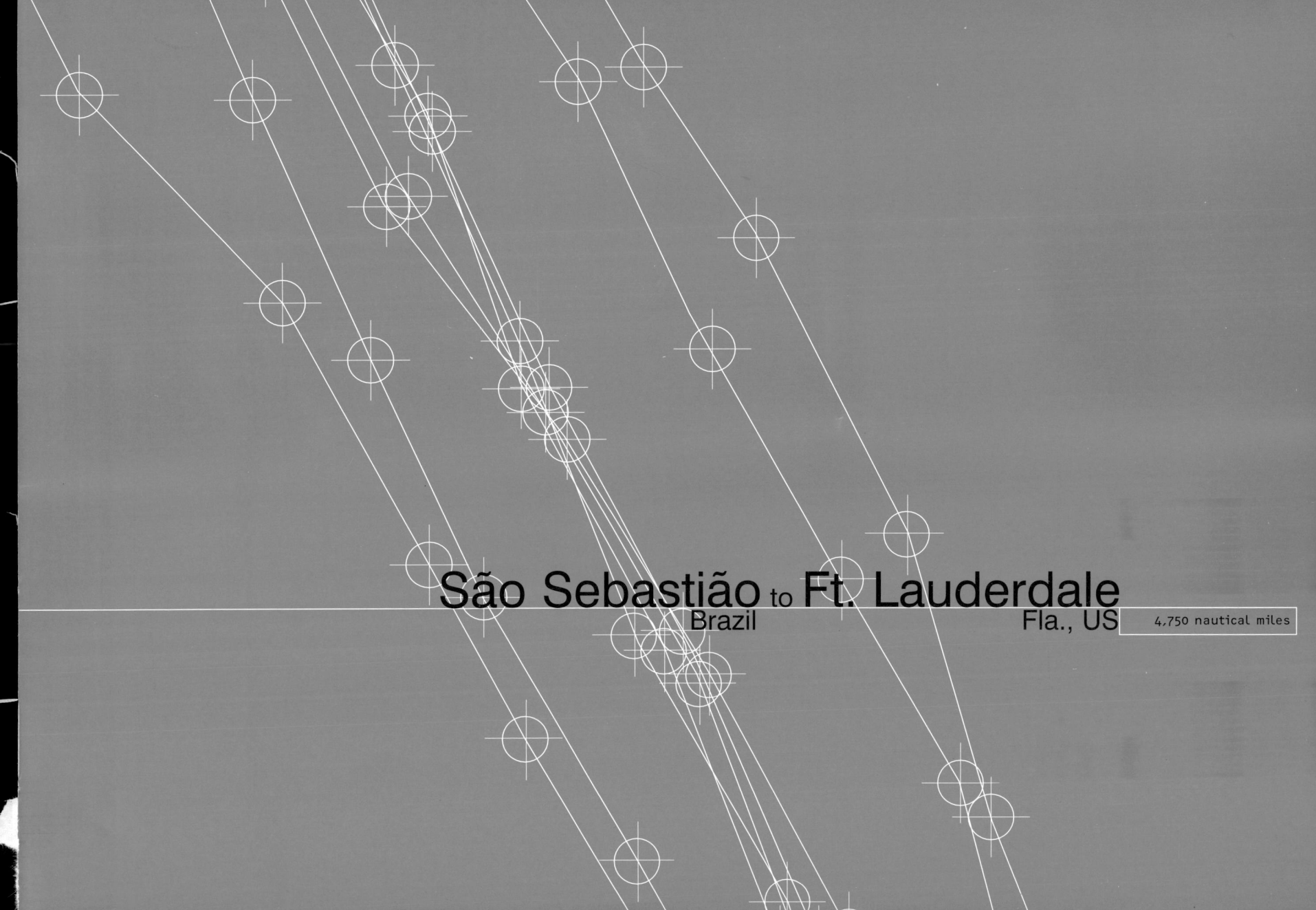

Leg 6: Prelude

Leg 5 had taken a toll on the fleet. Only seven of the nine boats officially finished the leg. Silk Cut and EF Education had both suffered catastrophic mast failures approaching Cape Horn and were forced to divert to the coastal town of Ushuaia, Argentina, for repairs. The EF Education team had a new mast waiting there for its boat when she arrived. The mast was installed and the women resumed racing.

The Silk Cut crew first tried a jury-rig to see if they could actually sail on. They found the speeds they were getting out of the reduced sail would get them to São Sebastião, Brazil, too late for the restart. The team decided the wisest course was to retire from the leg and motorsail into port so they would have time to replace their mast in time for the start of the next leg.

EF Education made a valiant effort to finish the leg. After first hitting two days of light winds followed by a gale that blew out a patched-up mainsail, it became clear to the EF Education crew that unless they motored as well, they would not get to port in time for the next leg's start. The determination and sheer grit of the EF women had captured the hearts and imagination of fans — email from around the world poured into the Whitbread Web site cheering them on.

Meanwhile, in São Sebastião, the Toshiba team would probably have been happy to trade places with either Silk Cut or EF Education. The team found itself the target of a serious Race Committee protest alleging the team had broken one of the cardinal race rules during Leg 5 — that the crew had turned the boat's engine on and motored, albeit in reverse.

Toshiba had finished Leg 5 in fifth place. On arrival, there was no hint that anything unusual had occurred. When a boat finishes a leg, the skipper and crew members must individually appear before a race official to submit their 'declaration' for the leg. Rules require that crew members report any incident that might constitute a violation of race rules. During declarations it was revealed that during Leg 5 the boat's engine had been turned on and the prop engaged in reverse in order to clear weed from the prop.

"The Race Committee became aware of the incident at 1500 on 28 February 1998 when the Person in Charge (Paul Standbridge) and one crew member recorded it on their declarations."

The Race Committee

The revelation sent shock waves through the Race Village. The Race Committee immediately protested the Toshiba team; the International Jury was again summoned to sit in judgement. The allegation left veterans of the race scratching their heads wondering what on Earth could have possessed the team to break the most fundamental rule of the race.

At the hearing, Toshiba skipper Paul Standbridge explained that the engine had been started when the crew could not loosen kelp which had stuck to the boat's keel and rudder. In order to free the kelp, they had finally started the engine and put the boat in reverse. However, the team had not notified the Race Committee immediately that the official seal on the boat's propeller shaft had been broken, as required by race rules. Nor had the crew photographed the broken seal before replacing it with a new seal, also as required in the rules. Most damning, no mention of the incident was recorded in the boat's log.

Standbridge characterised the string of omissions as unintentional mistakes by the crew. Regardless, the jury felt it had no choice but to disqualify the team from the leg. The decision meant that Toshiba would earn zero points for Leg 5, dropping her from fifth to sixth position overall. Each boat that finished behind her on the leg moved up one place.

Skipper Paul Standbridge was visibly shaken by the ruling, claiming it was overly harsh. "We are all very disappointed in the jury's ruling," he said after leaving the jury room. "Their decision

Leg 6: São Sebastião, Brazil, to Ft. Lauderdale, Fla., US

"As you wake up you grab around for your T-shirt to wipe the sweat that has accumulated on your body ... trying to get outside as fast as possible to get a gasp of that fine fresh air you missed for four hours."

Arend van Bergeijk, BrunelSunergy

The start of Leg 6 looked like a nautical extension of the Carnival festivities that had been on going since before the boats arrived. A large and unruly spectator fleet, described diplomatically in a WRO press release as "over-enthusiastic," churned up the waters and frustrated attempts by harbour police to herd them outside the restriction zone. Instead, a party atmosphere prevailed as these floating fans mixed with the Whitbread boats jockeying for start positions. Aboard Swedish Match, skipper Gunnar Krantz struggled to pilot his boat safely through the chaos. "The start line was absolutely full with spectator boats," Krantz recalled later. "Somehow the smallest police boats I have ever seen managed to clear the area enough for us to start. After that, all hell broke loose."

The 'hell' that Krantz reported was not gale winds but the return of the spectator boats. The wind all but disappeared after the start, and the fleet once again found itself surrounded by curious fans sailing and motoring around and across their paths as if they were on display. The light conditions prevailed until the boats inched their way south of Ilha Bela, 'Beautiful Island.' There, they finally hooked into a stiff breeze from the southwest that put the entire fleet into fast-forward. The boats, flying fractional spinnakers, began reaching in 28 knots of wind.

With the strong winds producing good speeds, navigators aboard each boat were beginning to plot their individual strategies — slowly the fleet began to split. Innovation Kvaerner and EF Language opted to stay closer to shore. Merit

is harsh. A communication error does not deserve disqualification."

While Standbridge was left to deal with the fallout from his boat's broken shaft seal, Merit Cup skipper Grant Dalton was dealing with a broken collarbone. During the last leg he had taken a nasty header down the companionway during rough weather. Dalton flew home to New Zealand to consult with his doctor. There was speculation that if surgery was required Dalton could be out of the race. Dalton was determined to be aboard when the boats left Brazil. When he returned from his long-distance doctor's visit, he claimed he had been given the green light to sail again. "I have already regained good mobility," Dalton said, moving his shoulder ever so slightly. "I will be able to steer and perform other lighter duties without any difficulty, but I don't expect to be grinding for a while. The doctors say that pain will remind me if I start overdoing things."

With only three days left to prepare for the start of Leg 6, EF Education finally arrived in São Sebastião. While the other teams had enjoyed two weeks of rest and Carnival festivities, the EF Education women had barely enough time to pack new sails and provisions aboard before heading to the starting line. "I am sure we will get one day off," said a wishful navigator Lynnath Beckley.

Cup plotted a course 22 miles farther offshore. Toshiba became the boat farthest offshore, where she found good wind.

The choices of course were few, so even though the boats were no longer sailing like a regatta fleet, they were still tightly bunched, by ocean-racing standards. Only 13 miles separated the boats from east to west by the second day. Sailing conditions were near to perfect for all the boats, with a respectable 28- to 30-knot southerly breeze allowing the crews to hoist their large masthead spinnakers. The lead changed hands several times over the next several days as the boats duelled along the short east/west axis.

Day 4 saw Innovation Kvaerner holding a narrow lead, with Silk Cut moving into second from sixth in just six hours of sailing. Toshiba was in third place. Some 30 miles to the east of the leader, Swedish Match had fallen to ninth place as skipper Krantz plotted a course he knew would cost him in the short run. His only concern was that he might have gone too far east. "It doesn't look too flash at the moment for Swedish Match," Krantz said that morning. "We may have overcooked it a bit when going east."

Across a 30-mile span, the fleet settled into three basic groups: Innovation Kvaerner, Silk Cut and BrunelSunergy to the west; Chessie Racing, Merit Cup, EF Education and EF Language in the middle; and Toshiba and Swedish Match to the east, with Swedish Match farthest east. This configuration put the women aboard EF Education in an unaccustomed position, just ahead of their male team members aboard EF Language.

The biggest problem the crews faced on this leg was heat. The hot and humid conditions ate away at crew morale and performance. "You just can't sleep inside the boat," Knut Frostad reported. He said temperatures belowdecks approached 50 C (120 F). "How nice it is to jump into a bunk that is already soaking wet from the sweat of the guy who slept there before you!"

Hugging the coastline of Brazil began to pay off handsomely for Silk Cut. She snatched the lead and then extended it on Day 6 to nearly 14 miles over Innovation Kvaerner. At one point, Silk Cut's inshore strategy took the yacht to within two miles of shore. Skipper Lawrie Smith was determined to build a cushion large enough to protect him from the approaching Doldrums. This leg held bad memories for Smith. While at the helm of Intrum Justitia in the last Whitbread, it was precisely at this point that Smith's luck turned sour. Then, as now, he held the lead. He saw his hopes dashed when Yamaha (with Ross Field at the helm) punched through the Doldrums ahead of him and left Smith and his crew sitting becalmed.

By Day 6, Paul Cayard was also looking ahead and had begun to close on the leaders. By now, Cayard was the 'danger man' as far as the other teams were concerned. Time and again in this race he had shown tenacity that kept any crew ahead of him always looking over their shoulders. In just the last 24 hours he had pushed his boat and crew hard, clawing his way to third place, 16 miles astern of the leader, Silk Cut.

Though the entire fleet was still experiencing good reaching conditions, they all knew it couldn't last. As the boats neared the equator, the question again was how thick the Doldrums area would be, and where to find its narrowest point. By Day 8 the fleet had entered the Doldrums, with each boat picking her way through this relatively windless zone. The prize for the first boat through was a respectable northeasterly trade wind. Yet for every boat in the fleet the path through the Doldrums was proving frustrating. The boats were finding it difficult to avoid squalls — the large black clouds the crews came to call "glue pots." If one of these squalls settled over a boat, she didn't move until the cloud moved on.

"The whole fleet is falling into potholes randomly, and we don't know what we can't see," a frustrated Cayard reported. "Every hour is spent watching the clouds," Knut Frostad wrote. "Will it rain? Where is it moving? How fast? Can we pass ahead or do we have to hike up behind? You just have to make sure you don't end up right in the middle! Some of the clouds are just too big, and you can't avoid them."

As the winds dropped, the already intolerable temperatures and suffocating humidity shot even higher. Crew after crew began reporting outbreaks of a heat-induced condition called 'gunwale bum' on some boats and 'spotty botty' on others. It was discreetly described by Grant Dalton as "most uncomfortable."

As the boats picked their way through the minefield of squalls, some boats gained and some lost ground. By Day 9, EF Language had closed to within four miles of Silk Cut. Innovation Kvaerner was seven miles farther back in third. All the boats had crossed the equator, which put them back in the Northern Hemisphere for the first time since Leg 1, the previous October. The bulk of the fleet was still fairly bunched up; positions shifted with every report. Gunnar Krantz's decision to keep Swedish Match the farthest east (and now north) of the rest of the fleet was finally beginning to pay off. Having been the last boat for most of the first week, Swedish Match was picking off the yachts ahead of her one at a time.

After wrestling her lead back from Toshiba, Silk Cut was overtaken by EF Language on Day 10. Cayard nosed his yacht to a three-mile lead over Lawrie Smith and his crew — at one point he extended his lead on Smith by over 20 miles. At this point, most of the boats had passed through the Doldrums. The dreaded zone had proven so narrow and weak that Silk Cut crewmember Adrian Stead said he suspected the Doldrums "were a figment of someone's imagination."

For other yachts, the 'black hole' squalls were proving just as devilish as the worst the Doldrums could hand out. BrunelSunergy had fought briefly into third, only to fall into a wind hole — before it freed her she was back in eighth position. Such dramatic slippage was not surprising when considering that even after sailing over 2,400 nautical miles, the fleet remained closely bunched. It did not take the loss or gain of more than a few miles to shift several positions.

Aboard EF Language, Cayard and his navigator, Mark Rudiger, had caught Silk Cut for the second day in a row. Now, Cayard was looking well ahead to the next waypoint, the island of Barbuda, which still lay about 1,000 miles away. "Should get there Thursday morning," Cayard wrote. "Then we will have a 1,200 mile run into Ft. Lauderdale." If Cayard could hold on to his lead after rounding Barbuda and win Leg 6, his overall total would be a tough-to-beat 622 points.

Lawrie Smith had other ideas. For the next couple of days Silk Cut stalked Cayard like a wolf, and as the two boats were rounding Barbuda, Smith took the lead from Cayard. EF Language had held too close inshore at Barbuda, expecting the wind to lift the boat. Instead, the wind headed EF Language. Silk Cut rolled through to the windward with her big masthead kite up, while Cayard had to change to a much smaller headsail.

Cayard had seen his strategy evaporate. "Frustrating," he wrote. "Came into Barbuda with a reacher on while Silk Cut got up high on the rhumb line [and] were able to carry spinnakers all the way... watching a 20-mile lead turn into a 15-mile deficit is not fun."

Cayard's strategy now was to make sure that his two overall point competitors, Merit Cup and Swedish Match, stayed behind him for the balance of this leg. As long as he finished ahead of them he would remain the overall points leader.

Aboard the Dutch boat, skipper Roy Heiner reported that not all the 'Happy Crew' were happy. Several had been stricken with the flu and quarantined to the bow in an effort to stop its spread to the rest of the crew. "Everyone showing early signs is locked in the bow," Heiner reported. "We trust this will work pretty well." Reading this, one could only imagine what it would be like to suffer from the flu while cooped up in the 'sauna' belowdecks.

With Silk Cut and EF Language battling for first place, Innovation Kvaerner held onto third, but Swedish Match was catching up fast. Grant Dalton and his Merit Cup crew were in fifth. Chessie Racing and Toshiba were slugging it out for sixth, while BrunelSunergy and EF Education brought up the rear of the fleet, roughly 200 miles back.

On the end of the day on 29 March, Day 15, it was Silk Cut first across the line in Ft. Lauderdale, Fla. It was a surprising four days earlier than expected and marked the first leg victory for Lawrie Smith and his crew. It was a heartening comeback for the team that had been forced to retire from the last leg. Just over an hour after she crossed the line, Cayard and his EF Language crew crossed in second. Swedish Match took third place almost four hours behind the leader.

It was a clearly depressed Grant Dalton who, after coming in fifth behind Innovation Kvaerner, said dockside, "I guess EF Language has the whole thing in the bag now barring accidents. We are now chasing for second and third position overall."

If anyone could have been more dejected than Dalton, it might have been Toshiba's skipper, Paul Standbridge. After suffering disqualification on the last leg, he needed a great showing on Leg 6 to get back into the race. It was not to be — standing dockside after arriving in seventh place, a red-eyed and exhausted Standbridge described himself as "shattered."

The leg ended with the arrival of BrunelSunergy and EF Education, a day and a half behind the leaders.

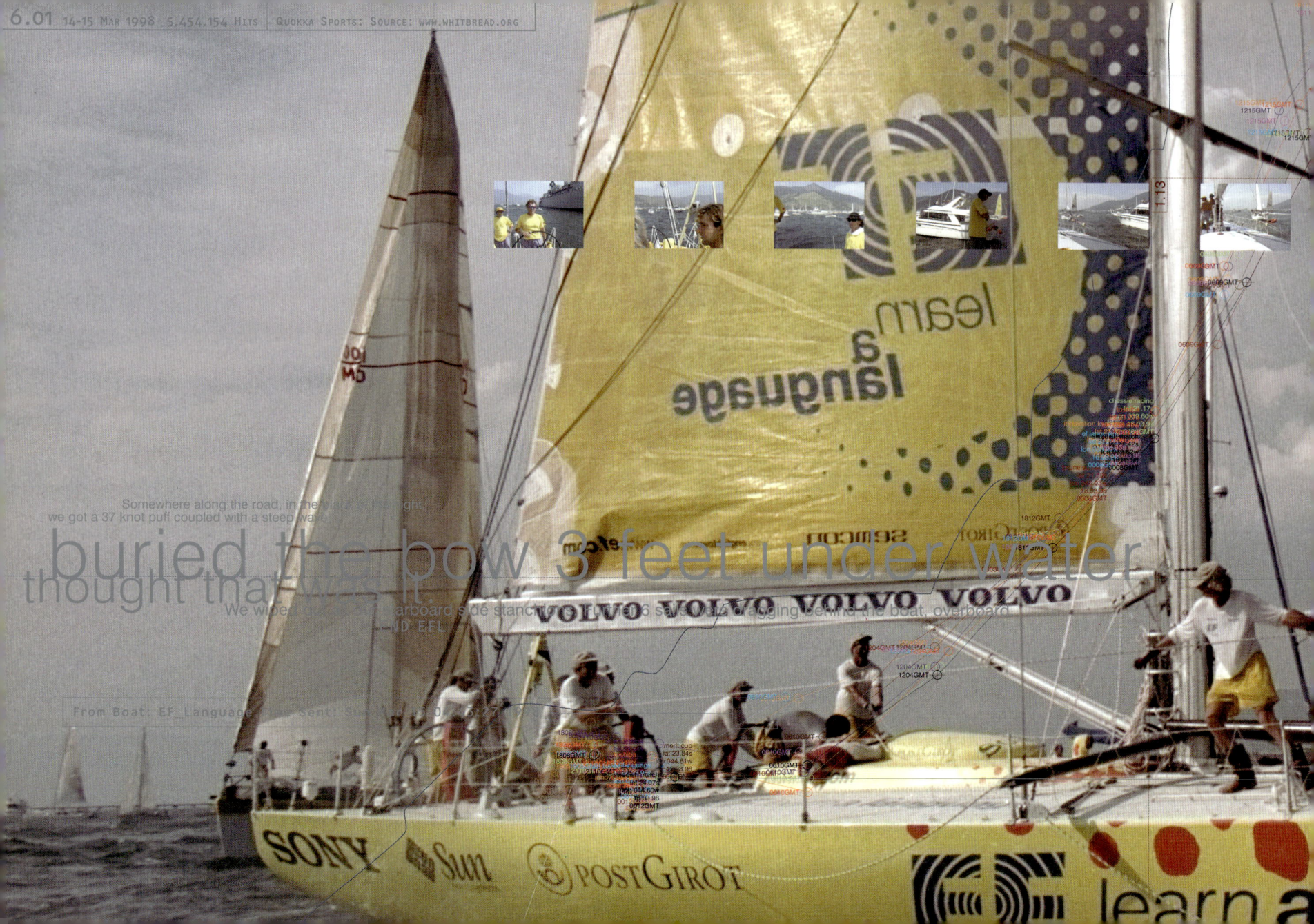

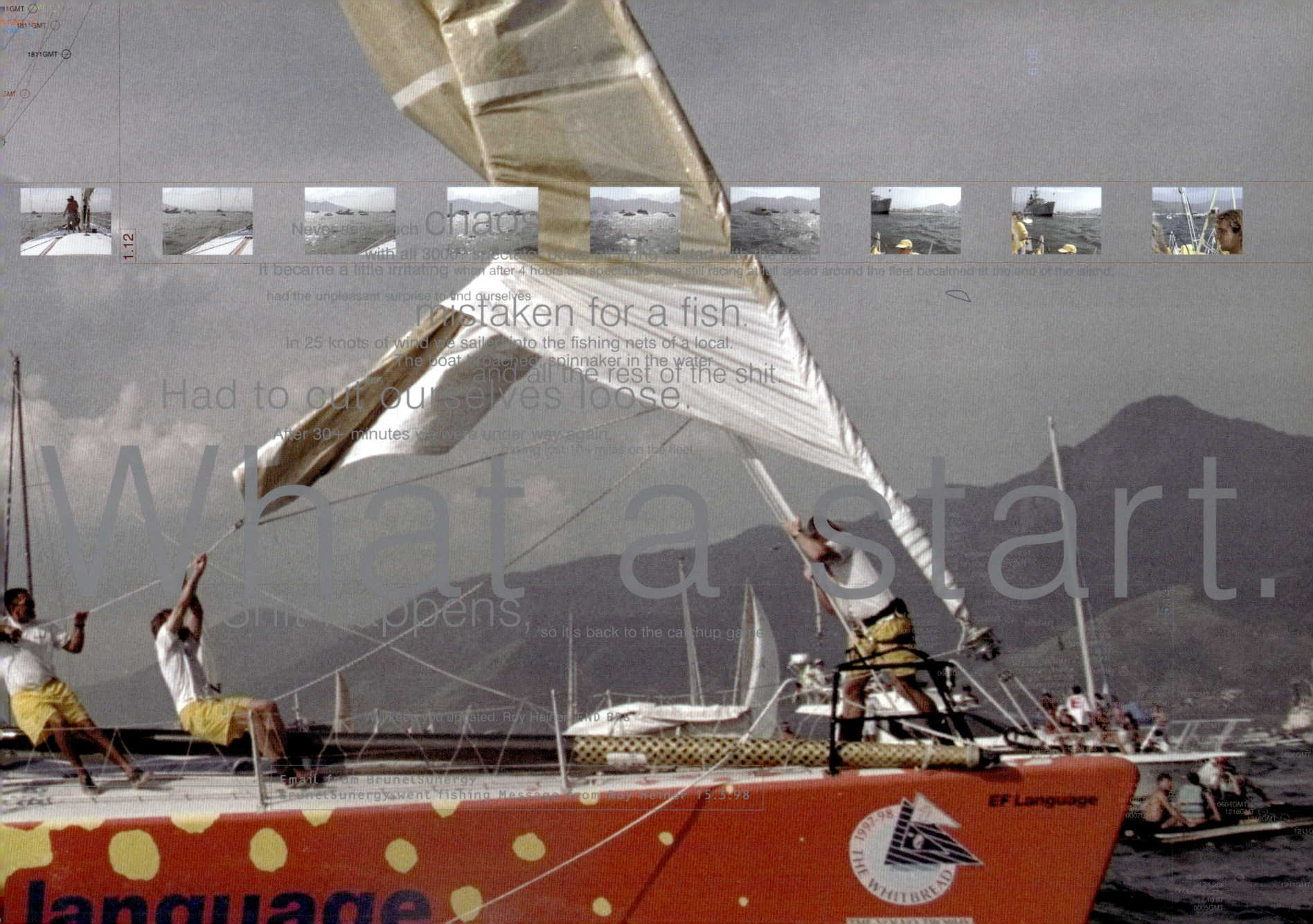

6.02 16-17 Mar 1998 11,372,638 Hits Quokka Sports: Source: www.whitbread.org

From Boat: BrunelSunergy   Mon Mar 16 03:34:10 1998

We all agreed not to complain about the heat on board, so when we say it is

another nice

From Boat: Toshiba Mon Mar 16 1998
I managed to slip into my bunk only to break into a 4 hour sweating session...

like sleeping in a sauna

Sean Clarkson - END TOS

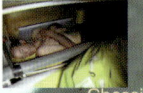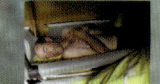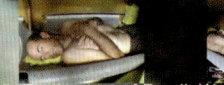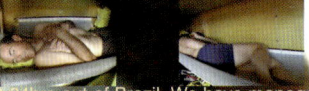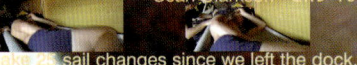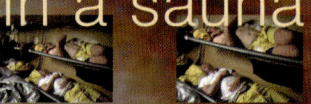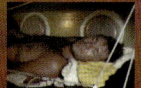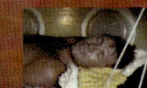

Chessie Racing has enjoyed the first 24hrs out of Brazil. We have managed to make 25 sail changes since we left the dock, and have **raised the heat index inside the boat to 105.7 degrees.**

Dave Scott Watch Captain, Chessie Racing END CHR   From Boat: Chessie Time Sent: Mon Mar 16 23:28:15 1998

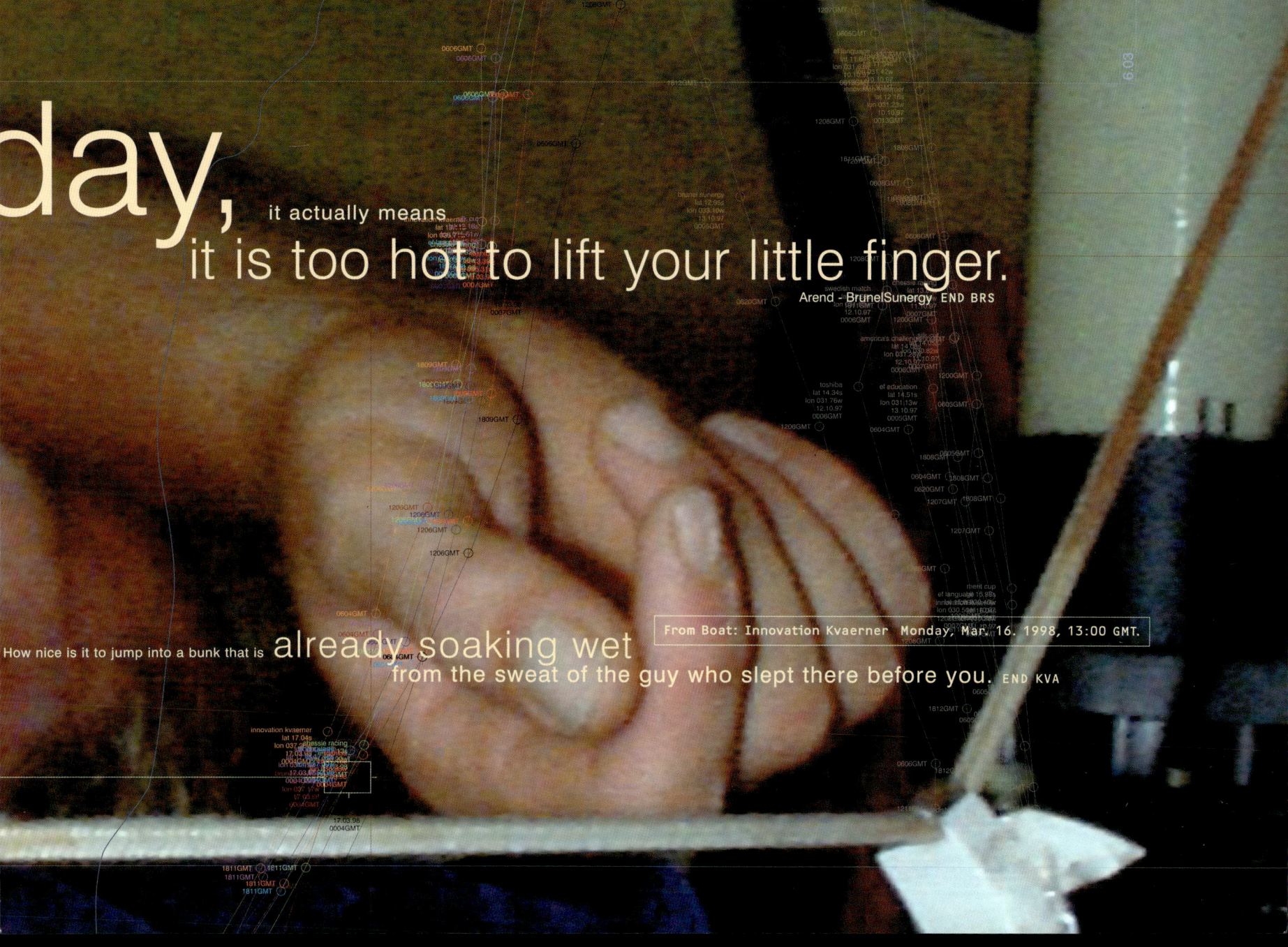

6.03 18-19 MAR 1998 10,939,981 HITS | QUOKKA SPORTS: SOURCE: WWW.WHITBREAD.ORG

One cloud sealed the fate for Chessie today.

Last night Chessie had to sail through a large black rain cloud. This doesn't sound too bad in itself. In fact a rain shower is a pleasant relief from the stifling heat. What is bad is the associated phenomena that comes along with the rain, like the 60 degree wind swing towards the coast of Brazil. The bald headed sail change to a jibtop (Reaching headsail), more header (unfavoured wind direction), wind dying to 4 knots. The tack and sail change to the whomper. Another sail change to the stays'l as the wind dies even more. The tack back and wind filling in again. Two trips up the mast to strop off various sails. Then finally the wind filling in from its old direction and back to our old sail combination. All this took place over 3 hours and the net loss was 13 miles. All of a sudden we went from the front of the pack to the back in one rain cloud.

Grant "Fuzz" Spanhake Watch Captain Chessie END CHR

From Boat: Chessie Time Sent: Wed Mar 18 17:15:50 1998
Wind Speed: 13 knots Boat Speed: 9 knots Temperature inside Chessie: 93 degrees

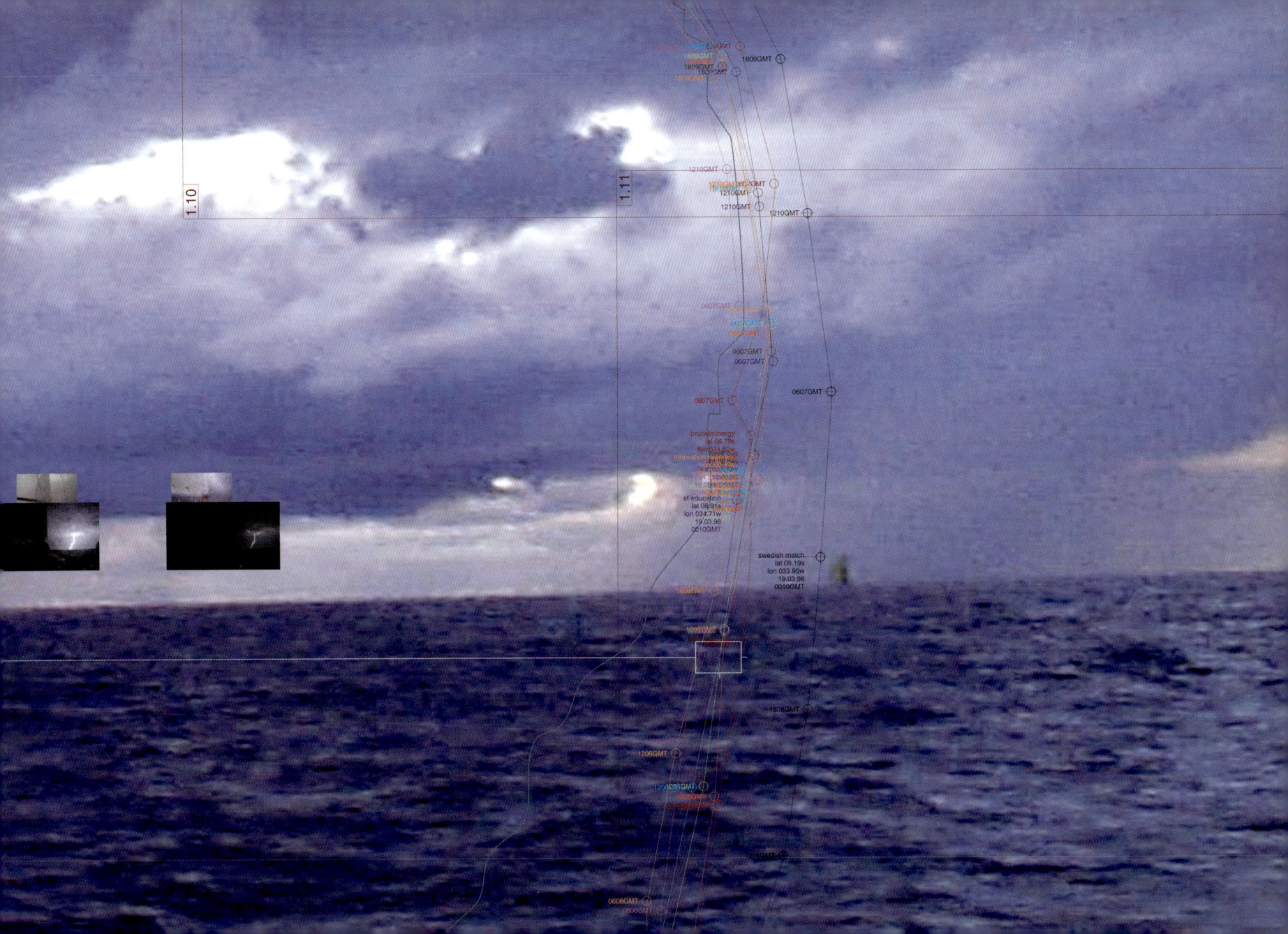

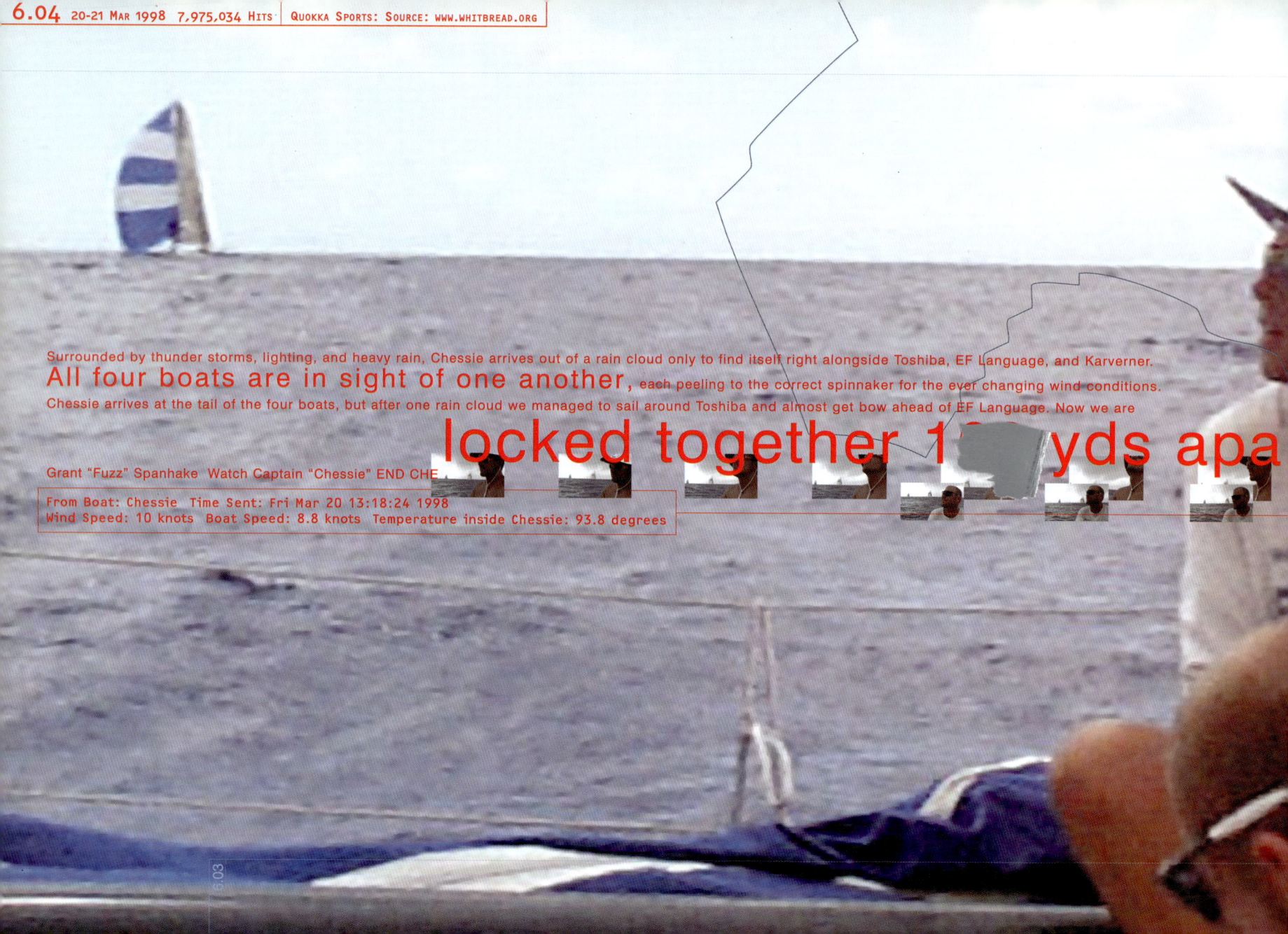

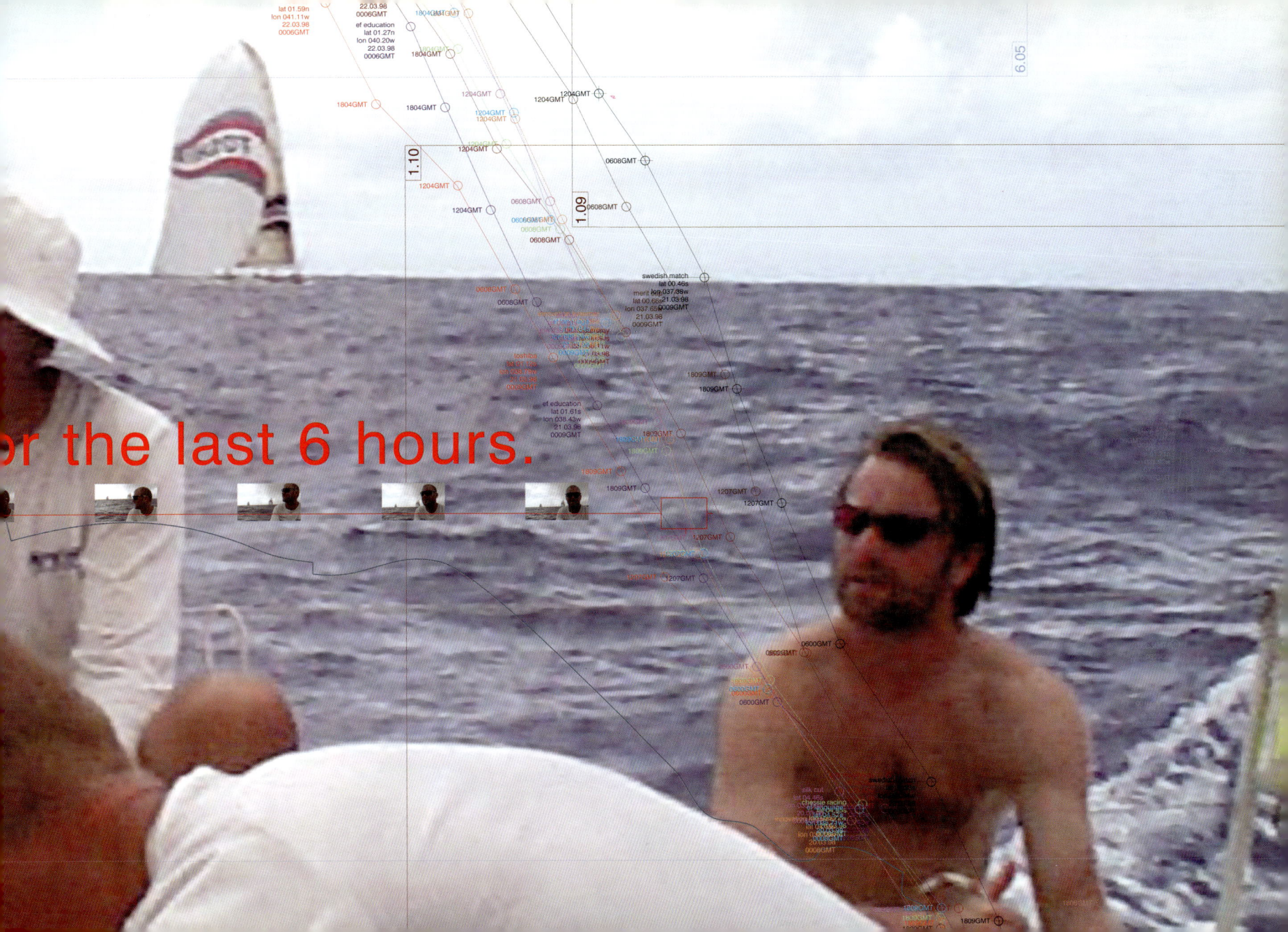

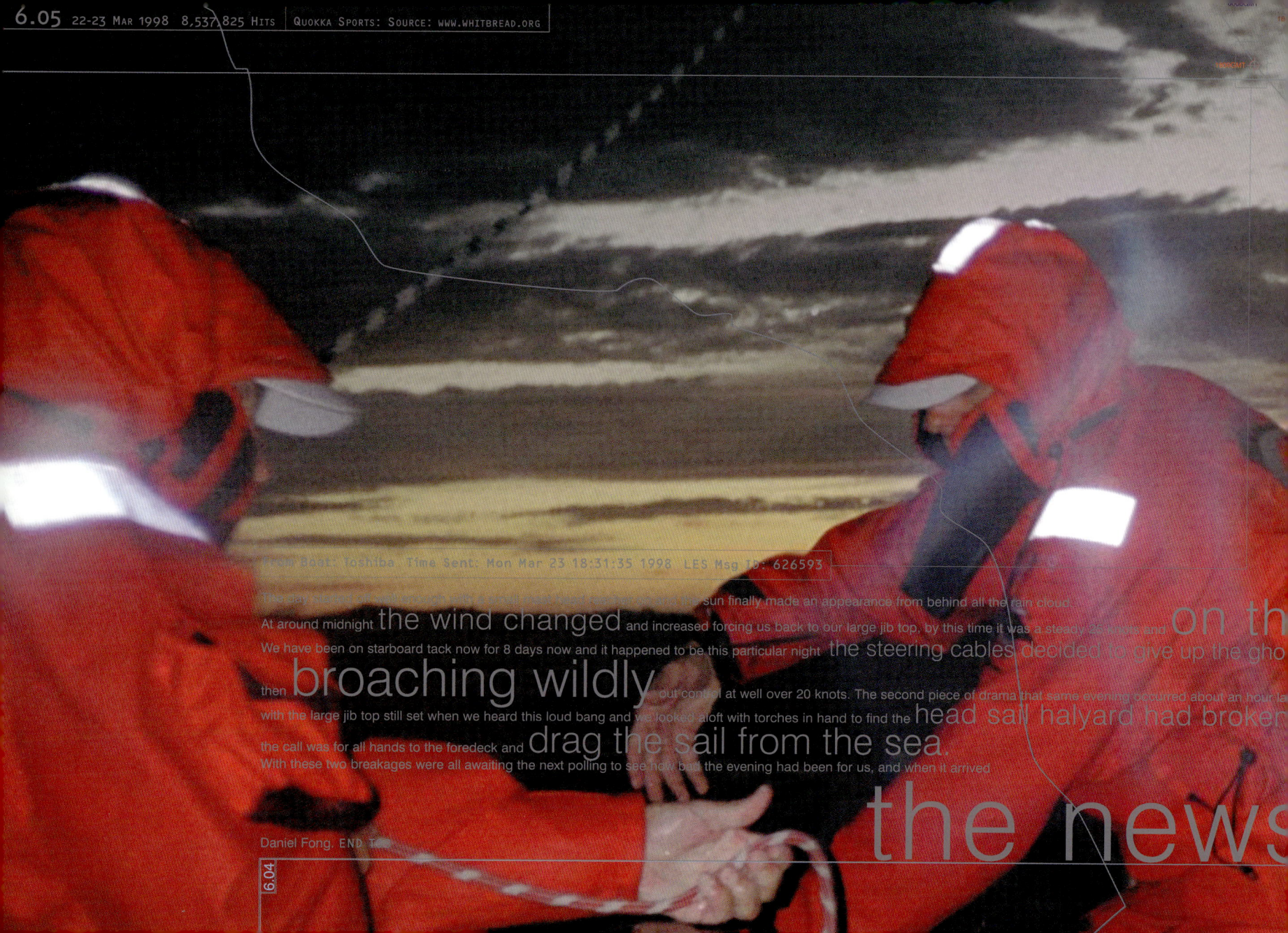

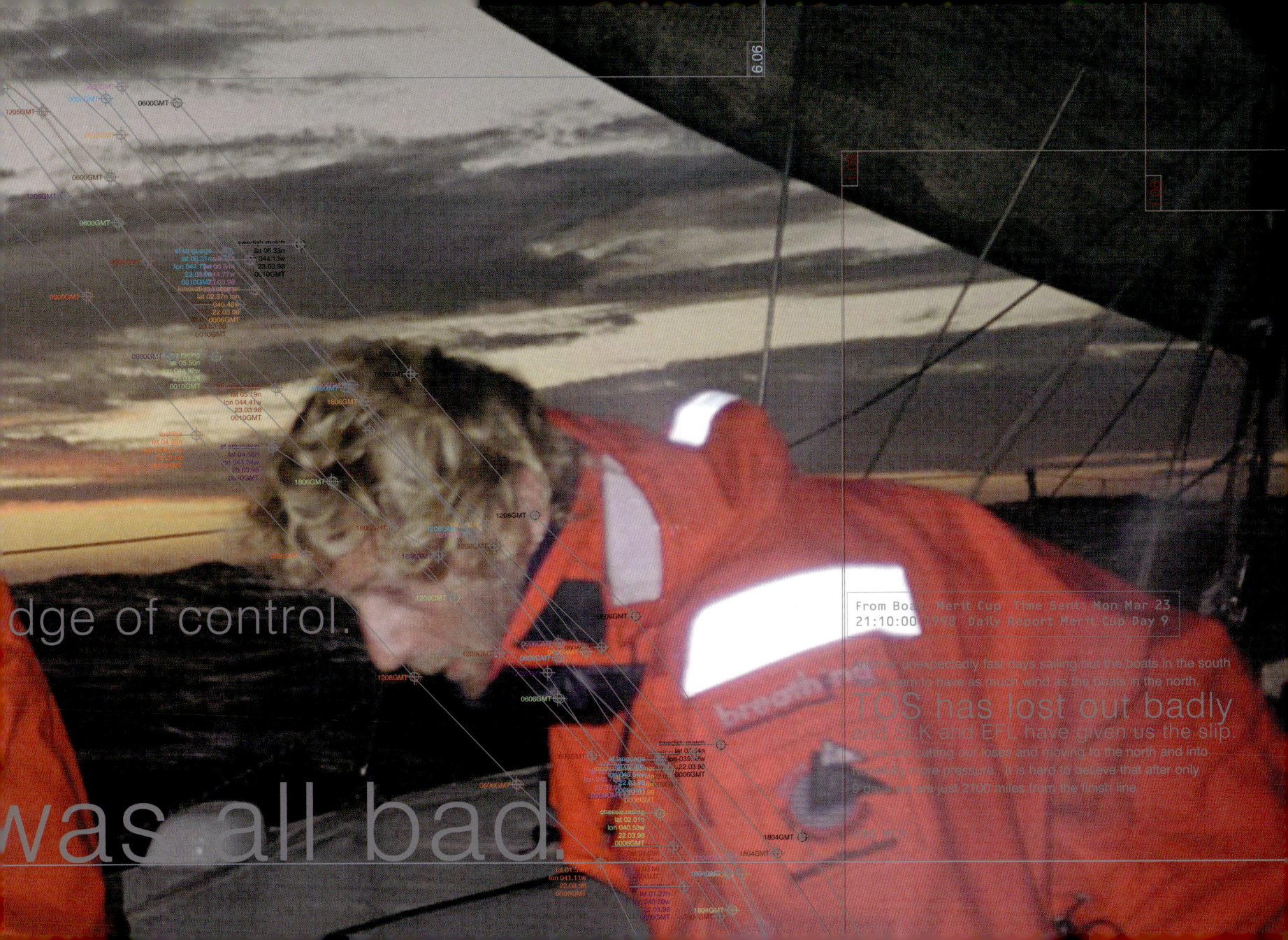

dge of control.

was all bad.

From Boat: Merit Cup Time Sent: Mon Mar 23 21:10:00 1998 Daily Report Merit Cup Day 9

After unexpectedly fast days sailing out the boats in the south seem to have as much wind as the boats in the north. TOS has lost out badly and SLK and EFL have given us the slip. We are cutting our loses and moving to the north and into hopefully more pressure. It is hard to believe that after only 9 days we are just 2100 miles from the finish line.

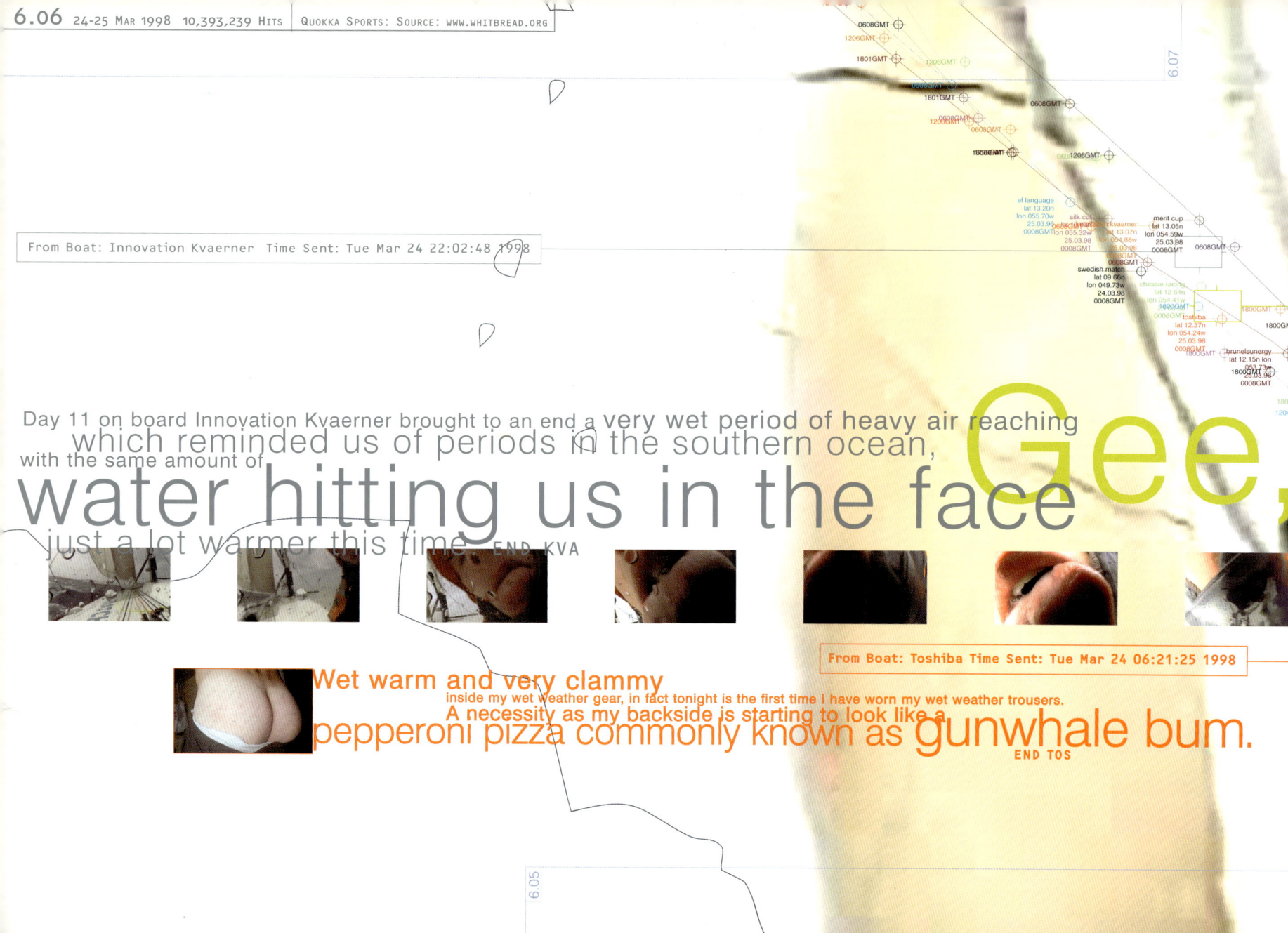

6.06 24-25 MAR 1998 10,393,239 HITS QUOKKA SPORTS: SOURCE: WWW.WHITBREAD.ORG

From Boat: Innovation Kvaerner Time Sent: Tue Mar 24 22:02:48 1998

Day 11 on board Innovation Kvaerner brought to an end a **very wet period of heavy air reaching** which reminded us of periods in the southern ocean, with the same amount of **water hitting us in the face** just a lot warmer this time. END KVA

Gee,

From Boat: Toshiba Time Sent: Tue Mar 24 06:21:25 1998

Wet warm and very clammy inside my wet weather gear, in fact tonight is the first time I have worn my wet weather trousers. A necessity as my backside is starting to look like a **pepperoni pizza commonly known as gunwhale bum.** END TOS

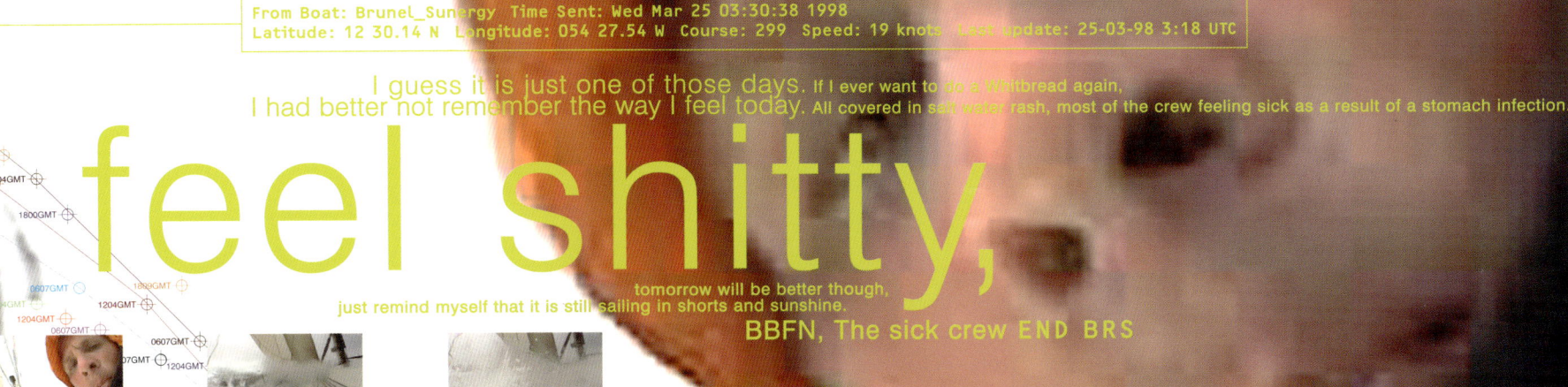

From Boat: Brunel_Sunergy Time Sent: Wed Mar 25 03:30:38 1998
Latitude: 12 30.14 N Longitude: 054 27.54 W Course: 299 Speed: 19 knots Last update: 25-03-98 3:18 UTC

I guess it is just one of those days. If I ever want to do a Whitbread again,
I had better not remember the way I feel today. All covered in salt water rash, most of the crew feeling sick as a result of a stomach infection.

feel shitty,

tomorrow will be better though,
just remind myself that it is still sailing in shorts and sunshine.

BBFN, The sick crew END BRS

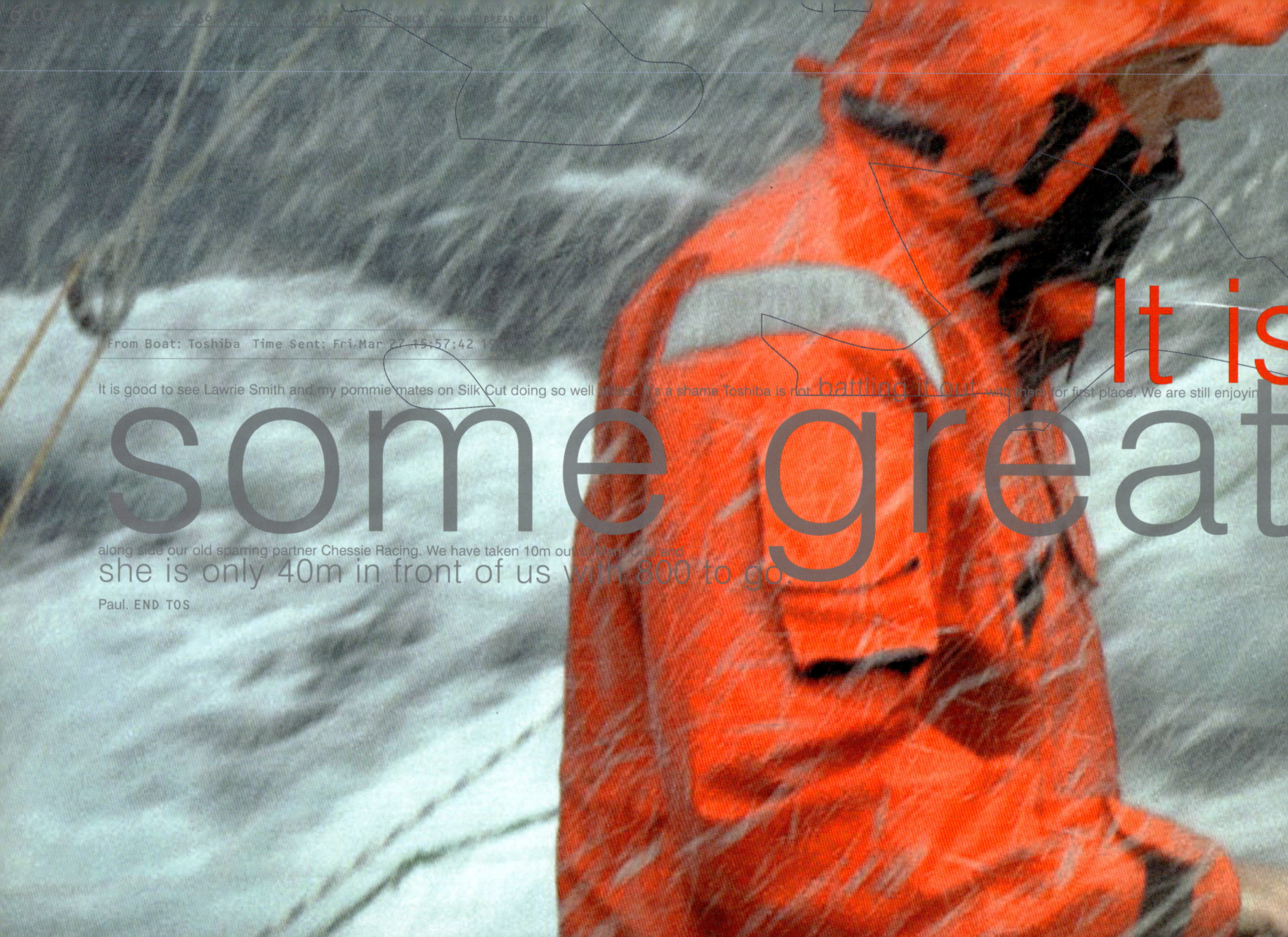

From Boat: Toshiba Time Sent: Fri.Mar 27 15:57:42 1998

It is good to see Lawrie Smith and my pommie mates on Silk Cut doing so well though it's a shame Toshiba is not battling it out with them for first place. We are still enjoying **It is some great** along side our old sparring partner Chessie Racing. We have taken 10m out of them today and she is only 40m in front of us with 800 to go.

Paul. END TOS

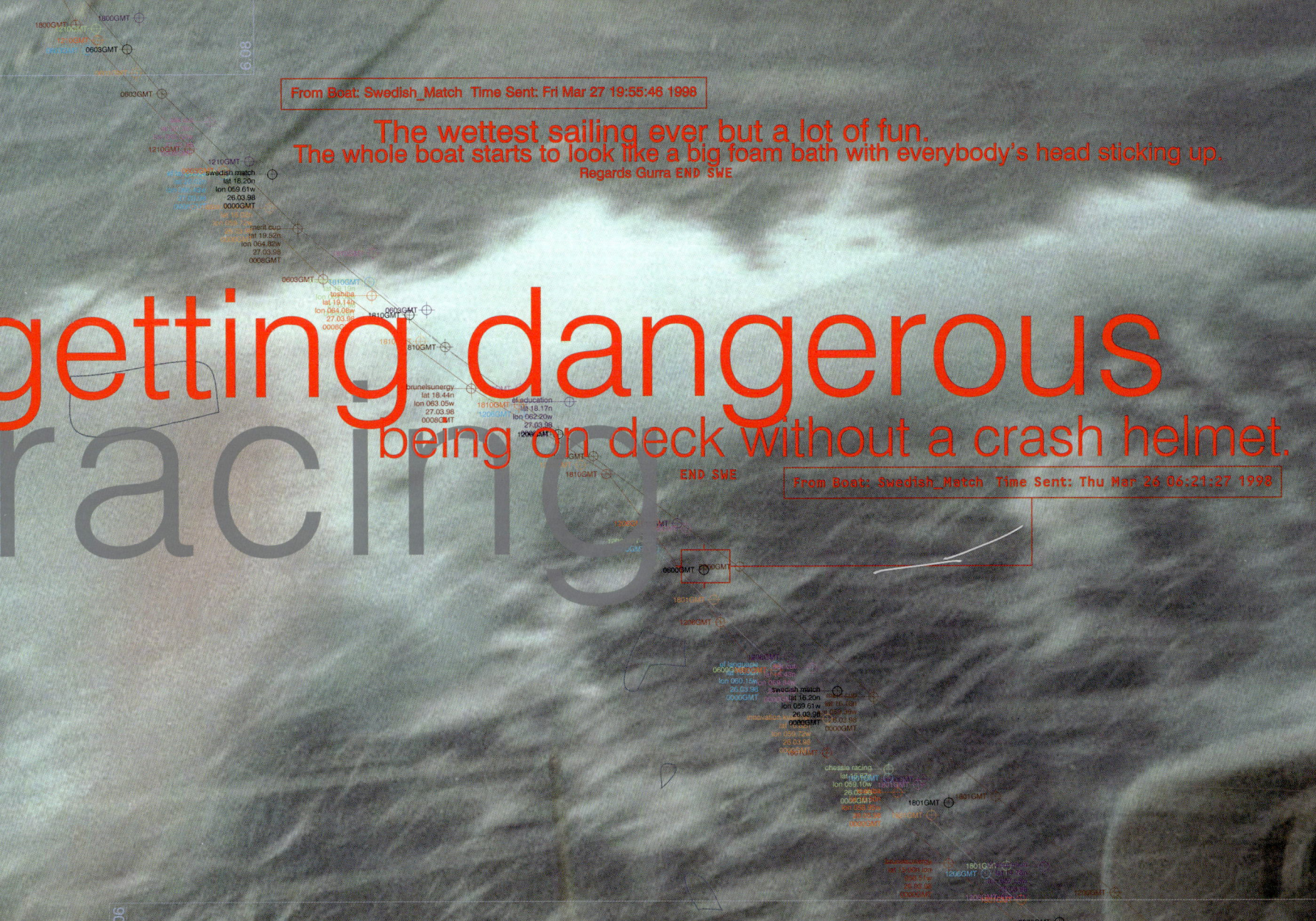

6.08 28-31 Mar 1998 13,731,871 Hits Quokka Sports: Source: www.whitbread.org

leg 6 leaderboard and status

pos	boat	elapsed time	points	totals
1	Silk Cut	14d+ 19:55:09	115	399
2	EF Language	14d+ 21:13:17	101	608
3	Swedish Match	14d+ 23:42:43	89	493
4	Innovation Kvaerner	15d+ 07:59:07	77	449
5	Merit Cup	15d+ 11:37:39	66	477
6	Chessie Racing	15d+ 19:39:12	55	454
7	Toshiba	15d+ 19:42:05	44	343
8	Brunel Sunergy	16d+ 08:41:35	33	248
9	EF Education	16d+ 10:40:30	22	148

From Boat: EF_Language Time Sent: Sat Mar 28 11:22:25 1998 LES Msg ID: 707158 Daily Report #1

Yesterday's frontal passing of the so called, "Discipated Front" was a little more than discipated. As Rudi wrote, we got slammed by 40 knots on the nose for an hour or two. The water is still 84F, so it was kind of fun stuff rattling, shaking, flapping, spray flying, lightening going off, thunder and all of us wrestling sails down on the deck and body slamming th

it was what we call a shi

to hold them down...
you know, boys like that kind of stuff.
END EFL PC

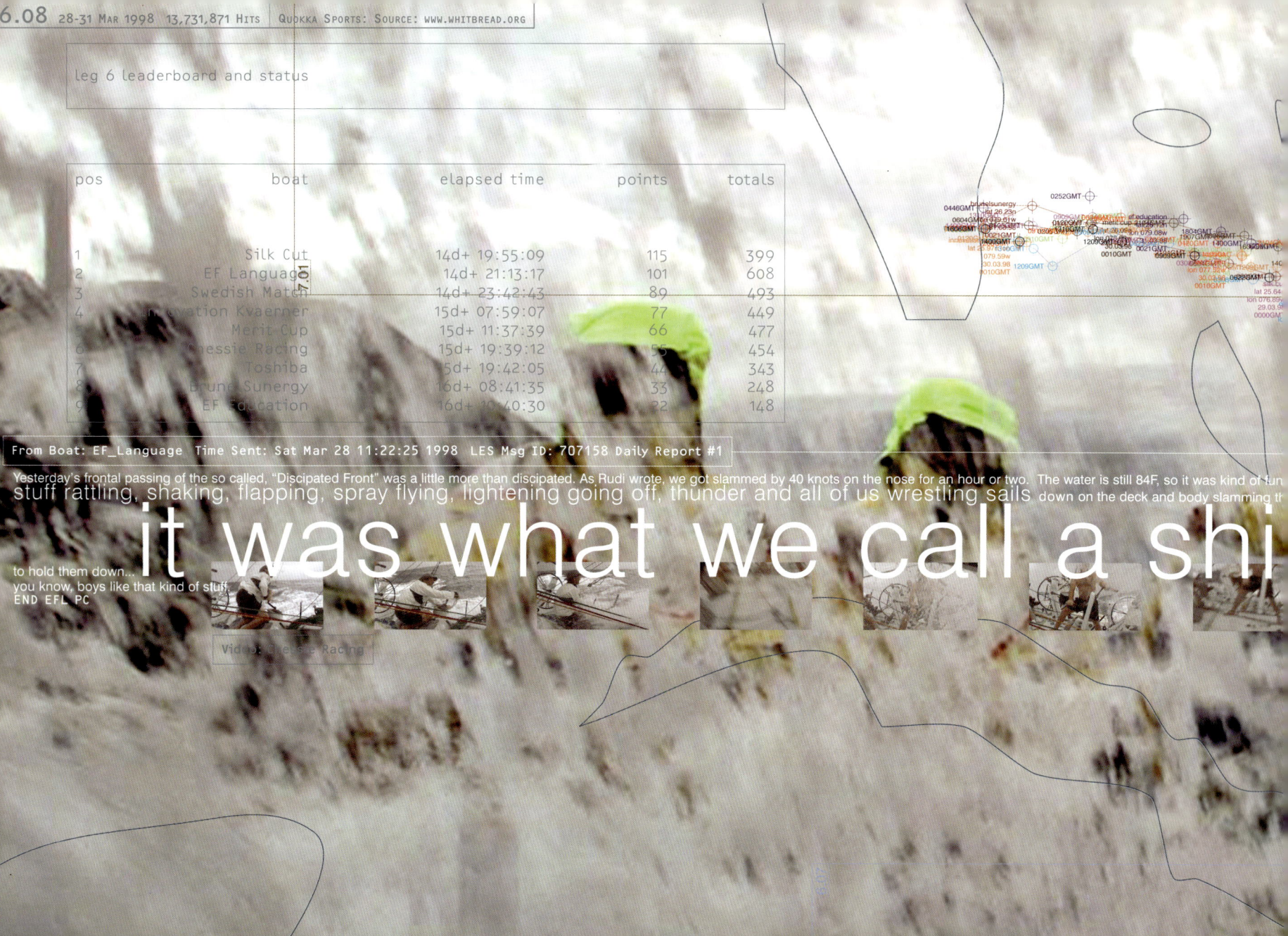

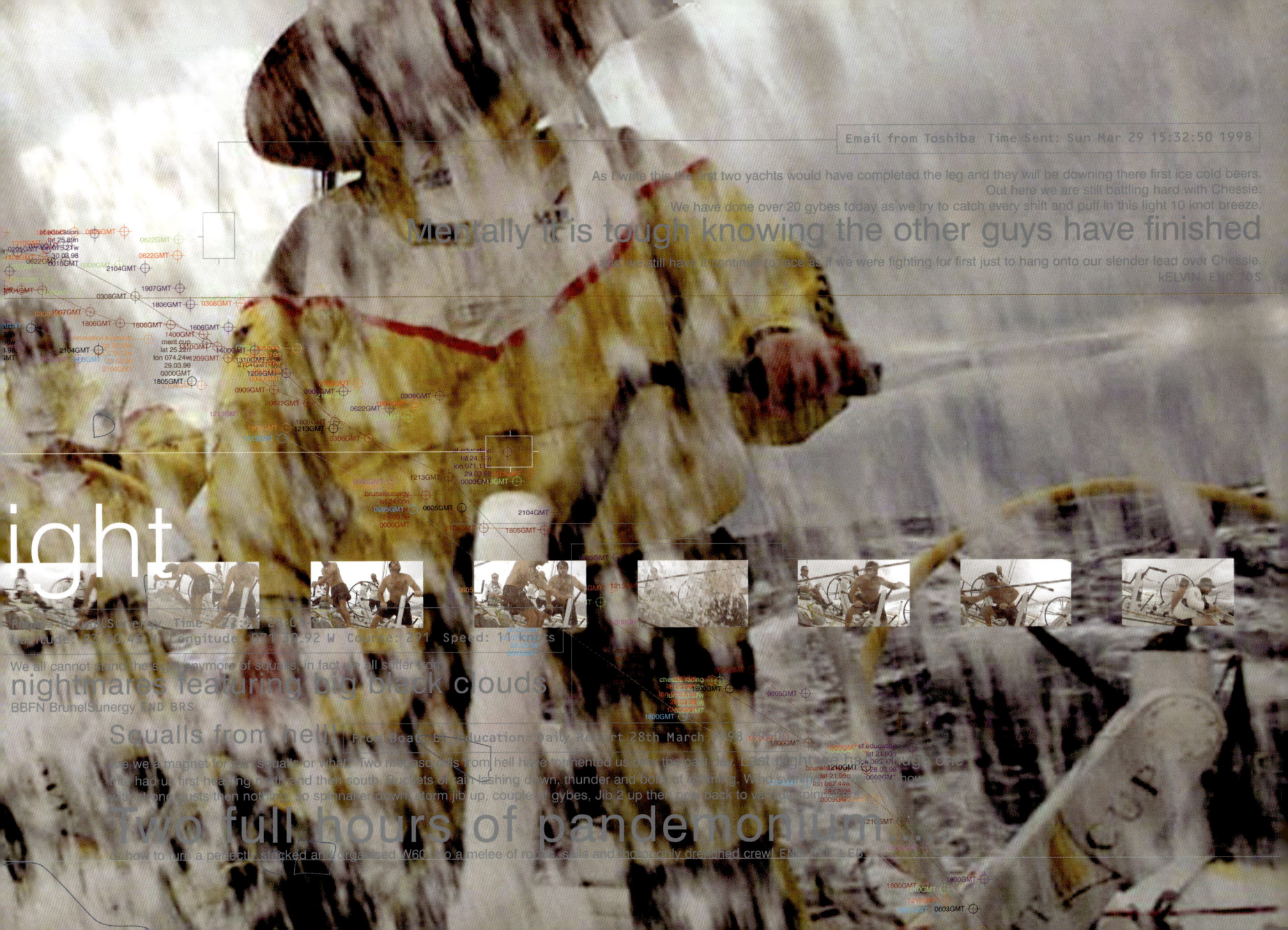

7.0.0 19 Apr – 22 Apr 1998   27,330,217 Hits | Quokka Sports: Source: www.whitbread.org

Leg 7

Distance:

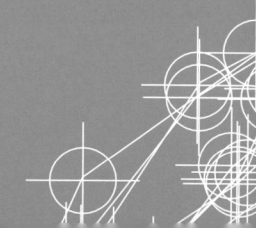

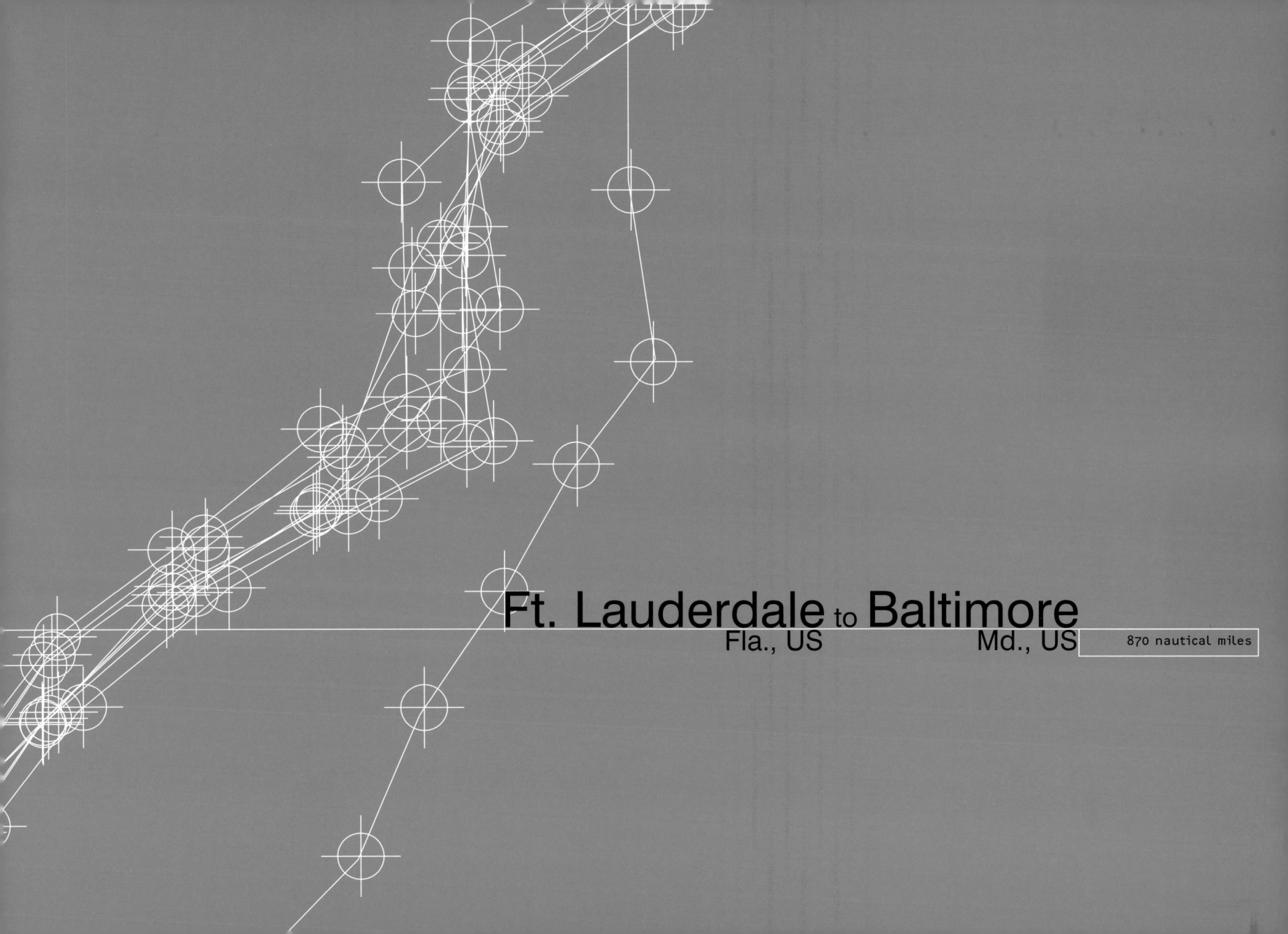

Leg 7: Prelude

The Ft. Lauderdale stopover marked the point where those behind in overall points had to stop kidding themselves. Only three legs remained, with two of them as the shortest legs of the race, offering the lowest point totals. Leg 7 would be an 870-mile sprint up the United States' East Coast, a trifle for these veterans of 7,000-mile-plus legs.

With 608 points now safely in the bank, EF Language had a comfortable lead, allowing Paul Cayard the luxury of sailing more conservatively on the legs ahead. Swedish Match was the closest rival with 493 points, and Gunnar Krantz and his crew had already proven themselves to be fierce and capable competitors. Cayard indicated that he would be keeping a close eye on Krantz for the rest of the race.

Meanwhile, things were still not clicking for the star-crossed Toshiba team. After a disastrous disqualification on the point-heavy Leg 5, and a poor seventh-place finish on the previous leg, Dennis Conner again stepped forward to take the helm. It was announced that skipper Paul Standbridge would stand down for Leg 7 to allow Conner to skipper. His departure would also make room aboard the boat for Mike Powers, a professional Chesapeake Bay pilot.

The area was familiar racing territory for Conner, though he had never sailed the Chesapeake. "I have always enjoyed racing in this part of the world," Conner said. "The challenge of the Gulf Stream ... coupled with the challenges of the Chesapeake" made this leg irresistible, he added.

After what they had already been through over the past seven months, a sprint up the East Coast of the United States had few of the skippers worried. Instead, it was the last stretch of Leg 7, the 130 miles up the Chesapeake Bay, that kept many of them awake at night. The Baltimore/Annapolis, Md., stopover had been added to the race for the first time, and the bay would expose the teams to a unique set of risks. Chesapeake recreational sailors posted plenty of warnings and advice to the crews on the Web site. They warned of the bay's notorious tides, constantly shifting sandbars, fluky wind patterns, GPS dead spots, and in particular the hundreds of crab pots floating like snares waiting to attach themselves to a boat's rudder or keel.

All this raised hopes with Chessie Racing fans. After all, this was Chessie's home port, where skipper George Collins sailed almost every weekend. Collins would again take personally the helm on this leg. Also, several of Chessie's crew were Baltimore or Annapolis natives, who had cut their teeth navigating their way through Crab Pot Alley.

The other teams were taking no chances. As the boats were pulled out of the water and readied for the leg, some of the teams sent their skippers and navigators ahead to Baltimore to reconnoitre the bay. Some chartered powerboats, some sailboats and a few even chartered planes and flew the length of the Chesapeake, charting it from the air. What they saw were plenty of opportunities to go aground or get tangled in anchored crab pots. "Anything could happen," said Gunnar Krantz, returning from a look at the bay.

The strategy for the trip up the coast seemed straightforward. "At the start we have the Gulf Stream," said Cayard. "A nice conveyor belt that everyone wants to get into early." EF Language's skipper was referring to the three- to four-knot current that moves warm water from the Gulf of Mexico north, nearly paralleling the East Coast of the United States.

For Swedish Match, a Leg 7 win was critical. With a second-place overall standing, it represented the team's final chance — slim as it was — to close the current 115-point gap to the lead. "It is a must-win leg for us," said Krantz, "and a must-do-bad leg for EF Language!"

Dennis Conner predicted a very close race up the coast, with the boats first into the Gulf Stream leading all the way to the entrance of the Chesapeake Bay. "It is logical to think that the guys who get around the gate first will be the first into the Gulf Stream," he said. "That's good for morale and puts more pressure on the people behind." However, Conner added, once the boats entered the bay the fleet would likely bunch up again, creating close racing conditions to the finish.

On 22 April, the fourth and final day of the leg, the fleet passed over the Chesapeake Bay Bridge Tunnel. The boats were now in the heart of Chesapeake Bay's 'danger zone' — an area notorious for its fish traps, lobster pots and sandbars. Adding to the confusion, the breeze turned fluky — at times 1.5 knots, then strengthening to eight to 10 knots.

The fleet became tightly bunched. Only one mile separated the four backmarkers: Chessie Racing, Merit Cup, Toshiba and EF Education. In the middle of the fleet, just over seven miles in front of Chessie Racing, sailed fourth-placed Innovation Kvaerner and fifth-placed Silk Cut.

BrunelSunergy was still leading with just 40 nautical miles to go to the finish line. Her lead continued to dwindle as Swedish Match and EF Language rushed up from behind. During the night, the 'blue boat' overtook Swedish Match to snatch second place, yet barely. Only three tenths of a nautical mile separated them at dawn. Both boats continued reeling in BrunelSunergy, taking almost two miles out of her lead in one hour that morning. BrunelSunergy was now just 11 miles in front of EF Language.

By this time the Toshiba team had managed to climb from last to eighth place by passing EF Education, then Conner began closing on Chessie Racing.

Within the Chesapeake Bay, furious match races raged as 'the race' broke down into several individual races. At the front, the hungry-for-a-win Dutch crew was determined that neither EF Language nor Swedish Match was going to steal this moment from them, even though both boats were now clearly visible astern and closing.

Cayard was desperately fighting to keep the only boat that had an outside chance of bumping him from first, Swedish Match, from passing. All day, the two boats match raced, while at the same time nibbling away at BrunelSunergy's lead. With just 20 miles to the finish, EF Language had closed to within 4.5 nautical miles of BrunelSunergy. Swedish Match was only eight-tenths of a mile behind EF Language.

Desperate to hold her lead, BrunelSunergy plotted a course down the middle of the bay. There, she found better wind than EF Language and Swedish Match, who had both tacked into the southern shore. Finding less wind there, they quickly tacked back out toward the centre. The moment gave BrunelSunergy just the breathing room she needed to hold off the two pursuers. Yet just as the Dutch team was approaching the harbour the winds shifted, and her speed began to fade as the two sails astern grew larger.

As this battle raged in the front, seven miles back another shooting match was going on between Innovation Kvaerner in fourth, and Silk Cut, just half a nautical mile behind. Both boats were in good wind and reporting boat speeds of 12.2 and 12.5 knots respectively.

Behind these two, Merit Cup, hometown favourite Chessie Racing and Dennis Conner's Toshiba were racing virtually side by side, vying for sixth place. Merit Cup was logging the best speed. A mile and a half behind eighth-placed Toshiba was EF Education in last place.

While these secondary battles were still being fought at the fleet's rear, up front BrunelSunergy pulled it off: Heiner and crew crossed the finish line to capture first place. They took the finish gun at 5 p.m. local time, 22 April, sailing dead downwind in 10 knots of breeze. It was an electric moment for both fans and crew as they revelled in the upset victory. Skipper Heiner was at the wheel, flanked by navigator Stuart Quarrie and meteorologist Frits Koek, as the boat crossed the line. Even before the gun went off, crewmembers began shaking hands and punching the air, beneath a full-bellied spinnaker. Heiner left the helm to another crewman so he could hug his fellow teammates. Bespectacled Stuart Quarrie turned to the press boat and blew kisses.

Twenty-one minutes later, Swedish Match crossed, having snatched second place back from EF Language by a mere 30 seconds. Cayard did not fall easily. Moments before the end, EF Language was on the attack, gybing every 60 to 90 seconds and forcing Swedish Match to do the same. "EFL refuses to let go behind us," Krantz reported.

Also fighting down to the wire were Innovation Kvaerner and Silk Cut. At the line, Innovation Kvaerner won the match race, capturing fourth place three and a half minutes ahead of the British team.

Attention then shifted to the battle between local favourite Chessie Racing and Toshiba. The two boats were wrestling over seventh place. With a podium finish no longer in the cards, Collins wanted to give Chessie fans something else to cheer about by beating Dennis Conner to the finish line. Conner was just as determined to see that didn't happen.

Toshiba had a healthy lead over Chessie as the two raced toward the Annapolis Bridge — it looked like the race was over. Then the unexpected happened. Even though Conner had taken the extra precaution of having a professional Chesapeake Bay pilot aboard, Toshiba suddenly lurched to a stop.

"We ran aground and they passed us," Conner said later. "Then we caught back up with them on the other side of the bridge and passed them again. It was pretty exciting. Once we came together on the other side of the Annapolis Bridge it was more like the America's Cup than The Whitbread," Conner claimed. "It's just too bad we weren't racing for first and second."

As the two combatants approached the finish line, Chessie Racing was cheered on by an enormous fleet of local boaters who had gathered to see 'their boys' complete a circumnavigation. When Toshiba crossed ahead of Chessie, it was only by moments. Only 10 seconds separated the two boats, the closest finish between two boats in Whitbread history.

Even though he did not win the match race, the spectacle of local boy Collins challenging sailing legend Dennis Conner was clearly a crowd-pleaser. It took a bit of the sting out of finishing eighth on the leg. "It was really thrilling. To sail that long together up the bay, it was exciting to be racing against a world legend like Dennis Conner," Collins said. "We nipped them in Ft. Lauderdale, and they nipped us here. But today he just had better boatspeed than we did."

EF Education finished ninth, less than two hours behind the leader. As soon as her skipper, Christine Guillou, stepped ashore, new problems developed for the Toshiba team.

Guillou filed a protest against Toshiba's skipper, alleging contravention of the International Regulations for Preventing Collisions At Sea (IRPCAS). She said that Conner had sailed recklessly the first night out of Ft. Lauderdale, Fla. Guillou said she was filing the protest because breaking those rules at night is a great risk. "I think it is important to respect this rule, so we have protested Toshiba," she said. She described the incident as happening when all the boats were gybing and crossing repeatedly. "All the boats were very close, you crossed other boats very often, so everyone has a lookout on deck, so it is impossible that they did not see us. It's a part of the race when you are very aware of what can happen."

In response, Conner said that as soon as he was made aware of Guillou's protest that night he had performed a 720-degree penalty turn in accordance with the rules. The turn allows a team that may have infringed upon one of the rules to exonerate itself. However, since it was dark at the time, there was no way to verify that Toshiba had actually made the penalty turn.

This would be Toshiba's third time in front of the International Jury, the team's second time in the dock as a defendant.

EF Education's complaint was effectively about a port-and-starboard incident — a boat on starboard tack has the right of way over a boat on port tack. It was not, however, specifically a port-and-starboard protest, because the incident took place after sunset, when IRPCAS rules apply. These rules, explained Whitbread Race Manager Michael Woods, say that "at night there can be no luffing — getting in the way of another boat's breeze. Next, when one boat overtakes another, the lead boat must maintain her course. This means the front boat cannot make defensive moves to try to prevent the second boat from overtaking. Effectively, that means no boat-to-boat match racing at night."

Even as the Toshiba team awaited a ruling from the International Jury, it was hit with yet another problem. Andrew Cape, Toshiba's navigator since the start of the race, resigned apparently without warning or explanation. Cape would only describe it as "a personal decision," elaborating only to the extent of saying that it had "been a very hard race and I have not especially enjoyed it."

Toshiba co-skipper Paul Standbridge said Cape's decision to leave the team was a complete surprise. "We had no prior discussions about this, not in Ft. Lauderdale, not during the leg. I learned about it when Dennis phoned me yesterday after he received Capie's fax." Standbridge described Cape's decision as a serious blow to the team, which now had less than two weeks to find and train a navigator for the last two legs.

As the team struggled with the loss of its navigator, the International Jury was considering EF Education's protest. After five hours of testimony and deliberation, the jury handed down a verdict declaring Toshiba and skipper Dennis Conner had indeed violated "Rule 12 (a) (i)" of the International Regulations for Preventing Collisions At Sea. The jury also found that Toshiba's 720-degree penalty turn was not "effective," as it was not performed as soon as possible after the incident, in the jury's opinion.

The jury penalised Toshiba two places on Leg 7, which pushed Toshiba back to last place for the leg.

EF Education's formal protest against Toshiba:

"During the first night of Leg 7, the 20th of April, at 01.35UTC, EF Education was sailing downwind (between 145.150TWA) on starboard tack. The wind was 18 knots from 170 degrees. Boat speed around 13 knots, heading 20.25 degrees, the fleet was still close with gibes and crossings. Before the incident, Toshiba was 0.5 miles to windward of EFE on a parallel course, both on starboard tack. EFE was monitoring them visually and on radar. As soon as we saw that they had gibed, we realised that the boats would cross close. Before the incident, one crew member on EFE was illuminating the main with a torch to make it clearly visible and another crewmember was whistling and hailing "STARBOARD" to make sure we were clearly noticed. Despite these actions by EFE, the two boats continued to get closer quickly without any sign of actions from Toshiba to avoid a collision. When the boats were within one boat length from each other, the helmsman on EFE had to alter course radically to avoid a collision.

"EFE passed very close behind the stern of Toshiba. In the dark, it was impossible for the crew of EFE to determine whether its spinnaker touched the backstay of Toshiba but it was close enough for it to have happened. EFE estimates that the boats were less than half a boat length apart when they finally crossed.

"Within seconds of the incident we hailed 'PROTEST,' displayed the protest flag and around ten minutes after the incident we notified Toshiba via Inmarsat C of our intention to protest — this message was also copied to the Race Committee."

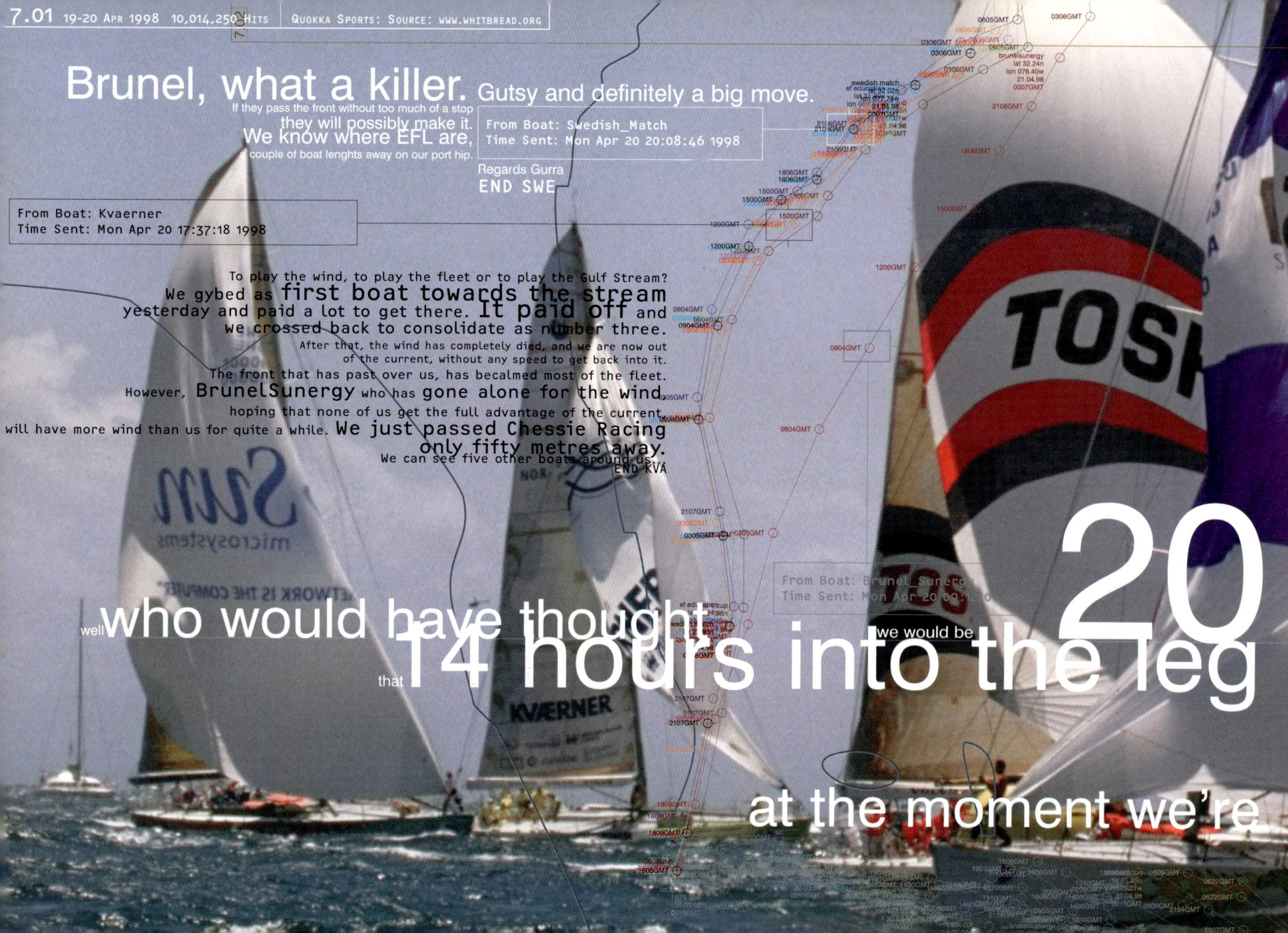

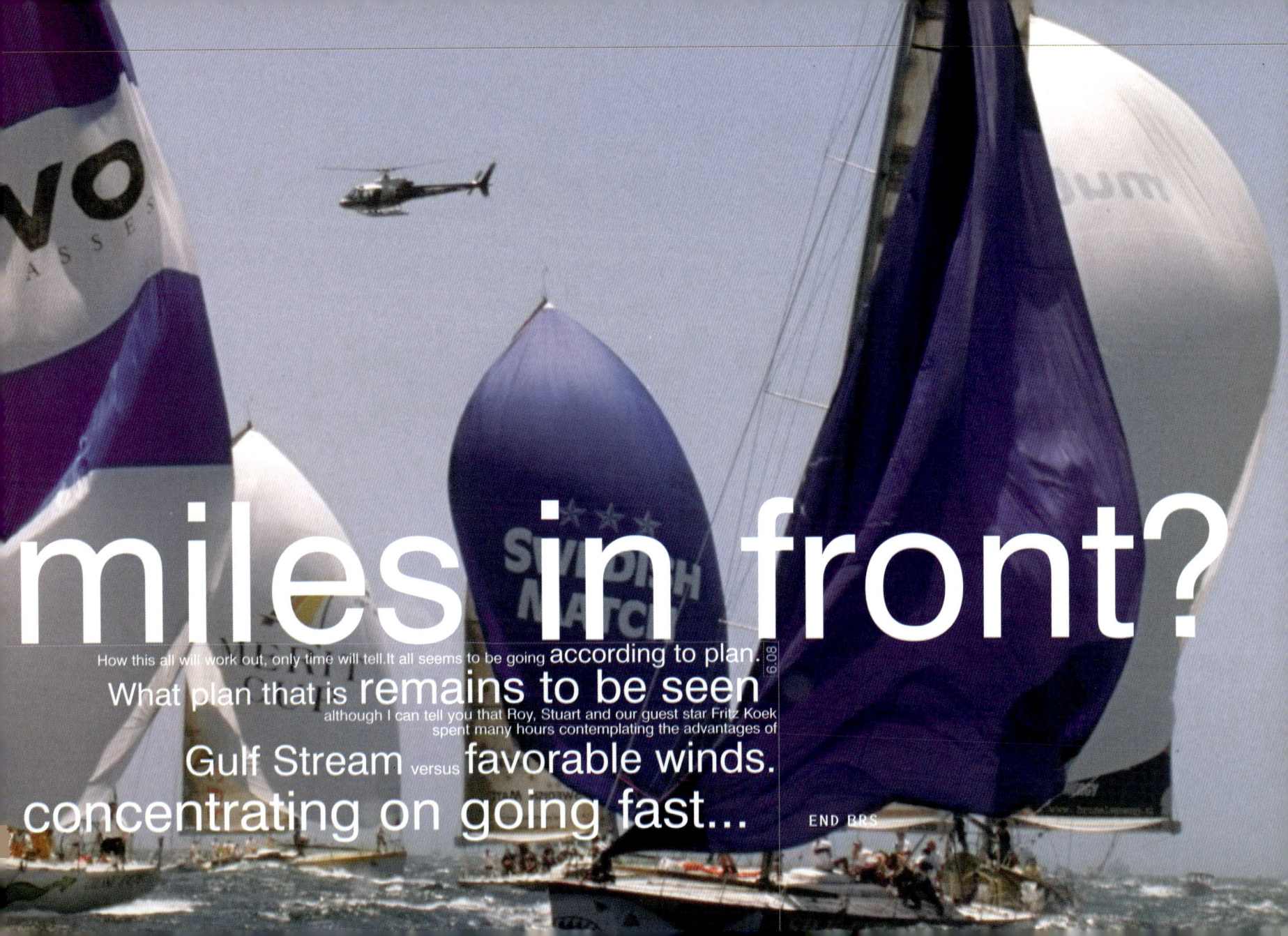

miles in front?

How this all will work out, only time will tell. It all seems to be going **according to plan.**
What plan that is remains to be seen
although I can tell you that Roy, Stuart and our guest star Fritz Koek
spent many hours contemplating the advantages of
Gulf Stream versus **favorable winds.**
concentrating on going fast...

END BRS

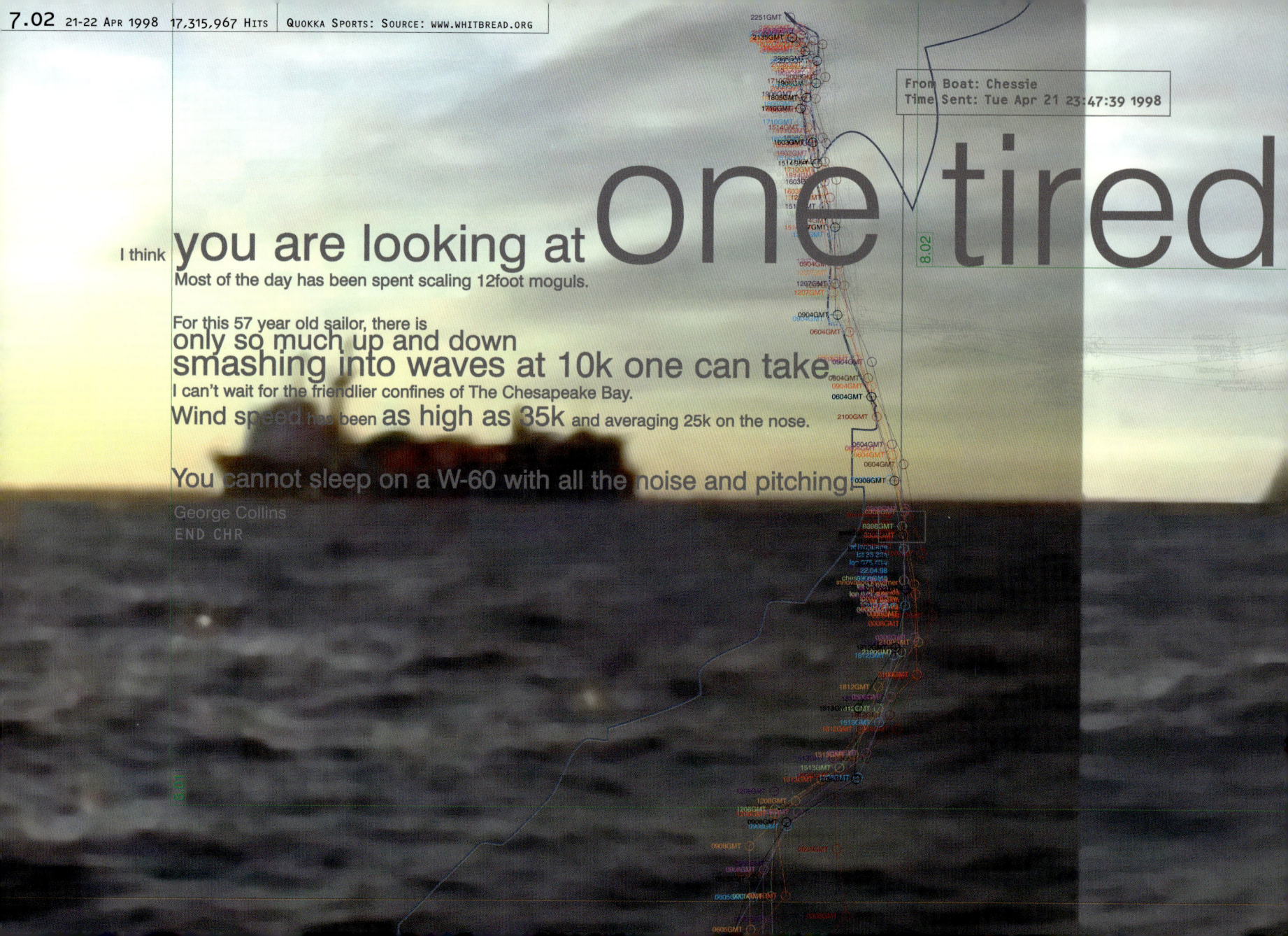

fleet.

leg 7 leaderboard and status

pos	boat	elapsed time	points	totals
1	BrunelSunergy	3d+ 03:59:39	105	353
2	Swedish Match	3d+ 04:20:24	92	585
3	EF Language	3d+ 04:20:54	81	689
4	Innovation Kvaerner	3d+ 04:58:36	70	519
5	Silk Cut	3d+ 05:02:07	60	459
6	Merit Cup	3d+ 05:21:44	50	527
7	Chessie Racing	3d+ 05:30:53	40	494
8	EF Education	3d+ 05:39:54	30	178
9	Toshiba*	3d+ 05:30:43	20	354

*two-place penalty

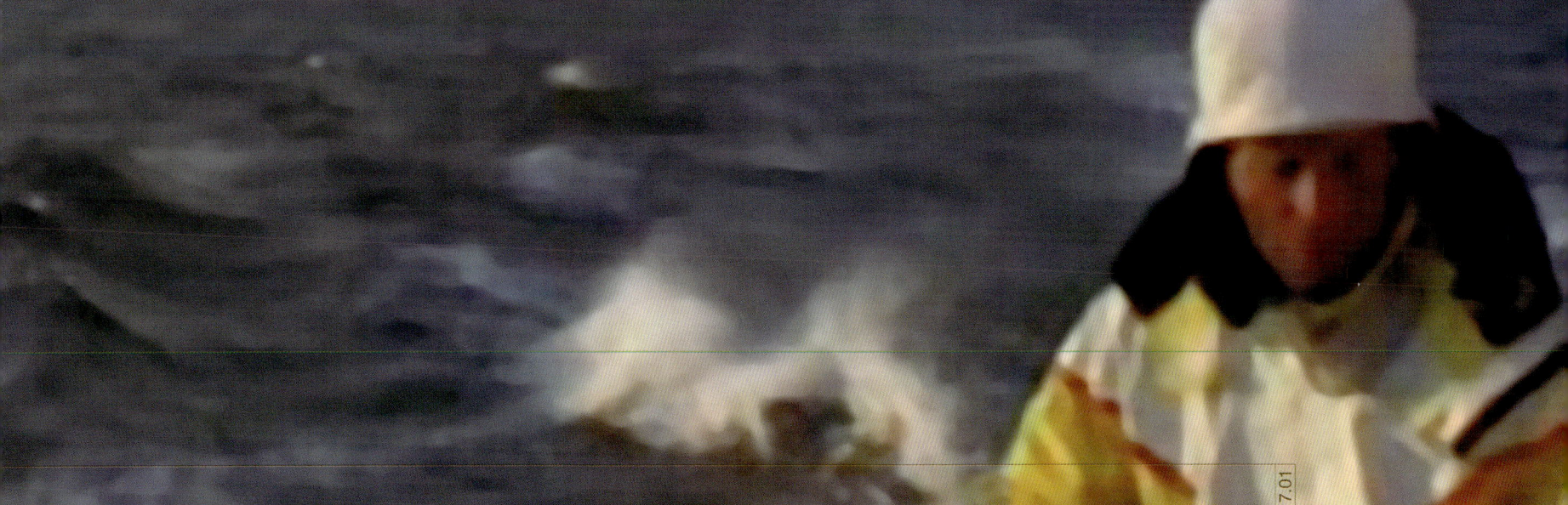

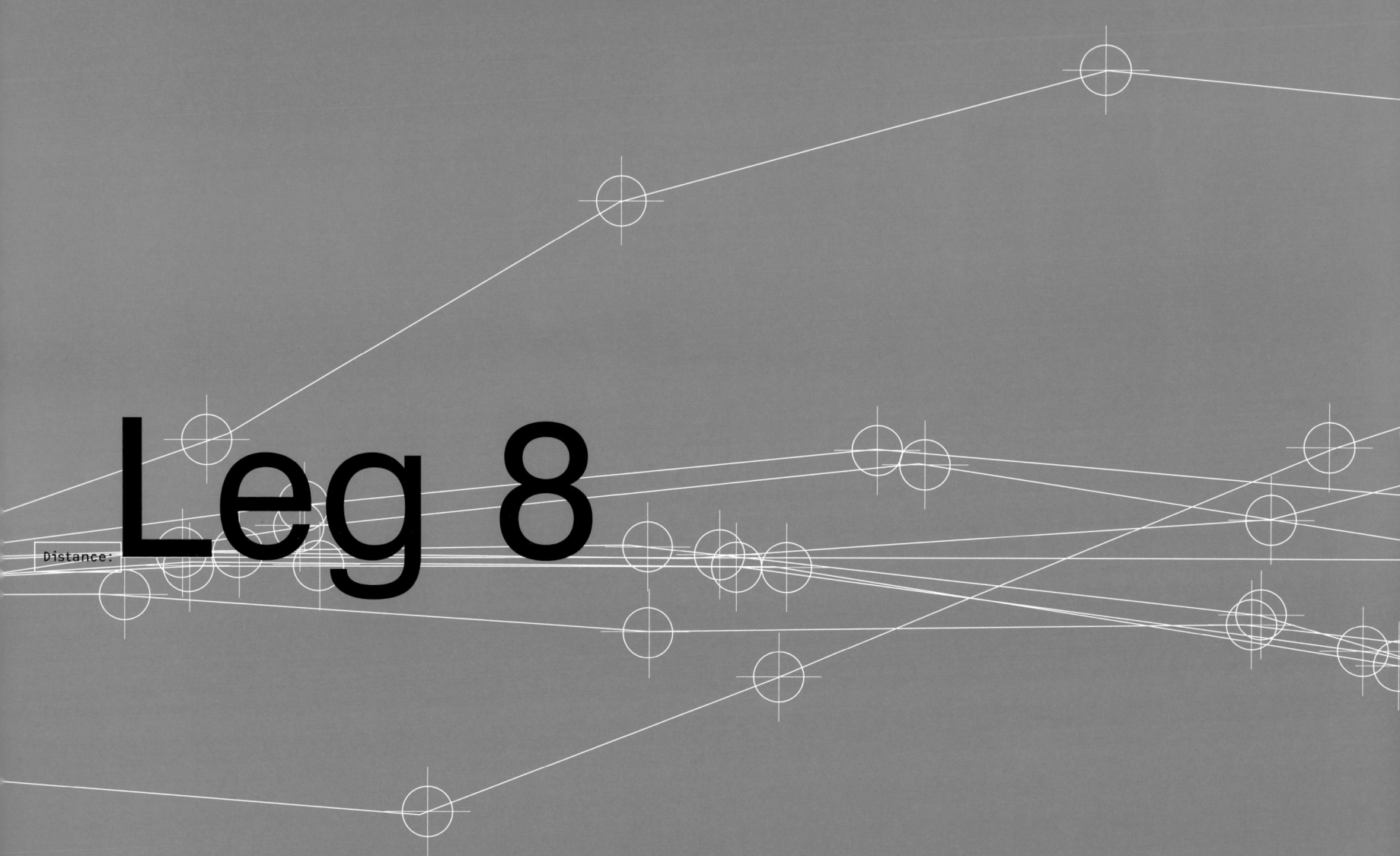

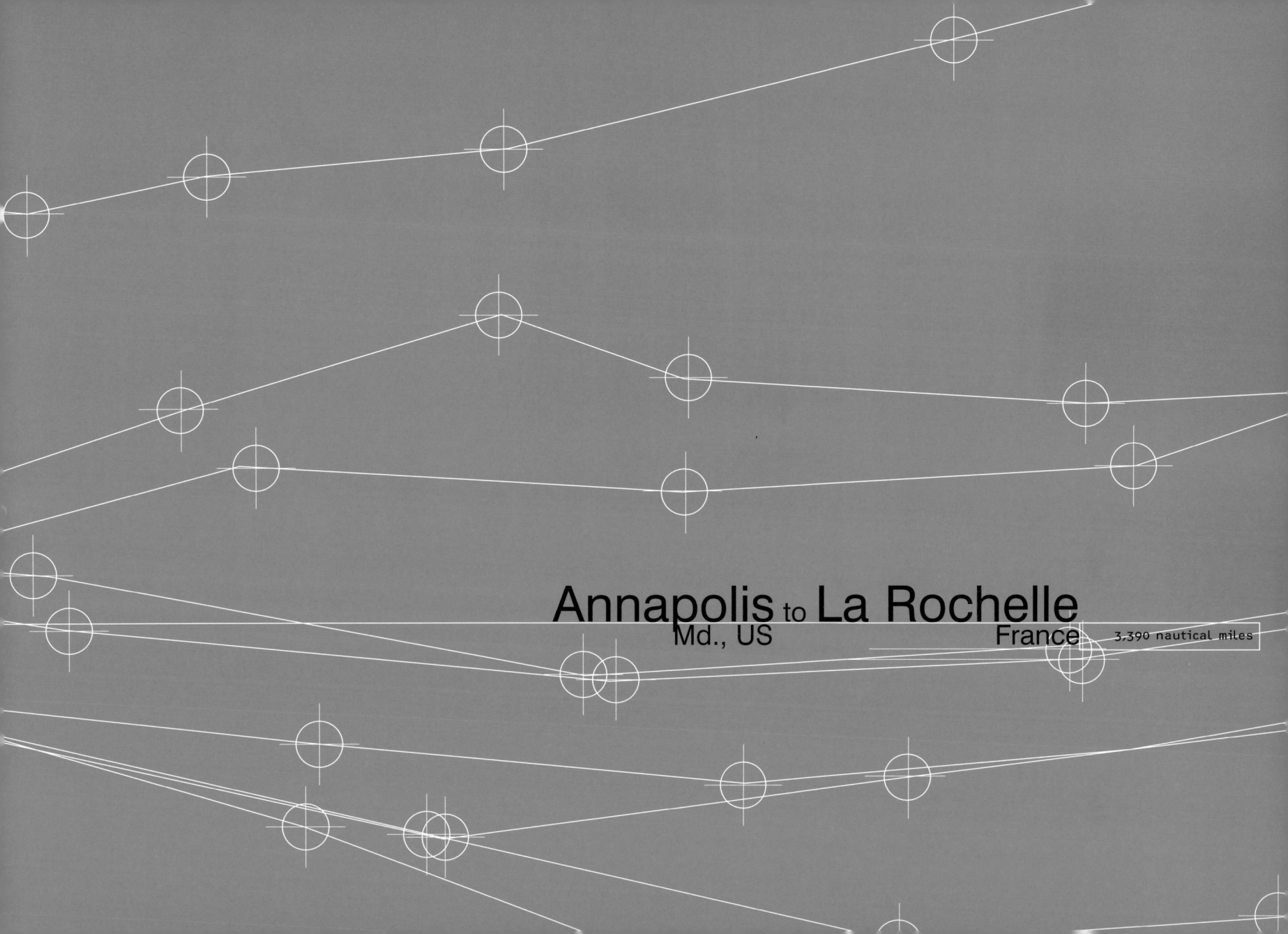

Leg 8: Prelude

If the Toshiba team thought their disqualification for Leg 5 was bad, the outcome of Leg 7 must have seemed a close second. First the International Jury ruled that an EF Education protest against Toshiba was valid, penalising the team two places in the leg standings. This shoved the boat to dead last for the leg. Then the team's navigator, Andrew Cape, resigned without warning. It left the team scrambling to fill the second most important slot onboard.

There were still two legs to sail. Within 48 hours of Cape's resignation, the team announced that Murray Ross was on a plane flying from New Zealand to Baltimore to fill Toshiba's empty navigator's chair. In his early 50s, Ross was no stranger to The Whitbread. He had sailed in both the 1985-86 and 1989-90 Whitbread races, and consulted for New Zealand Endeavour and Yamaha during the 1993-94 race. Prior to the start of this Whitbread, he worked as a training coach for Innovation Kvaerner.

Though the sudden departure of Cape sent shockwaves through the team, Dennis Conner put the best possible face on the situation. "I have known Murray for a while and welcome him to the team," Conner said. "He is the best replacement in the world for the yacht Toshiba. With Murray on board I am optimistic about our chances for a podium position in the remaining two legs."

Before the next leg could start, the W60s had to move. They had finished Leg 7 in Baltimore, Md.; they would start Leg 8 outside the 'Sailing Capital of the United States,' Annapolis. On 30 April, the boats led the Fleet Parade of Sail down the Chesapeake to their new berths. There, they prepared for the restart.

Leg 8 would take the fleet back into freezing temperatures. The boats would pass through the area of the North Atlantic where the Titanic had been sunk by an iceberg. With spring warmth creeping into the Labrador pack-ice, it had begun breaking up, meaning icebergs had started their annual migration south toward the Grand Banks. Frits Koek, meteorologist for BrunelSunergy, said he expected to see ice. "There is some ice coming down the Labrador Current," he said. He estimated the fleet should encounter icebergs beginning at around 45 N. Race officials, always concerned that the single-minded competitors would put themselves in harm's way to gain a few miles, decided to impose a 'leave to port' limit on the fleet. They set a northern latitude boundary at 46 N.

The race's overall points leader, EF Language, was now sitting on a comfortable 104-point lead over second-placed Swedish Match. This fact imposed an unusual strategic dilemma for Cayard. After the misery Gunnar Krantz and his crew gave Cayard in their drag race up Chesapeake Bay, he could not take Swedish Match for granted. "We will obviously keep a close eye on Swedish Match," Cayard said. His navigator, Mark Rudiger, said they would dog the Swedish Match yacht every inch of the way to France. Cayard's biggest fear was that Swedish Match could break away from him. If Swedish Match came in first, and EF Language got stuck in traffic and was pushed far back into the fleet, the combination would put Swedish Match in solid contention for first place. Cayard and Rudiger were determined not to let Krantz out of their sight.

Skipper Krantz, of course, had other ideas. "We have a slim chance [to win the race]," Krantz said. "It's a game of putting the throttle all the way down but not taking too many risks."

Fifty-eight points behind Swedish Match and 162 points behind EF Language, Merit Cup skipper Grant Dalton had given up any hope of capturing first place. He still had a shot at second, though. Aboard fifth-place Chessie Racing, George Collins decided to step back off the boat to let a younger man, John Kostecki, skipper the difficult North Atlantic leg.

The once-favoured Toshiba team was now far back in seventh place overall. Skipper Standbridge was hungry for a winning leg. The weight of two adverse jury rulings followed by the last-minute navigator change had the odds-makers wondering what could be left of crew morale. Most were betting that Toshiba would sail another lacklustre leg.

The all-woman EF Education crew got a shot of star power with the addition of a world-famous single-handed French sailor, Isabelle Autissier. La Rochelle, France, was Autissier's home town — an added incentive for the team to show well on this leg. A question remained: Would Autissier be any advantage to the team? After all, this would be her first appearance in a Whitbread race, and she had never sailed a W60 before.

Leg 8: Annapolis, Md., US, to La Rochelle, France

"After coming this far maybe all we did is find out that The Whitbread is actually all about not being able to run away and hide from it all."

Arend van Bergeijk, BrunelSunergy

Under clear sunny skies, with winds out of the south-southwest at eight knots, the nine W60s prepared to set sail on Leg 8. More than 2,000 spectator boats lined the course, sometimes five deep, herded into position by a no-nonsense fleet of US Coast Guard vessels determined that this would not be a re-run of the chaotic São Sebastiao start. On shore, over 50,000 people participating in the charitable Bay Bridge Walk swelled the already substantial crowd.

When the starting cannon sounded, Toshiba led the pack on port tack, with Chessie Racing by her side. The rest of the fleet crossed on starboard. With light winds, the fleet was only making six to seven knots.

Toshiba was first under the Bay Bridge, which acted as a big wind screen for the fleet, slowing them considerably. At the back of the fleet along with sister ship EF Education was EF Language. "I screwed up the start," Cayard wrote. "I got a little low, got tangled up with my girlfriends [EF Education]." This was no time to be stuck in the back of the fleet. If Swedish Match won both legs, EF Language had to finish above sixth place in the final two legs in order to maintain her overall first position.

Just over three hours and roughly 25 miles from the start, Cayard's worst nightmare was taking shape. While he struggled to make up for his sloppy start, Swedish Match was leading the nine-boat fleet down the Chesapeake Bay. Chessie Racing was second and Toshiba third as nightfall settled over the competitors. When the sun came up the next morning, Chessie had overtaken Swedish Match and was leading.

Cayard, frantic to catch up with Swedish Match, had pushed his crew all night. He had closed the distance to his nearest rival by 1.3 miles during the night. Cayard explained that the team paid a high price to repair the damage the poor start had caused. "We have been in our full-race watch system all night," Cayard reported that morning. "This means we are pretty tired after getting about two hours' sleep each."

By midday on Day 2, EF Language had clawed herself past Swedish Match and taken the lead, with Swedish Match three-tenths of a mile to the rear. Former leader Chessie Racing was back where EF Language had been six hours earlier, in third, eight-tenths of a mile behind the new leader.

While the crew aboard EF Language was in top form, certain of the boat's important equipment was not. Cayard reported that the boat's watermaker had failed. Just to make life interesting, the spare watermaker also didn't seem to want to work. Cayard began considering his alternatives. He could pull into Halifax for repairs, but that would mean letting Swedish Match get away. He could sail on, betting that his crew could get one of the two units working again. Cayard decided to continue on. Off-duty crewmembers immediately broke out the emergency hand-held watermakers and began pumping. It was painful work, resulting in less than four litres of water for every six hours of pumping. The crew also rigged a rain-catcher at the foot of the mast.

Cayard continued to shadow Swedish Match as Gunnar Krantz headed north. Cayard said he personally favoured a more southern route. Nevertheless, he had to remind himself that his goal on this leg was not so much winning, but making sure Swedish Match did not get away from him. "We will stay right with Swedish Match for better or for worse," Cayard reported. "But, it is frustrating to watch the whole fleet sailing off to the south."

Unencumbered by similar complications, Paul Standbridge was free to set the course his new navigator, Murray Ross, felt would get them to France first. The course he set was a middle course, not too far north, not too far south. It was a course that kept Toshiba in the strongest part of the remaining Gulf Stream current, and it seemed to work. Toshiba began moving up. The yacht had been back in eighth place as the fleet left the Chesapeake Bay, but Standbridge had driven the yacht to second.

Day 4 began a frustrating week for the fleet, as positions began to change rapidly. The boats approached the delimited northern zone, with Swedish Match going the farthest north. She lost the edge of the Gulf Stream, falling from second to dead last. Watching this unfold, Cayard held back, staying 48 miles to the windward of Swedish Match. Pulling away had a price: Cayard lost contact with his arch-rival. Yet following Krantz had already cost Cayard — EF Language was now in seventh place. He could only hope that Krantz's bad luck up north was continuing.

Krantz saw a silver lining in his last-place position. "We are working hard to get a separation with EFL and have managed to sneak away a little to the north," he wrote.

The fleet was now beam reaching in 25- to 30-knot winds, making for rough and wet sailing. Aboard Toshiba, things were going unusually well for the team that had seen nothing but trouble up until now. The boat had secured a firm hold on second place by the morning of Day 5. Keeping her in the Gulf Stream had given Standbridge just the edge he needed. "At times we have had up to 5 knots [of current]," wrote Standbridge. "We have done about 1,000 miles with about 2,500 to go."

The real drama was still between Swedish Match and EF Language. The two were currently in sixth and seventh places; EF Language finally had Swedish Match back on her radar screen. "Hopefully we help with getting the hit numbers up on the web site," Krantz wrote, referring to the match race between him and Cayard. Krantz reported that he was sailing in 18 to 20 knots of breeze from 165 degrees. EF Language was never far away. "EFL obviously wants to keep close and is heading our way," Krantz said.

It was a nautical game of cat and mouse, with the cat purring. "We have finally gotten the clamps back on Swedish Match after they gave us a head fake two days ago and escaped," wrote Cayard. "The problem is that we are both very far north and are now being squeezed by the ice on the north side and uncooperative wind on the southeast — making it hard for us to get east around the icebergs."

Those 'bergs' were rapidly becoming a major concern. Earlier that day, the Whitbread Race Office issued a warning that the US Coast Guard had informed them an iceberg had strayed out of the race's 'prohibited zone,' and was situated at 45.40 N / 48.00 W.

Finally, the warmth of the Gulf Stream had run its course. The crews reported that they were all climbing into their "woollies and wellies" (rubber boots). As the cold air from the north hit the last of the warm Gulf Stream waters, it produced thick fog. "We have got almost everything on that we brought; gloves hats and layers," Cayard reported that night. "Tonight the wind is 15 knots from 150 [magnetic] with a fairly smooth sea, so we are not getting too wet." Ten miles back, Swedish Match was complaining about the fog. "It is very foggy and the water temperature has dropped to 9 degrees C," wrote Krantz. "We will have constant radar watch and night goggles on with infrared light. We only have to watch out for logs, containers, whales, icebergs and other ships."

Up front the lead had changed several times, but for all of Day 5, Merit Cup held the front spot. That night, Merit Cup struggled to maintain her lead, then she slipped into second behind Toshiba. Suddenly, for some reason the crew could not squeeze any speed from the boat. Something was wrong.

"Just after dark last night the boat shuddered and we felt a vibration," Grant Dalton reported. "By torchlight, we checked keel, rudder and propeller through the inspection windows but couldn't see anything wrapped around them. But there was obviously something wrong because when the breeze strengthened we couldn't get any more than 11 knots out of the boat. We got out the searchlight and hooked Jared Henderson to a trapeze and put him over the side. In the murk, he could see a shadow

Leg 7: Ft. Lauderdale, Fla., US, to Baltimore, Md., US

"Some of the more violent drop offs are so violent it sounds like breaking glass in a car accident. I will be surprised if one or more boats don't sustain a little damage."
— EF Language navigator, Mark Rudiger

It was a perfect Florida afternoon on 19 April 1998, as the fleet lined up for the start of Leg 7. A stiff warm breeze blew out of the southeast at 20 knots. The sun was out, as was an impressive armada of spectator boats. Conner took the helm aboard Toshiba and had the best start, as the fleet crossed the starting line under spinnakers and full mains. At the final mark, Chessie Racing was leading. After rounding the mark, the boats peeled to reaching spinnakers, and headed out to sea in search of the Gulf Stream.

By the second day, boat after boat had staked out its own spot in the current and had settled down for a two-day ride north — all but one boat, that is. BrunelSunergy kept sailing east. By this time, the Dutch team was known for thumbing its collective nose at conventional wisdom and pursuing radical strategies — sometimes to advantage, but more often not. As the rest of the fleet settled into the middle of the Gulf Stream, BrunelSunergy sailed on, finally positioning herself at the far eastern edge of the current.

Skipper Roy Heiner and his navigator, Stuart Quarrie, were guessing that they would find better wind direction and flatter seas farther east — and it looked like they were right. Almost immediately, the rest of the fleet was hit by 20- to 25-knot headwinds. This was no trivial matter for the boats now positioned in the centre of the current. When the wind blows hard against the Gulf Stream current, very rough seas result — seas that pound right on the nose. The combination makes for most unpleasant sailing as the yachts hobbyhorse on the troubled seas.

Quarrie's gamble of staying on the eastern edge of the Gulf Stream to avoid this misery paid off. While the rest of the fleet slogged upwind in heavy seas, Heiner and his team had smoother and faster sailing. Yet BrunelSunergy's flyer was not without risk. By going farther to the east than the rest of the fleet, they were sacrificing some of the Gulf Stream's northerly momentum. The boat also ran the risk of falling into one of the many eddies that swirl along the edge of the Gulf Stream, any one of which could trap her in a current that pushed south.

Almost immediately the other skippers saw the wisdom in Heiner's move. Skipper Krantz wrote from Swedish Match, currently in third, "Brunel, what a killer. Gutsy and definitely a big move." Paul Cayard also took note. "Brunel has made a bold move to run east of the stream and the cold eddies that have adverse current." Even though the other skippers were admiring, it was too late to do anything about it. The leg was too short to correct these kinds of mistakes. The boats had placed their bets, and now had to make the best of their decisions.

EF Education was making her best showing yet in the race, holding to fourth place. The boat was less than six nautical miles behind Swedish Match, and eight miles behind her sister ship, EF Language. Following close on EF Education's transom was Chessie Racing. Chessie had held the lead briefly after the start, then fell back to fifth. Her skipper, George Collins, desperately wanted a podium finish in hometown Baltimore just like the one Grant Dalton got in his home port, Auckland. He had an uphill climb now. Behind him, Merit Cup was in sixth, followed by Silk Cut and Innovation Kvaerner.

The big surprise was Toshiba, which by the end of the second day was sailing in dead last, over 50 nautical miles behind the leader. "It's not a pretty picture," Dennis Conner wrote that day. "I have realised it's not as much fun writing email when you are behind and not feeling your best."

Heiner and his crew were now 20 miles ahead of Swedish Match and 22 miles ahead of EF Language. While BrunelSunergy extended her lead, the rest of the fleet was left beating against the wind-whipped Gulf Stream current. "Crash bang shudder! We are beating in the Gulf Stream with 3-4 knots of current under us and 22 knots of [head] wind," wrote Adrian Stead from Silk Cut. "It is very unpleasant and I am being thrown around the navstation while I type this."

On Innovation Kvaerner the crew reported that even getting sleep was proving difficult. "Sleeping in the bunks is like a roller-coaster ride at the fairground," a member of the crew reported. "You lie there with your feet forward and suddenly your stomach goes light as the bow leaps off a wave into the unknown. You brace yourself for impact — will it be soft, hard or boat-breaking? More often than not it's the middle one as the boat lands once more."

The tightly packed bunch in the middle of the fleet got the worst of it. Aboard sixth-placed Merit Cup, Grant Dalton complained, "A bit hard to type this today as I'm trying to wedge myself into the navstation as the boat leaps off waves in the Gulf Stream." Still in last place, Toshiba's Conner observed that the conditions were neither unusual nor unexpected. "The Gulf Stream has never been a very pleasant place to be in a 22-knot northerly," he wrote in response to all the complaining. "The waves are square and the boat makes quite a noise as it crashes off the top and falls to the bottom of the trough."

Conditions were so rough that several of the teams reported seasoned hands were suffering from seasickness.

By Day 3, BrunelSunergy had parlayed their dramatic flyer into a 40-nautical-mile lead. That lead began to dwindle as the teams began to peel out of the punishing Gulf Stream headwinds and turned toward the Chesapeake. BrunelSunergy, no longer having a wind-angle advantage over the other boats, began losing ground. In particular, second-placed Swedish Match quickly began chewing up the miles between her and the Dutch boat.

on the keel and something flapping. We stopped the boat and drifted back and a very dead seal broke the surface. He had wrapped himself around the keel."

Several of the leading boats reported sighting icebergs. "We just had visual contact with a twin-peaked iceberg, about 1 nm wide at 9 a.m. this morning," Innovation Kvaerner skipper Frostad reported. "We passed gently about 6-7 nm to leeward. As the crew had their eyes wide open focusing on the berg, two big whales came up alongside the boat."

If the far northern route chosen by Swedish Match (and by default, EF Language as well) was proving a bad choice, the southern route was no better. Silk Cut and Chessie Racing had selected the extreme southerly side of the course. Silk Cut had slipped back to eighth place early on Day 5, and was losing ground to Chessie Racing, which was dead last. The centre route chosen by Toshiba was proving to be the winning choice.

By the end of the ninth day at sea, the fleet was stretched across 142 miles of the North Atlantic, with Toshiba in the lead, followed 7 miles behind by Merit Cup. At the back of the fleet, 136 miles and 142 miles respectively behind the leader were Silk Cut and Chessie Racing.

Early on the morning of the tenth day, now free of the dead seal, Merit Cup had wrestled the lead back from Toshiba. Even a mid-day collision with a whale did not slow Merit Cup. In third place was EF Education, in one of her best showings of the race. This was familiar territory for Isabelle Autissier, who had sailed the Atlantic alone many times. This time she had eleven 'helpers' aboard.

A mile behind the EF Education crew, their counterparts aboard EF Language led Swedish Match by 20 miles. Being so far ahead of Swedish Match was worrying Cayard, who said in a satellite phone interview that he was seriously considering slowing down. "It would be easier for me to be three miles behind him and just following him wherever he goes," said Cayard. "That's the way for me to have the lowest risk of him putting a lot of boats between the two of us."

Conditions in the North Atlantic continued to affect fleet positions despite best-laid strategies. A high-pressure area stretching north to south between the fleet and the French coast created a 'choking ridge' that slowed the leaders. Two boats, Silk Cut and Chessie Racing, positioned farther north than the other boats in the fleet, were able to skirt around the edge of the ridge. Silk Cut, which had spent days languishing 180 miles behind the leaders, made a sudden rush around the fleet's northern side. On the morning of 14 May, she suddenly appeared in second just eight miles behind the leader, Toshiba. Chessie Racing moved from dead last into third place, while EF Education slipped to fourth. Merit Cup dropped to fifth, and EF Language and Swedish Match continued their kabuki dance back in sixth and seventh place.

As the boats approached the French coast and the finish line, the race for the lead had become a battle between two Brits, Lawrie Smith and Paul Standbridge. Both the Silk Cut and Toshiba teams were hungry for a first-place finish. Both had been favoured before the race; both had disappointed. A first in La Rochelle would go a long way toward repairing the injured egos on board. Standbridge had sailed an almost flawless leg, making the right choices from the beginning, then staying out of trouble along the way.

Even Cayard, consumed with his own concerns, was watching Toshiba's excellent run. "I am watching the battle up front between Toshiba and Silk, just as you are," Cayard wrote in his daily email. "Toshiba has sailed an excellent race. First they positioned themselves correctly in the Gulf Stream, then they stayed far enough away from the high pressure off Nova Scotia, something Silk did not do. Always in the lead or very close to it, Toshiba has made about five correct decisions in a row on a very tricky leg. I think they deserve to win this one."

It was a long time coming, but win they did. At eight minutes shy of 13 days at sea, the Toshiba team crossed the line in La Rochelle to claim their first leg victory of the race. Team members could be seen cavorting on deck as the boat inched across the line in an extremely light evening breeze. Just 10 minutes later, Silk Cut finished to take second place.

Dockside, Standbridge was quick to give credit to Murray Ross, who had replaced their original navigator just days before leaving. "We were very fortunate to get Murray Ross at short notice," said Standbridge. "He fitted in very well with the crew and did a very good job, and we're very grateful to him."

Chessie Racing bagged her fourth third place win of the race. The women on EF Education captured fourth in La Rochelle, their best showing of the race. Earlier that evening, as Merit Cup struggled to catch EF Education, a dolphin crashed into Merit Cup's rudder, which had already been damaged earlier in a collision with a whale. A tired and frustrated Grant Dalton said all he wanted to do was to reach La Rochelle and get his boat out of the water for repairs.

Sticking to his 'stay close to Swedish Match' strategy, Paul Cayard piloted EF Language across the line in sixth. Swedish Match crossed almost three hours later. To have a chance at an overall first, Swedish Match had needed to come in first on the last two legs, then have EF Language do badly on both legs. With her disappointing seventh behind EF Language, the race for first place in this Whitbread was over. Krantz's first dockside comments were directed at his winning rival. "Congratulations to EF Language," he said. "They deserve to win. They have done a tremendous job."

Cayard and his crew now had an unassailable hold on first place. Cayard said he had found the just-finished leg one of the most difficult in the race. "This was a hard leg for us because we had to have a special position," he said. "We had to stay close to Swedish Match and minimise any risk to seal winning The Whitbread. It was unexciting and boring, but it was the thing to do."

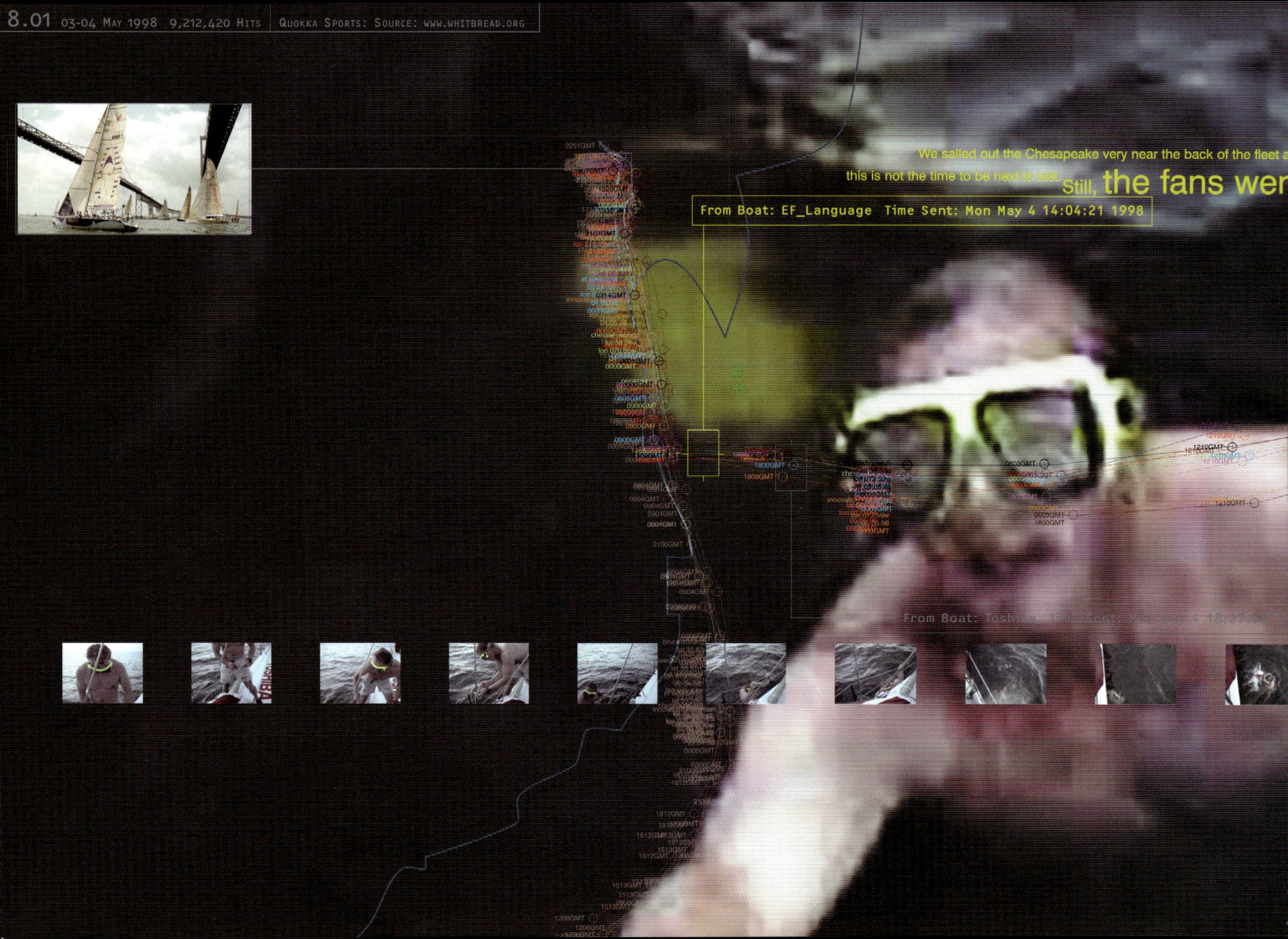

bad start by yours truly, live on TV.

unbelievable.

There must have been 5000 boats out there. Anyone who saw the sight had to be in awe. So I ate that piece of humble pie, sailing around all afternoon in the back of the pack, waved to everyone I could see, and pressed on. END EFL

Toshiba got caught in a fish trap.
We could not fully clear it until daybreak 5 hrs later when Sean went over the side with a knife. Our thanks to Sean.

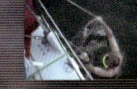 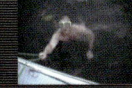 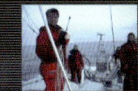 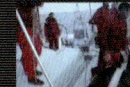 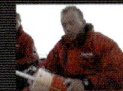 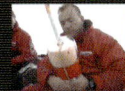 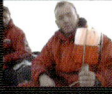

END TOS

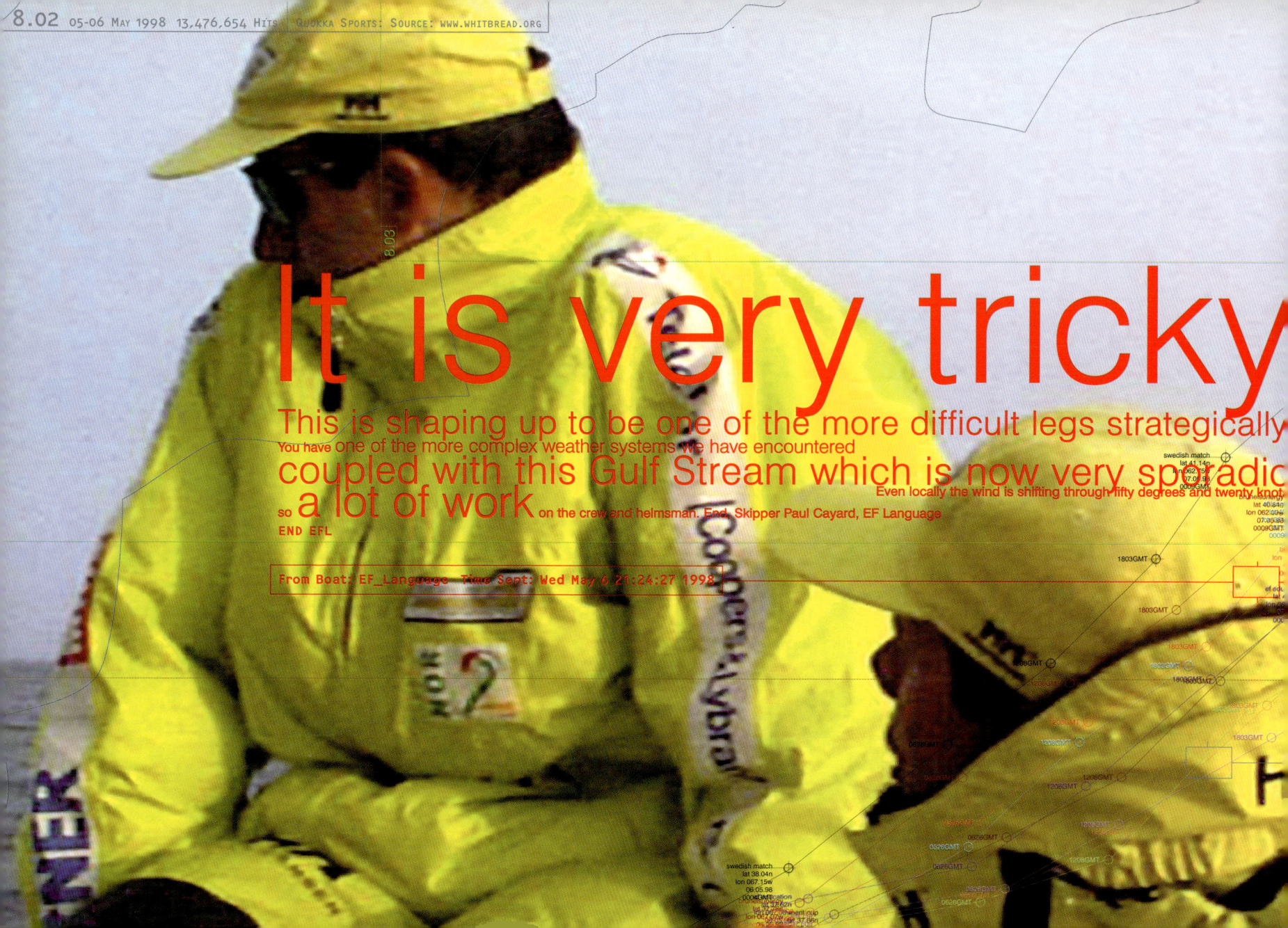

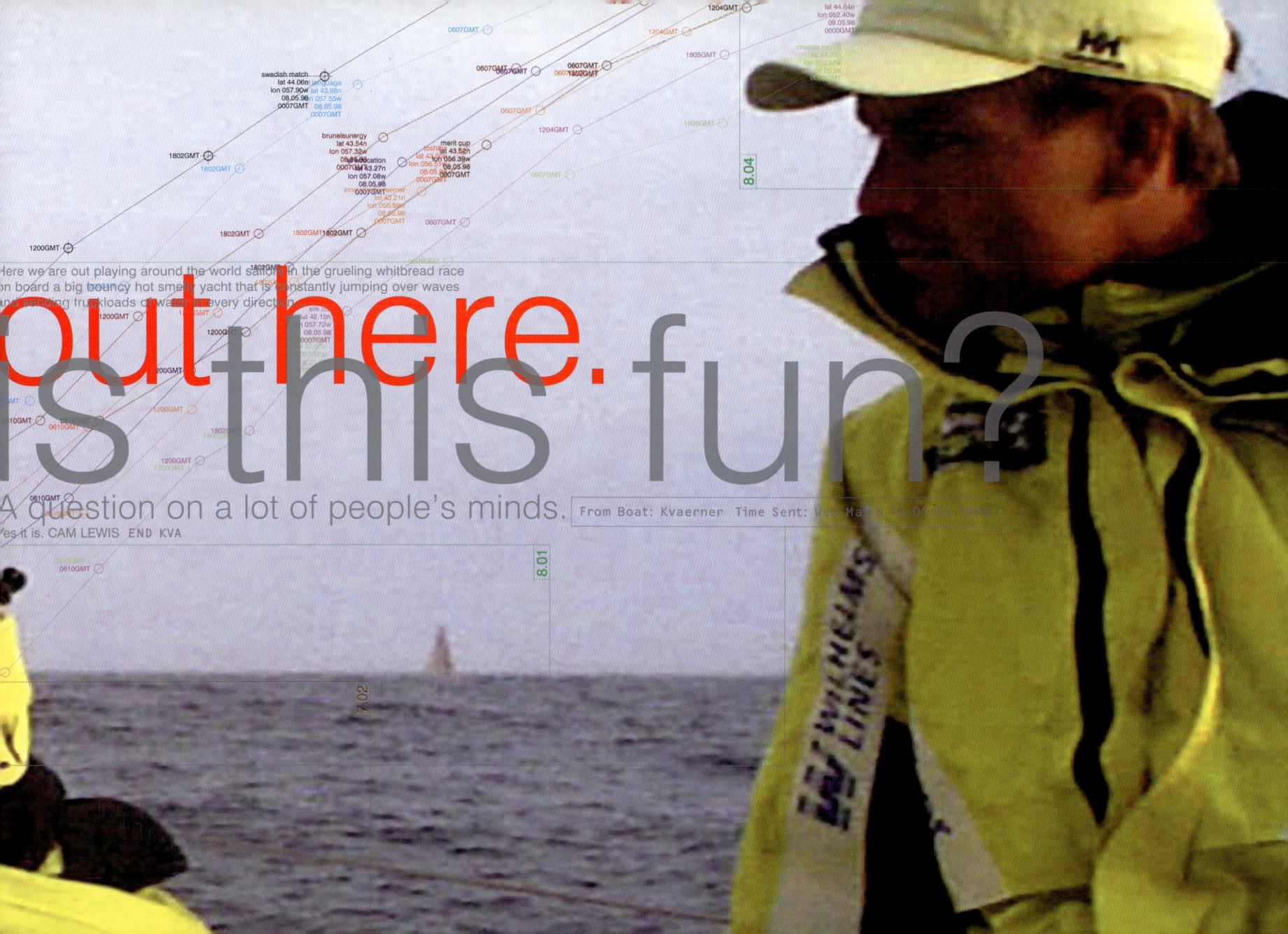

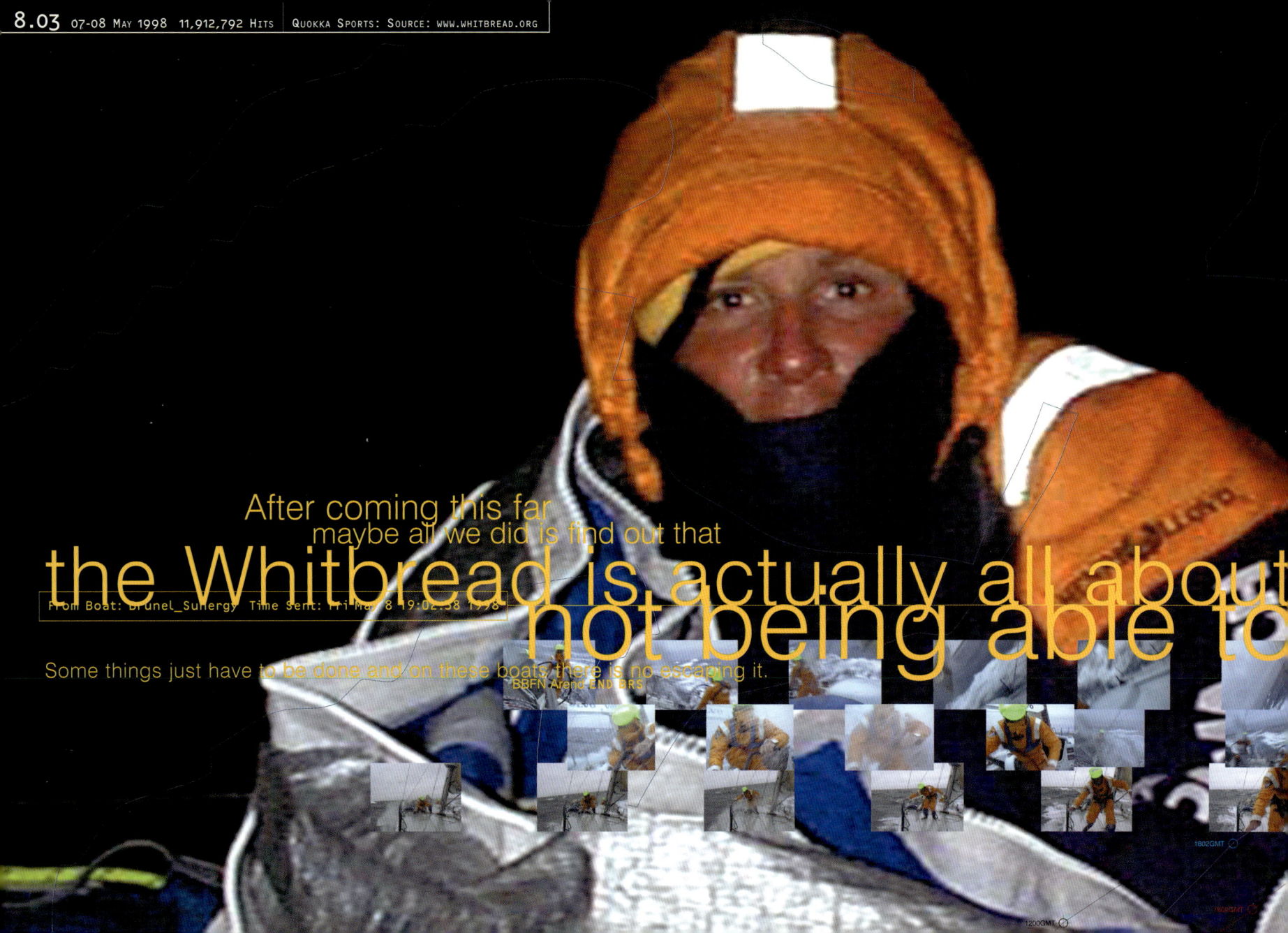

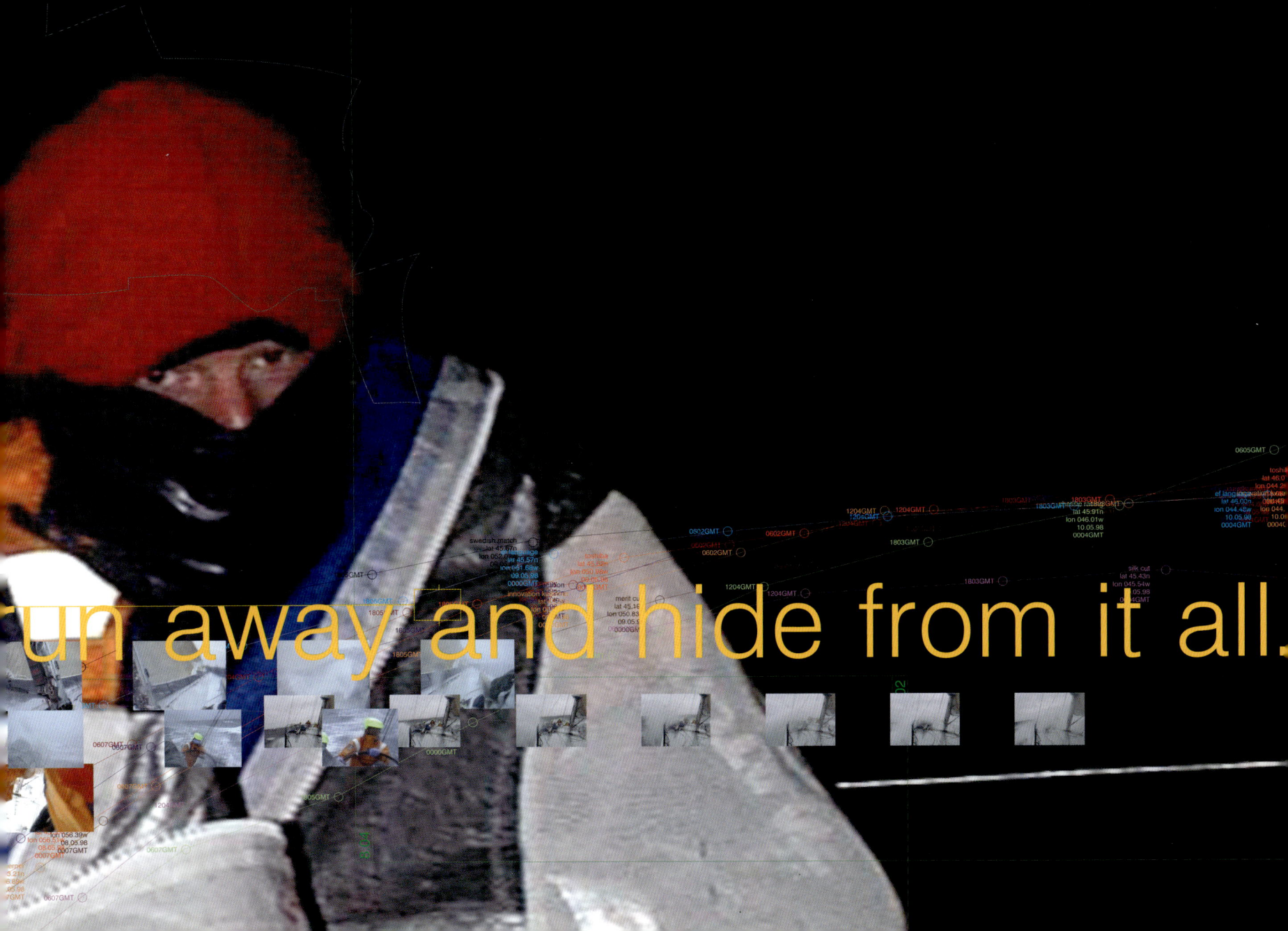

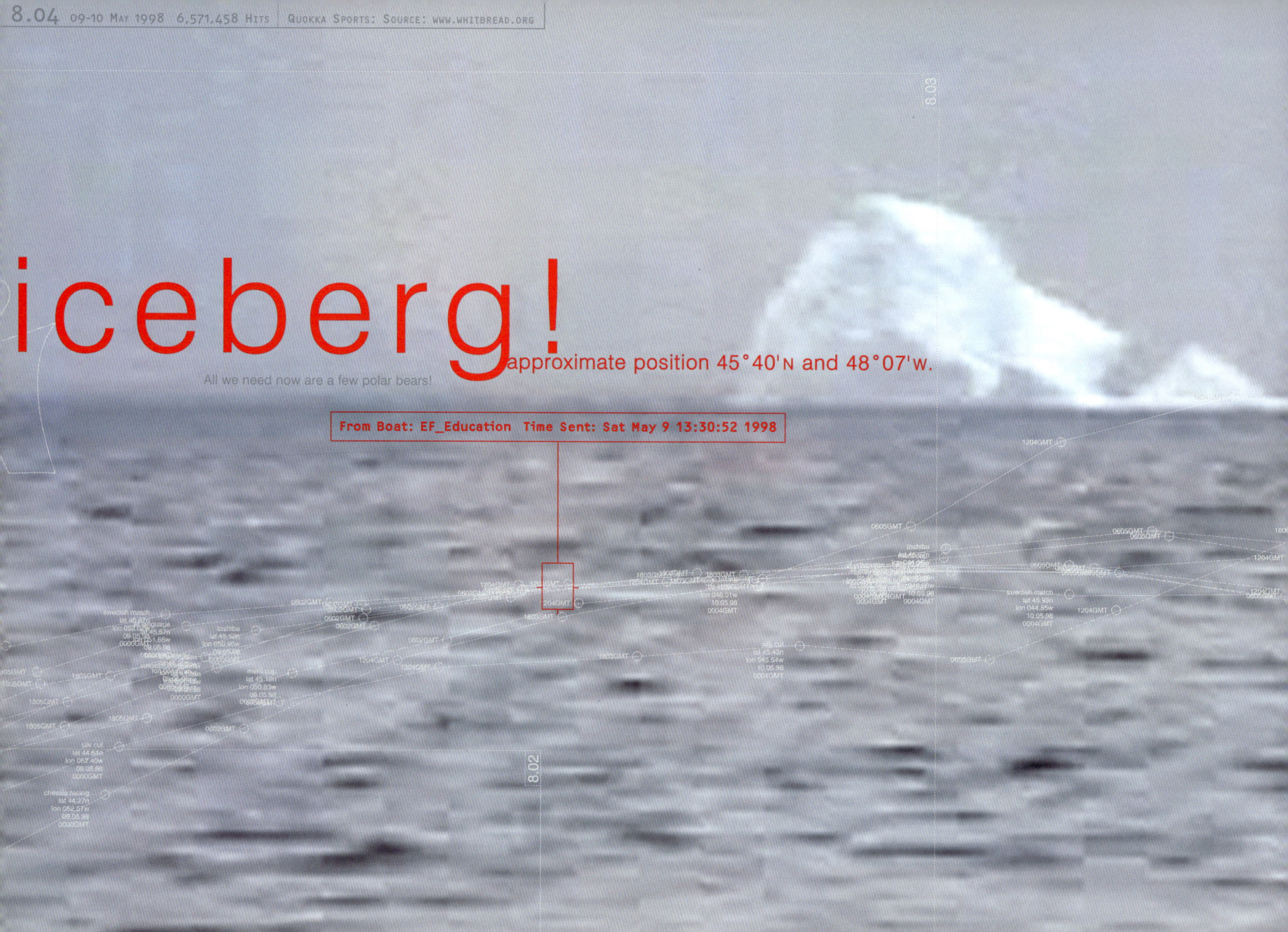

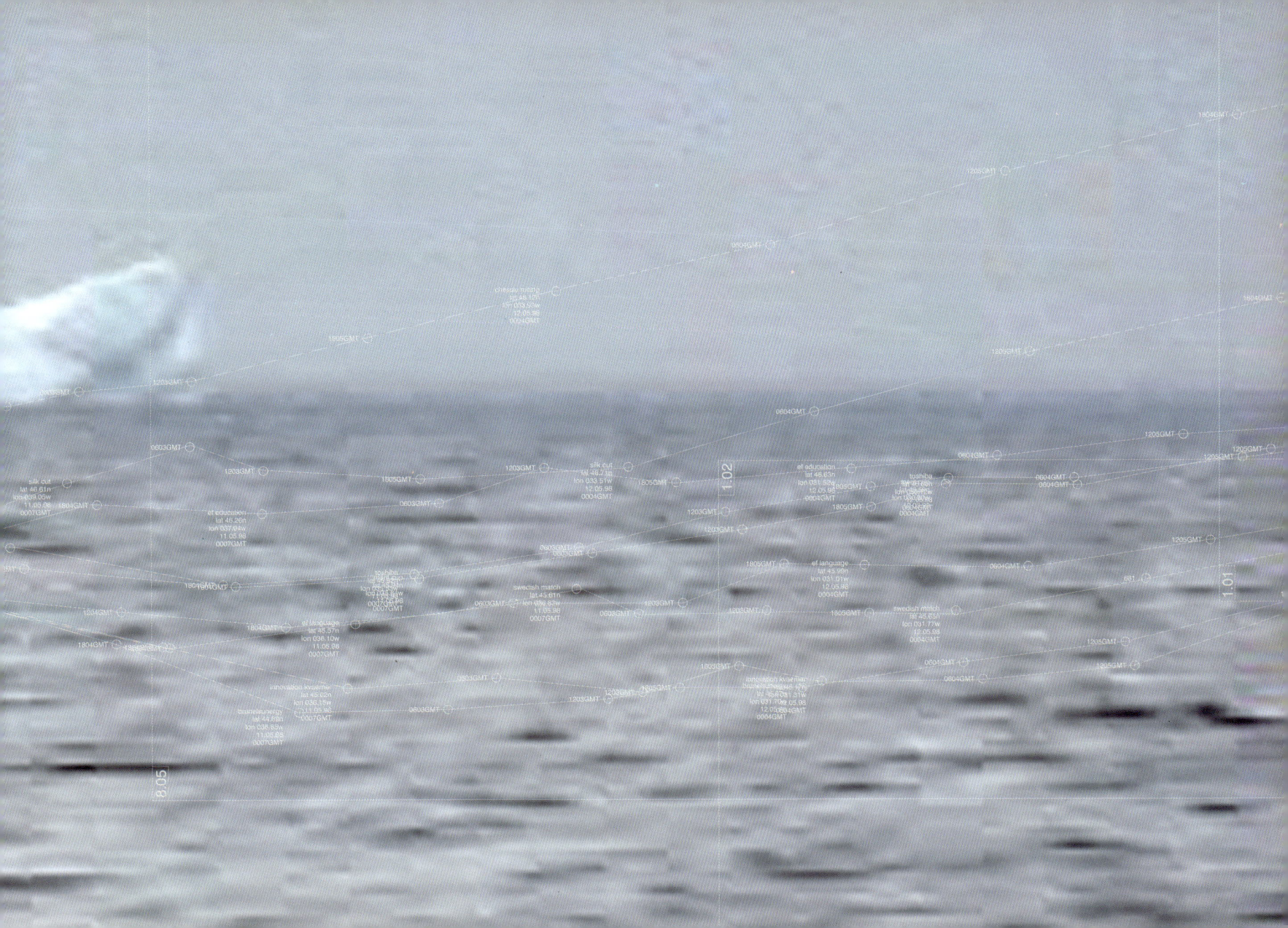

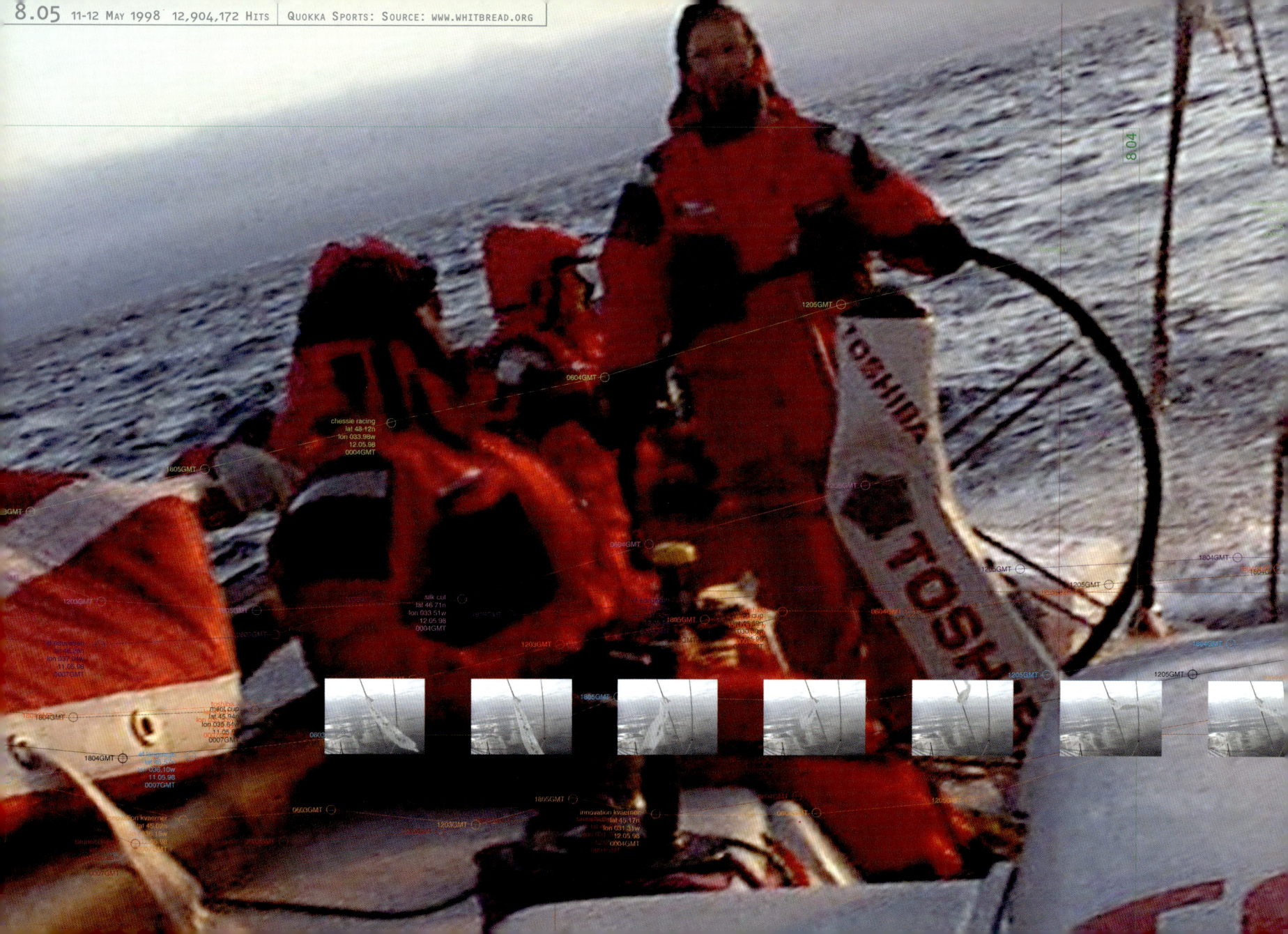

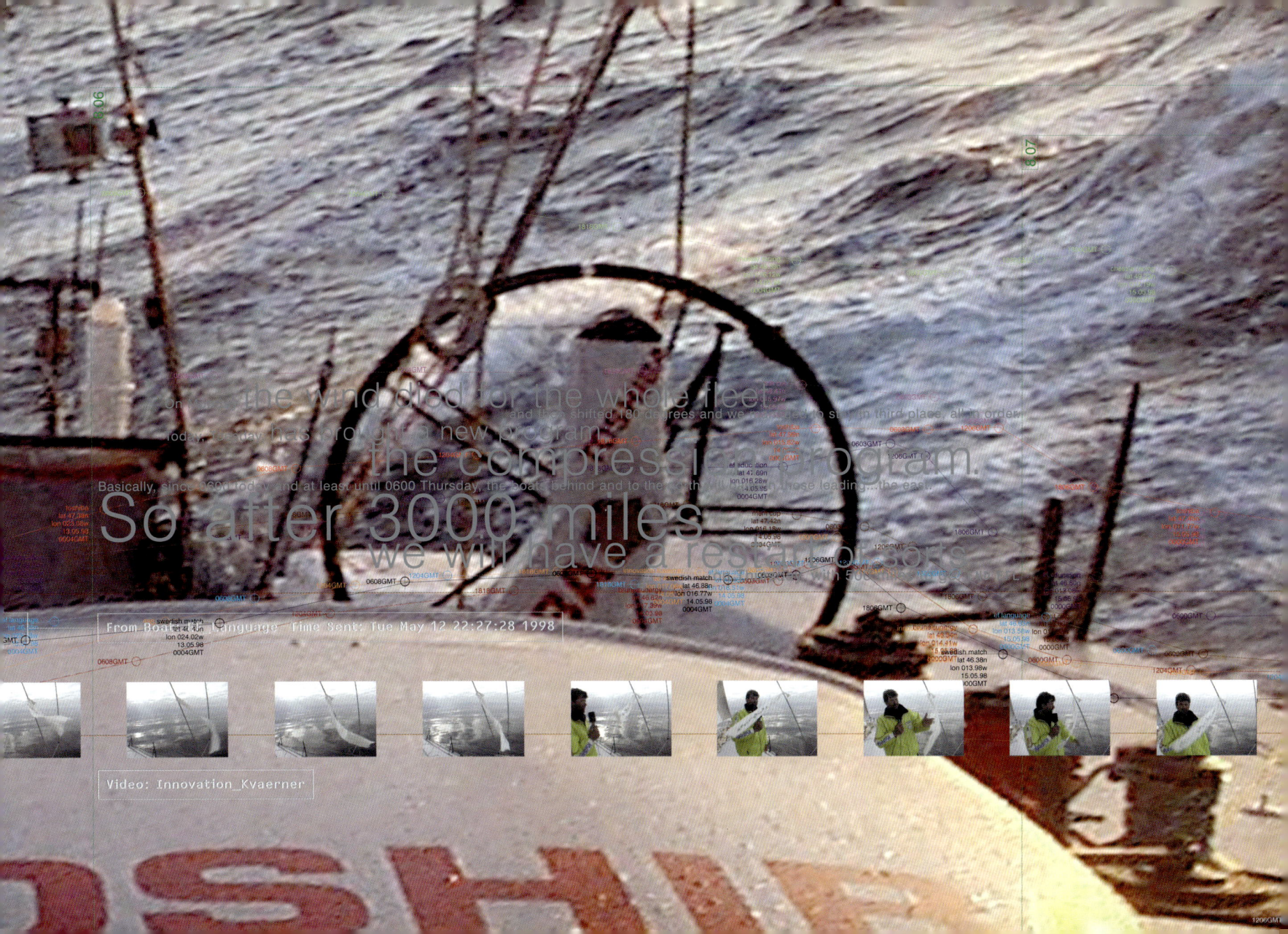

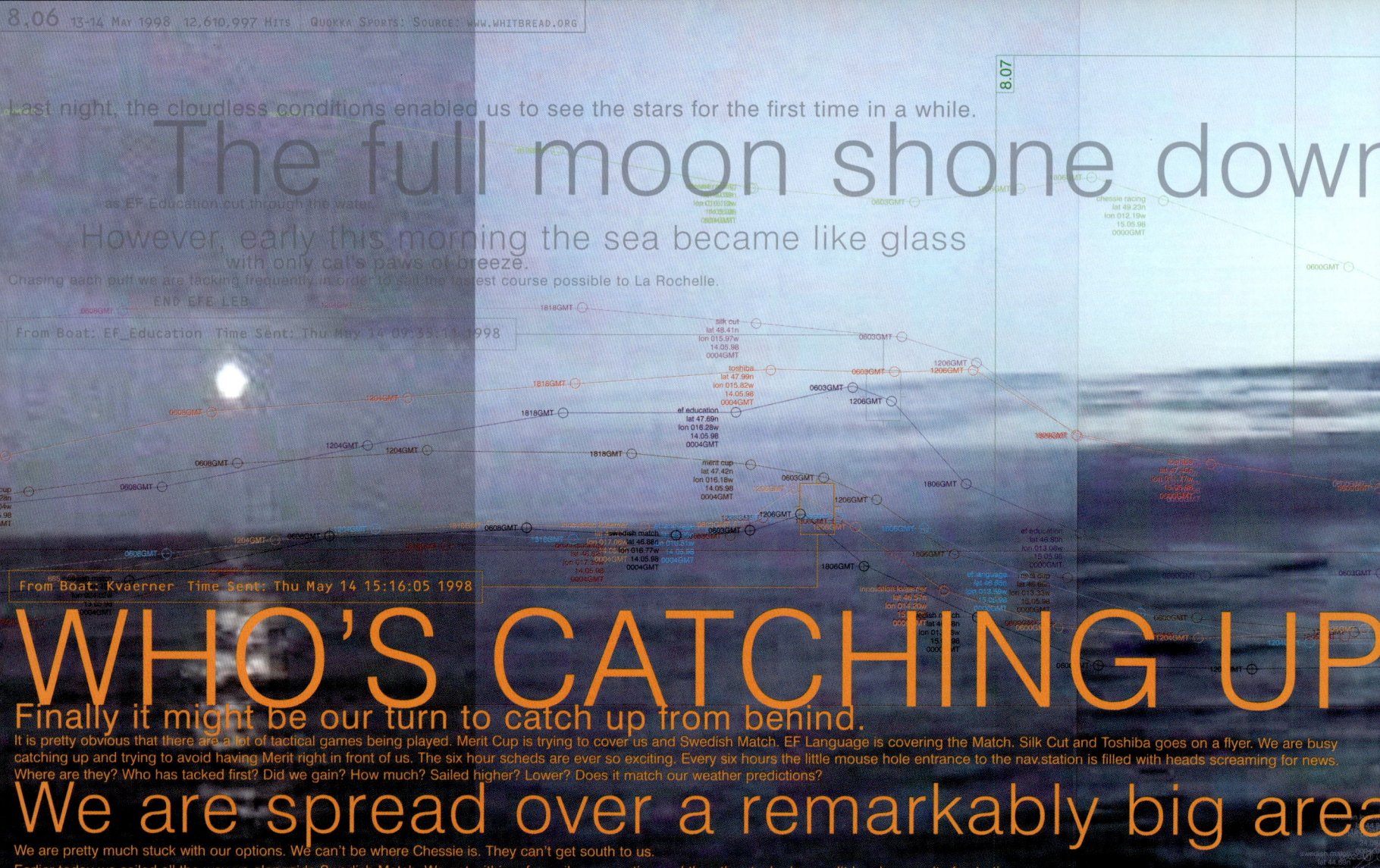

8.06 13-14 May 1998 12,610,997 Hits Quokka Sports: Source: www.whitbread.org

Last night, the cloudless conditions enabled us to see the stars for the first time in a while.

The full moon shone down

as EF Education cut through the water.

However, early this morning the sea became like glass

with only cat's paws of breeze.

Chasing each puff we are tacking frequently in order to sail the fastest course possible to La Rochelle.

END EFE LEB

From Boat: EF_Education Time Sent: Thu May 14 09:35:11 1998

From Boat: Kvaerner Time Sent: Thu May 14 15:16:05 1998

WHO'S CATCHING UP

Finally it might be our turn to catch up from behind.

It is pretty obvious that there are a lot of tactical games being played. Merit Cup is trying to cover us and Swedish Match. EF Language is covering the Match. Silk Cut and Toshiba goes on a flyer. We are busy catching up and trying to avoid having Merit right in front of us. The six hour scheds are ever so exciting. Every six hours the little mouse hole entrance to the nav station is filled with heads screaming for news. Where are they? Who has tacked first? Did we gain? How much? Sailed higher? Lower? Does it match our weather predictions?

We are spread over a remarkably big area

We are pretty much stuck with our options. We can't be where Chessie is. They can't get south to us.
Earlier today we sailed all the way up alongside Swedish Match. We got within a few miles separation and then they tacked away. It has been quite frustrating.
All the best from Knut F. and crew onboard the Lime Dragon

END KVA

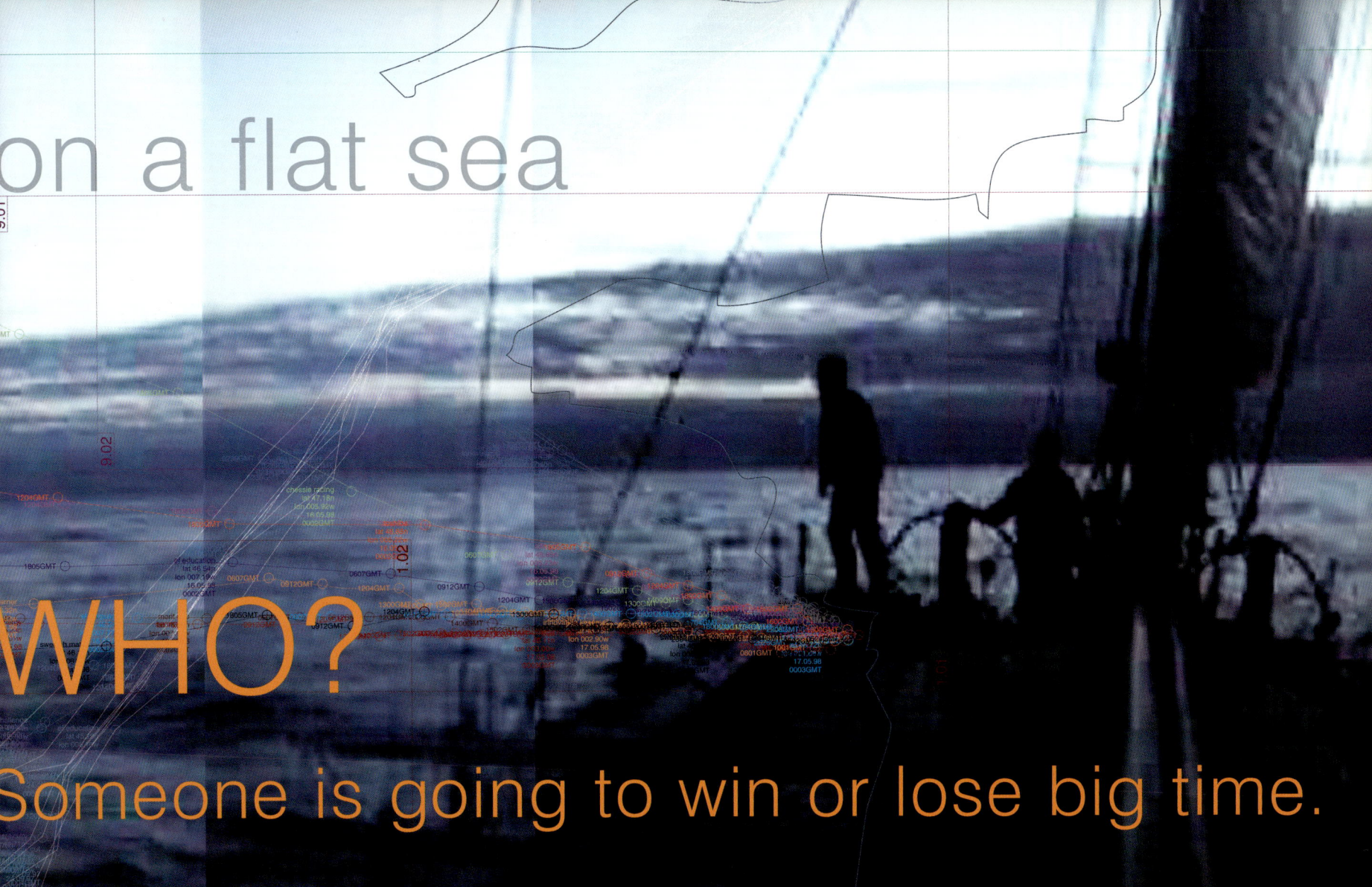

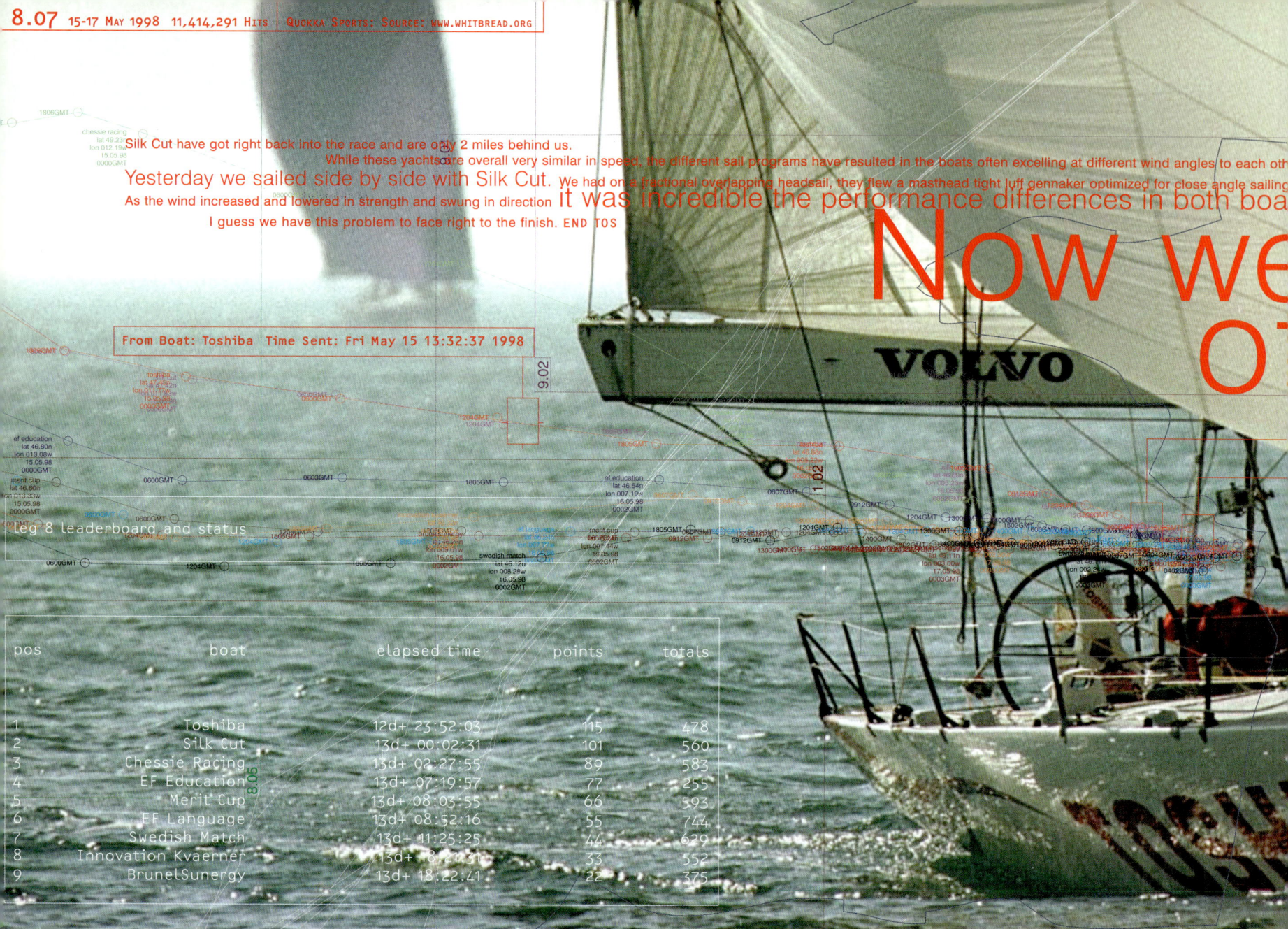

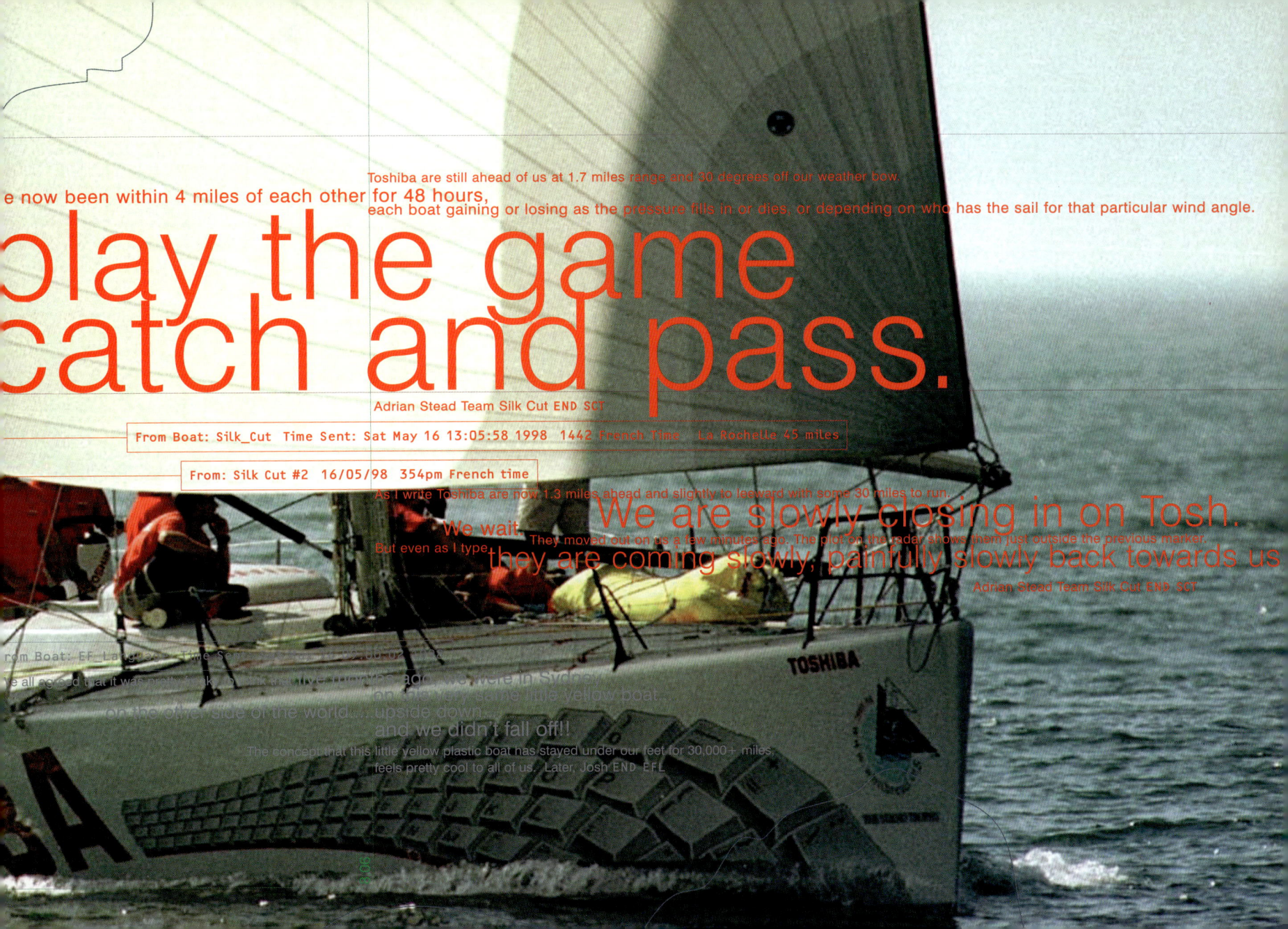

Toshiba are still ahead of us at 1.7 miles range and 30 degrees off our weather bow.
e now been within 4 miles of each other for 48 hours, each boat gaining or losing as the pressure fills in or dies, or depending on who has the sail for that particular wind angle.

play the game
catch and pass.

Adrian Stead Team Silk Cut END SCT

From Boat: Silk_Cut Time Sent: Sat May 16 13:05:58 1998 1442 French Time La Rochelle 45 miles

From: Silk Cut #2 16/05/98 354pm French time

As I write Toshiba are now 1.3 miles ahead and slightly to leeward with some 30 miles to run.
We wait. **We are slowly closing in on Tosh.**
They moved out on us a few minutes ago. The plot on the radar shows them just outside the previous marker.
But even as I type **they are coming slowly, painfully slowly back towards us**

Adrian Stead Team Silk Cut END SCT

rom Boat: EF_La
e all agreed that it was pretty freaky. Just five minutes ago we were in Sydney
on the very same yellow boat...
on the other side of the world... upside down...
and we didn't fall off!!
The concept that this little yellow plastic boat has stayed under our feet for 30,000+ miles,
feels pretty cool to all of us. Later, Josh END EFL

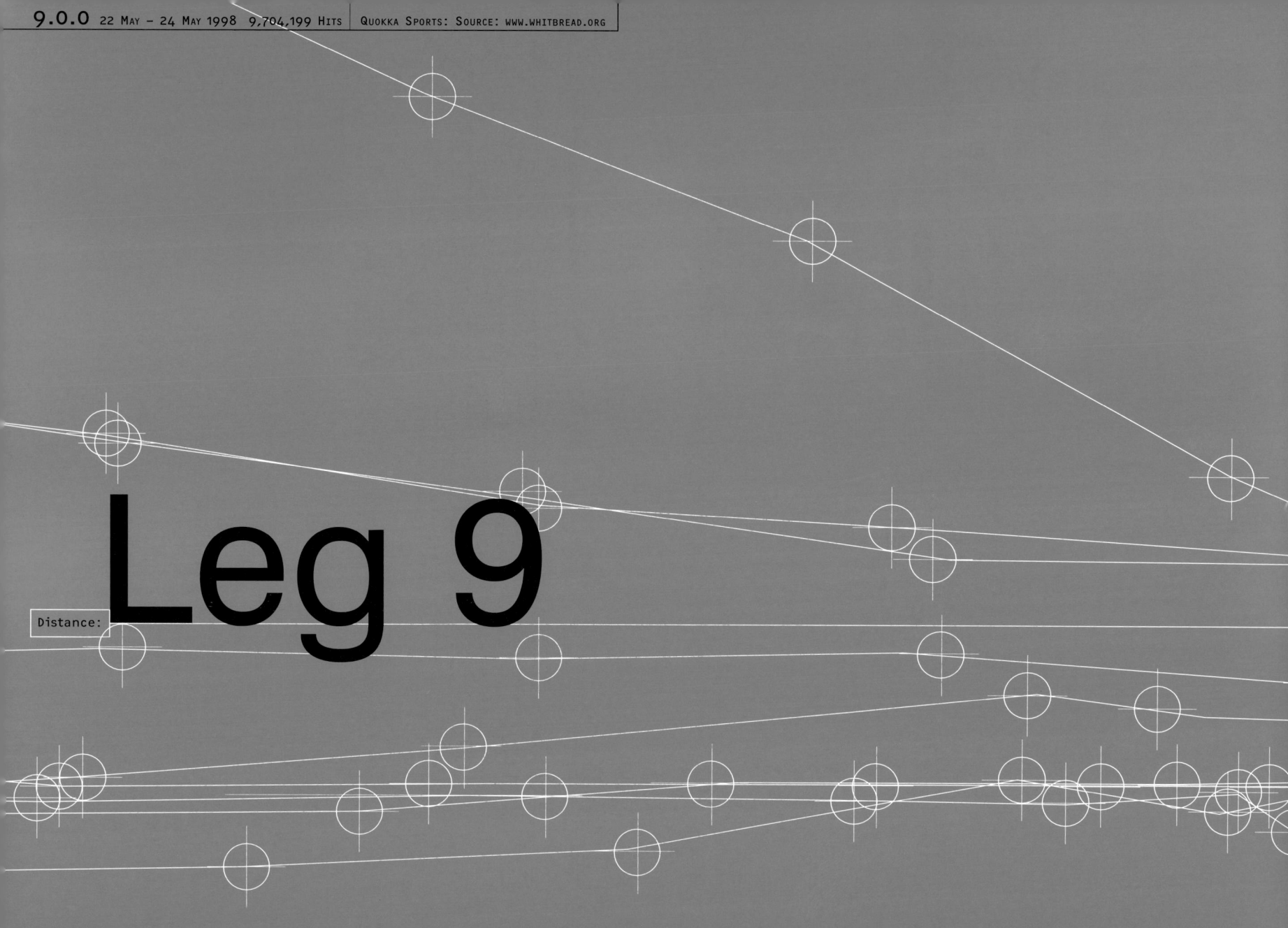

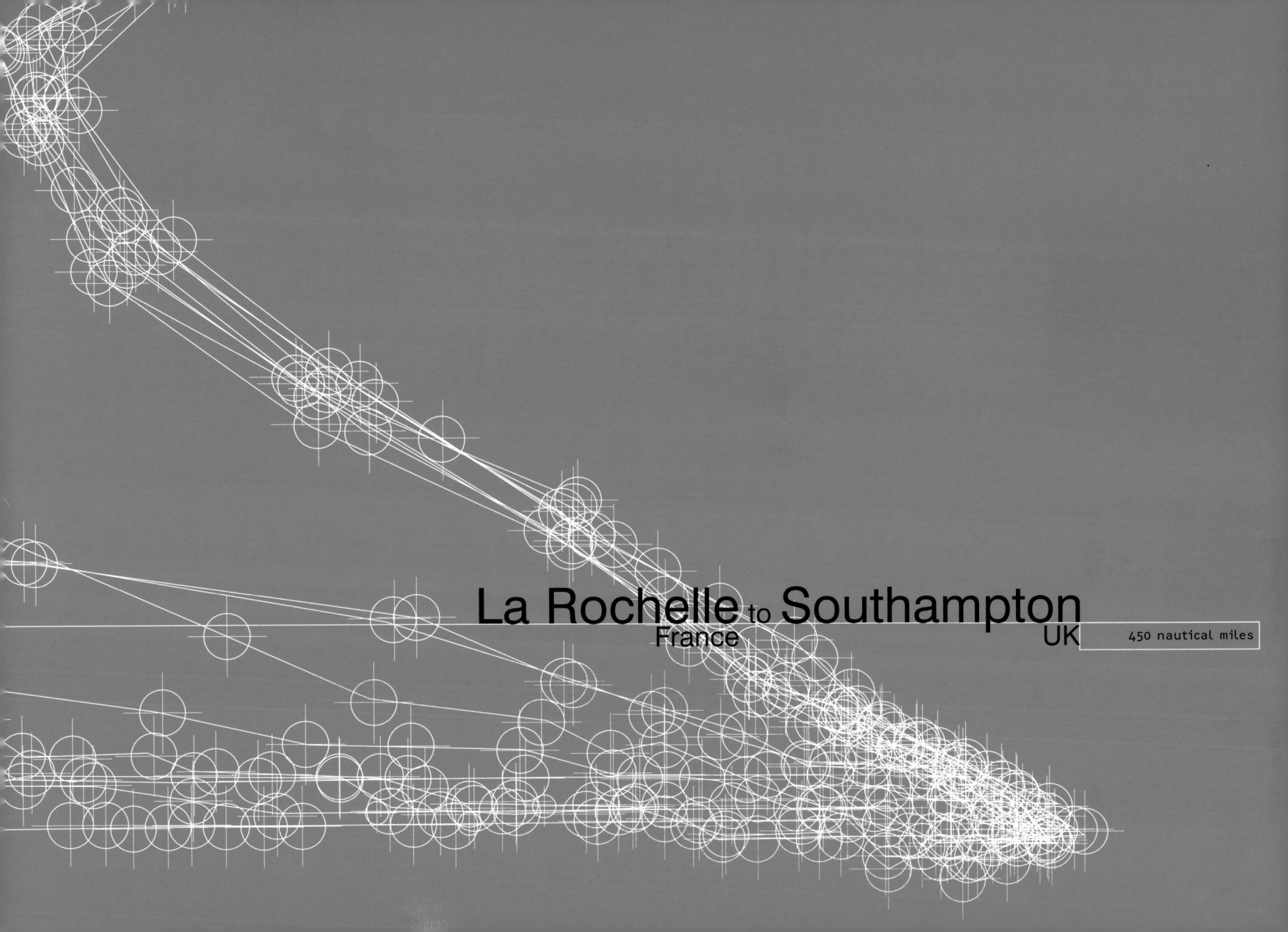

Leg 9: Prelude

As the boats prepared for the final 450 miles of the race — the dash from La Rochelle, France, to Southampton, UK — it was time to take stock of new realities. First place was no longer available. Even if she came in dead last on this leg, EF Language would be the winner of the 1997-98 Whitbread Round The World Race for the Volvo Trophy. The contest was now for second and third place. For some, even this was out of reach. Toshiba had bagged 115 points by taking first place on Leg 8, but that was not enough to erase all the setbacks the team had suffered on earlier legs. She remained in seventh place overall.

Silk Cut, finishing second on Leg 8, had earned 101 points and moved up into fifth place overall. This gave Lawrie Smith and his crew a realistic shot at overall third; they were just 33 points behind the current third-place holder, Merit Cup. Chessie Racing, third across the line in the penultimate leg, was even closer, just 10 points behind Merit Cup. However, Chessie's skipper, John Kostecki, said his sights were set on second place. "We have a chance for second place overall and that is what we have looked for," he stated.

The current second-place holder, Swedish Match, was not going to be easy to bump from that slot. For the No. 2 spot, it was going to be a battle royal between Swedish Match, Merit Cup and Chessie Racing. "We have improved our lot," said Merit Cup's skipper, Grant Dalton, as he reflected on the final leg. "Chessie Racing now has to beat us by two places, and we have to beat Swedish Match by four. It's going to be a bit of a ding-dong in the next leg."

That meant even before Cayard was added into the equation, the leg ahead was shaping up into a fierce test of the teams. Even though he had already won the race, Cayard made it clear he had no intention of letting the others fight this leg out alone. "We will try to finish The Whitbread as we started it," Cayard said. "First in, last out."

Leg 9: La Rochelle, France, to Southampton, UK

"For me this produces a mixture of joy and sadness — this has been one of the best experiences of my life and I, for one, will be sorry to see the demise of the Whitbread family."

BrunelSunergy navigator, Stuart Quarrie

With eight starts under their belts, the nine crews were greased and ready to go when the start was signalled. They attacked the starting line in a sudden burst. Spectators weren't sure if the boats had jumped the line or if they hadn't heard the gun go off. There was no mistake — the starting gun had misfired. Luckily, the crews pay little attention to the gun. Instead, they rely on the official start flag. When it's up, they race.

Nevertheless, it was still a confusing start for the teams. As the fleet picked its way through the spectator boats, a rash of protests were filed. Chessie Racing and Innovation Kvaerner both stated their intention to protest Toshiba, which they claimed entered a prohibited area during the start.

Silk Cut indicated a possible protest against EF Language, claiming that one of that team's support boats got in Silk Cut's way during the start. EF Language herself was forced to wave off one of her own support craft around the same time, when it got between EF Language and much-needed wind.

Chessie Racing indicated they might also file a protest against Toshiba for an undisclosed incident at the Chanchardon Beacon.

That would all have to be sorted out once the leg was over. Right now, the order of business was getting to Southampton — fast. As the boats hit the open seas, Toshiba led the fleet, followed by Innovation Kvaerner, Merit Cup, BrunelSunergy, Swedish Match, EF Education, EF Language, Chessie Racing and Silk Cut.

It was clear from the beginning that this would be a 'take-no-prisoners' race to the finish. No longer did the teams have to worry about preserving either the crew or boat for future legs. "We are going to use every little piece of energy we can drag out of our bodies. There is just going to be nothing left in Southampton," promised Knut Frostad, skipper of Innovation Kvaerner.

The crews knew the cost of pushing a W60 to the limit was breakage. "Last night we heard a big bang from the rig," emailed Frostad, "and as we lighted the rig up with a torch we found a 1.5-metre-long horizontal rip in our mainsail. We had no other choice than to get the sail down as it continued to rip further as we were watching it."

It happened at a crucial time for the team. "We were fighting with Silk Cut for second position with a good distance to Chessie Racing, the fourth boat at that time," wrote Frostad. The time it took sailmakers to repair the sail caused the team to drop from second to last place. "It was a big disappointment for us as we had shown very good speed since the start yesterday, and were constantly gaining on the boats around us. However, fixing broken parts quickly has been and is one of our strengths, and now more than ever we deserve to get back up in the lead."

Hours after the start, BrunelSunergy had moved into the lead, leading some to wonder if another upset victory was in the making. A member of the Dutch crew reported that no one on board was off duty on this leg. It was all hands on deck, all the time. "Sleeping on the rail in 25+ knots in reaching conditions is definitely no pleasure cruise," wrote crewman Arend van Bergeijk. "The boat inside looks ghostly empty as we hardly brought anything this leg. For instance, our toolbox contains the bare minimum: a hacksaw because it is compulsory and a hammer because Roy says he can fix everything with that."

Even in the heat of competition, the salt-encrusted Whitbread veterans were getting sentimental as the end approached. "Southampton is beckoning together with home and a return to what most consider normal," said BrunelSunergy's navigator, Stuart Quarrie, the first night out of La Rochelle. "For me this produces a mixture of joy and sadness — this has been one of the best experiences of my life and I for one will be sorry to see the demise of the Whitbread family who have become such great friends over the past few months."

On the overall leader, EF Language, skipper Paul Cayard was also in a reflective mood that night. "It definitely feels like the end is near and a lot of thoughts are going through my mind as to what we have been through in the last nine months."

Sentimentality wasn't the only thing on the racers' minds: Aboard sixth-place Silk Cut, Lawrie Smith and crew were determined to be first back to their home. "Southampton is our home port and we're determined to be waiting on the dock for the other blokes," Smith said. "There is still everything to play for, and tonight as the breeze drops off you'll see us all jostling for position and hoping that Silk Cut gets the new breeze first."

With a total of 450 nautical miles in this leg, and a fleet of W60s capable of eating nearly that much mileage in a single day, there was little time for the crews to plot subtle strategies. This was a drag race, pure and simple. For the first two-thirds of the leg, the boats switched positions almost hourly. Finally, with fewer than 135 miles to the finish, positions began to solidify. However, the boats remained so close that the leg leaders had only a tenuous hold on their positions. Less than one mile separated the four leading boats: Merit Cup, EF Language, Silk Cut and BrunelSunergy. Toshiba was 1.6 miles behind the leader in fifth, followed by Innovation Kvaerner 2.1 miles back, in sixth. Chessie Racing was seventh, 3.8 miles back, while Swedish Match was seeing her hopes for an overall second vanish as she followed 4.5 miles behind in eighth place. Each crew felt the final miles ticking off under their hulls, and each was determined to move up the ladder one last time.

Three hours later, with 104 miles to go, Swedish Match had edged her way into sixth place, gaining 2.2 miles on the leader, BrunelSunergy. Swedish Match was showing the fastest average speed in the fleet, 12 knots, compared with just under 11 knots for the fleet as a whole. Chessie Racing had slipped to eighth. The team's dream of second place was now little more than that — a dream.

After three more hours of sailing, BrunelSunergy lost first place to Merit Cup. There was only 75 nautical miles left to the entrance of the Solent. At this point, race organisers required the fleet to make a 25-mile detour — a loop around the buoys off Poole and Christchurch. This had nothing to do with the race and everything to do with public relations. Race organisers and sponsors had told fans and media to expect the first boats to finish between noon and 2 p.m. Southampton time, but the boats were early.

The extra miles offered a chance for Swedish Match and Silk Cut to close their gaps with the leaders. They would have to be fast about it, because once into the Solent, wind and currents could lock everyone into position for the finish.

EF Language was now in third, just half a mile behind BrunelSunergy, which was nearly neck and neck with Merit Cup. Silk Cut was in fourth, nine-tenths of a mile behind the leader, as her mostly British crew began to benefit from local knowledge. Swedish Match was stuck in fifth, with Innovation Kvaerner bearing down on her.

Another three hours of sailing saw the determined Innovation Kvaerner crew clawing three places up the ladder to third. Less than 60 miles remained to the finish line, and the fleet was lining up to enter the Solent. If the boats entered in their current order, it would be Merit Cup, EF Language, Innovation Kvaerner and Swedish Match, all within one mile of each other. Before the W60s could get to the Solent, however, there was one more disappointment for the Swedish Match team. Lawrie Smith and his Silk

Cut team snuck up from behind and snatched fourth place from them.

As the boats entered the Solent, Smith and his crew kept the pressure on. A hotly contested match race over third place commenced between Silk Cut and Innovation Kvaerner. Silk Cut briefly took third away from Innovation Kvaerner with just 10 miles to go to the finish. Then, as the fleet was within six miles of the finish, Frostad and his crew snatched third back from Silk Cut, pushing Smith and his team into fourth. Behind them, Swedish Match was fighting to get above fifth, nearly five miles behind the leaders.

The first boats to enter the Solent did so on a slack tide — the last boats to enter were not so lucky. They not only had to struggle in lighter winds but also were hit with an outgoing tide. EF Education was the last boat to enter the Solent. By the time she was at the Hurst Narrows, which marks the entrance to the Solent, the tide had become so strong and the winds so weak she almost had to drop anchor to keep from being pushed backward. The yacht had been only seven miles behind the leader, but her late entry into the Solent would shove her ultimate finish time back by three hours.

Meanwhile, up front, with less than three nautical miles to the finish, Cayard was giving Grant Dalton and his crew one last run for their money. The going was slow as the W60s beat upwind. Merit Cup was in the lead by barely one-tenth of a mile. Dalton bent on as much sail as possible — heeled over, the boat pounded into headwinds as Dalton searched for every ounce of potential, inching away from Cayard. With less than two miles to sail, Dalton had extended his lead to six-tenths of a mile over EF Language.

To cheers, Merit Cup crossed the finish line first on the final leg of the 1997-98 Whitbread, locking up second place overall for the team. EF Language finished immediately behind her to capture second place on the leg, confirming her overall first. Innovation Kvaerner, having fought her way back from last place, crossed third. Silk Cut finished fourth, which did not provide the team enough points to make it into the top three overall. Instead, the yacht held fifth overall.

Though the Swedish Match team had been favoured to place second in the race, her fifth-place finish on the final leg shoved her to third overall.

The Final Word

At their final news conference in Southampton, the skippers were decidedly reflective. Ten tired, sunburnt racers faced the media one more time. Dennis Conner joined his co-skipper Paul Standbridge for the news conference. The first order of business was to let bygones be bygones. All the protests filed at the start of the last leg were dropped, as a tone of conciliation replaced the cutthroat competitiveness these skippers normally display.

"We are not filing a protest," the often-taciturn Lawrie Smith explained. "Silk Cut was planning a protest because at the start of the race one of EF's [support] boats came straight across us and made us gybe. And at the time you get very annoyed, but afterwards you settle down. I guess it's not their fault."

Taking Smith's lead, Innovation Kvaerner's Knut Frostad explained his team was also dropping their complaint. "We were protesting Toshiba for sailing outside the prohibited area — whether it was legal or not legal to be in. But we are not protesting, and the race is over, so have a nice day."

When asked about the protests, even Toshiba's normally combative co-skipper, Dennis Conner, was magnanimous, brushing aside the opportunity to quibble. Instead, he lavished praise on the skippers who had beaten him. "I would like to congratulate Grant [Dalton] on sailing a wonderful leg. He deserves the win," Conner said. He then went on to praise Paul Cayard. "I have been a fan of his for a long time. I think that it's time in sailing that he got this well-deserved victory, and so, good on you, Paul."

That's not to say there were not obvious open wounds. The race had not turned out as expected for Smith, whose well-financed Silk Cut team finished fifth overall — a long way from the first- or second-place showing most handicappers were betting on. It was a somewhat defensive Smith who fielded questions from reporters. "I think you will find that if we did half-decent on the leg when we broke our mast," a stone-faced Smith said, "we would have come second."

Meanwhile, the unexpected winner of the race, Paul Cayard, made it a point not to rub salt into the wounds of the other skippers. He said that winning the race was a great honour for any professional sailor. "It's a special moment for sure," Cayard said. "Going around the world on a sailboat, when your whole life has been sailing, is a big deal. And then to win the race was extra special, and I am sure it has not all sunk in yet. I know from having been in a lot of big races that it takes a certain amount of luck to do what we did on EF Language."

Cayard then went on to compliment his fellow racers. "A race isn't worth winning unless the people you are racing against are really tough and very good. We have a full lineup here of highly credentialed skippers and crews and support teams, and that makes the victory worth winning."

Swedish Match's skipper, Gunnar Krantz, was taking home both a third-place trophy and a lot of regrets. When Swedish Match came in fifth on Leg 9, it knocked her out of second overall into third. Krantz said that finishing third was better than not being on the podium at all, but that it wasn't what he had expected. "All in all, I am bitterly disappointed," he said. "Somehow we made a great start in the race, we caught up in the middle and we made a few mistakes in the end."

Krantz then turned to Cayard and Dalton. "Congratulations to Grant for second place and to Paul for winning. It's been a great race — 32,000 miles is over."

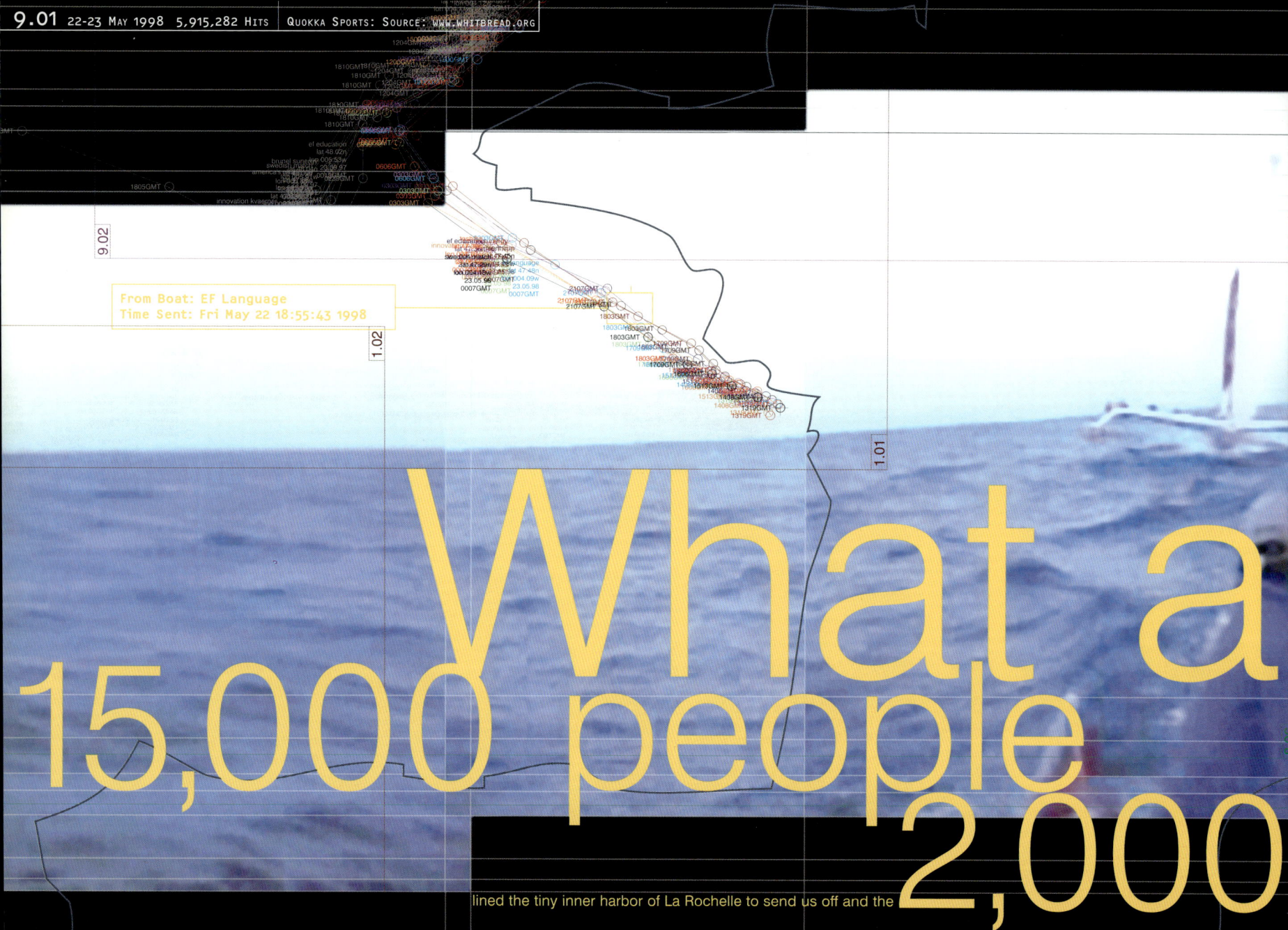

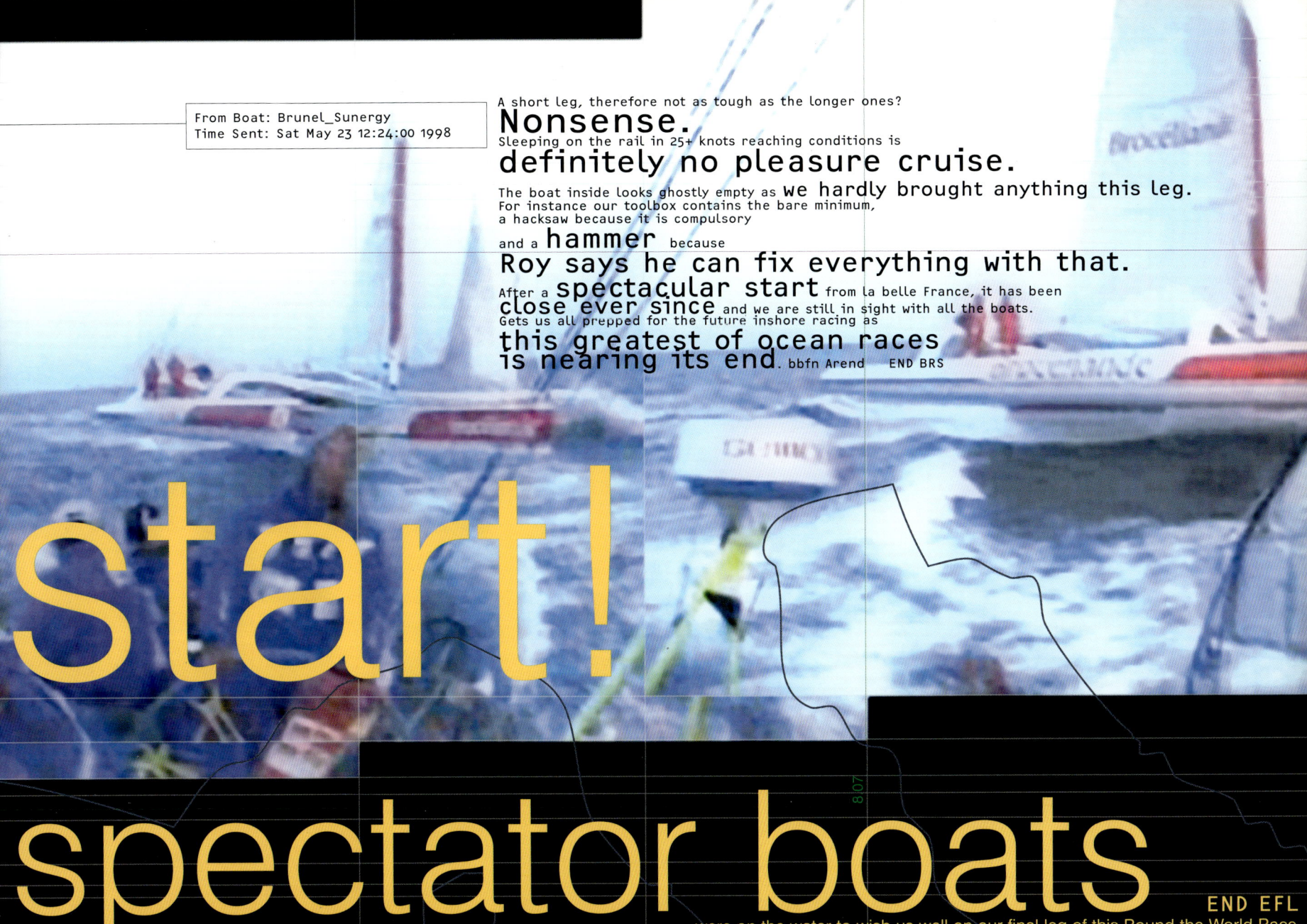

From Boat: Brunel_Sunergy
Time Sent: Sat May 23 12:24:00 1998

A short leg, therefore not as tough as the longer ones? **Nonsense.** Sleeping on the rail in 25+ knots reaching conditions is **definitely no pleasure cruise.** The boat inside looks ghostly empty as **we hardly brought anything this leg.** For instance our toolbox contains the bare minimum, a hacksaw because it is compulsory and a **hammer** because **Roy says he can fix everything with that.** After a **spectacular start** from la belle France, it has been **close ever since** and we are still in sight with all the boats. Gets us all prepped for the future inshore racing as **this greatest of ocean races is nearing its end.** bbfn Arend   END BRS

start!

spectator boats were on the water to wish us well on our final leg of this Round the World Race.

END EFL

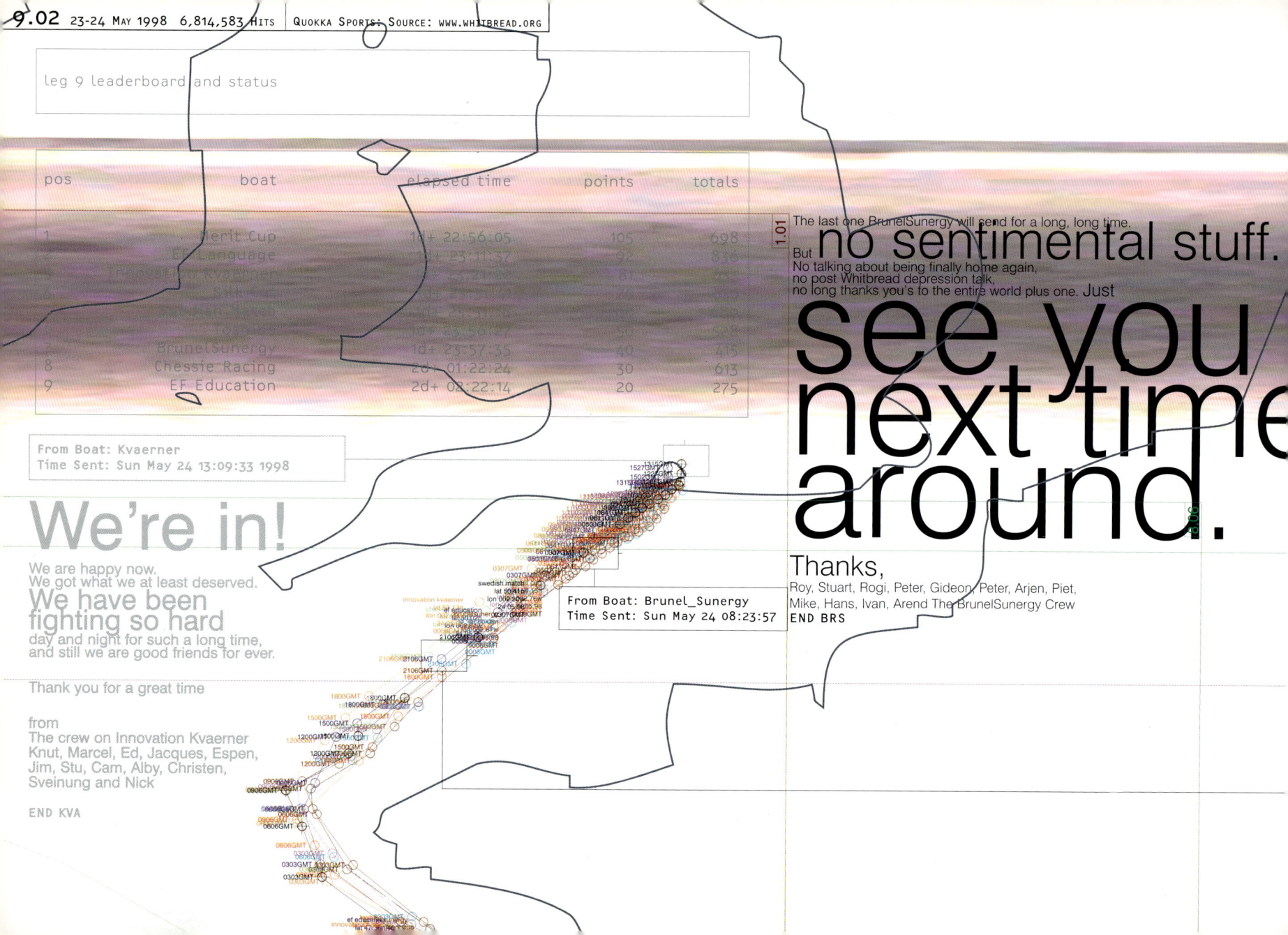

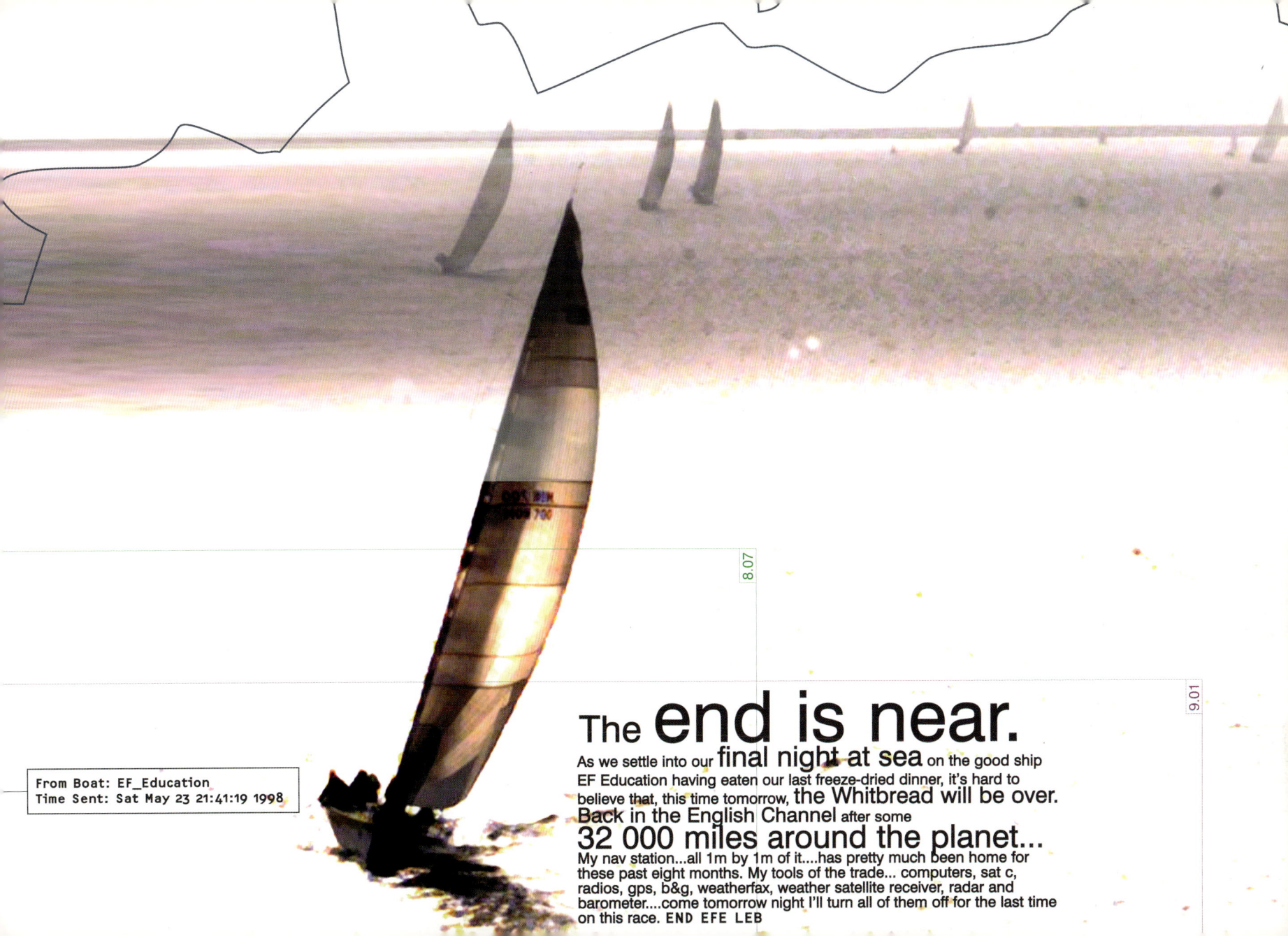

From Boat: EF_Education
Time Sent: Sat May 23 21:41:19 1998

The end is near.

As we settle into our **final night at sea** on the good ship EF Education having eaten our last freeze-dried dinner, it's hard to believe that, this time tomorrow, **the Whitbread will be over.** **Back in the English Channel** after some **32 000 miles around the planet...** My nav station...all 1m by 1m of it....has pretty much been home for these past eight months. My tools of the trade... computers, sat c, radios, gps, b&g, weatherfax, weather satellite receiver, radar and barometer....come tomorrow night I'll turn all of them off for the last time on this race. END EFE LEB

10.01 | 24 May 1998 | 3,788,917 Hits | Quokka Sports: Source: www.whitbread.org

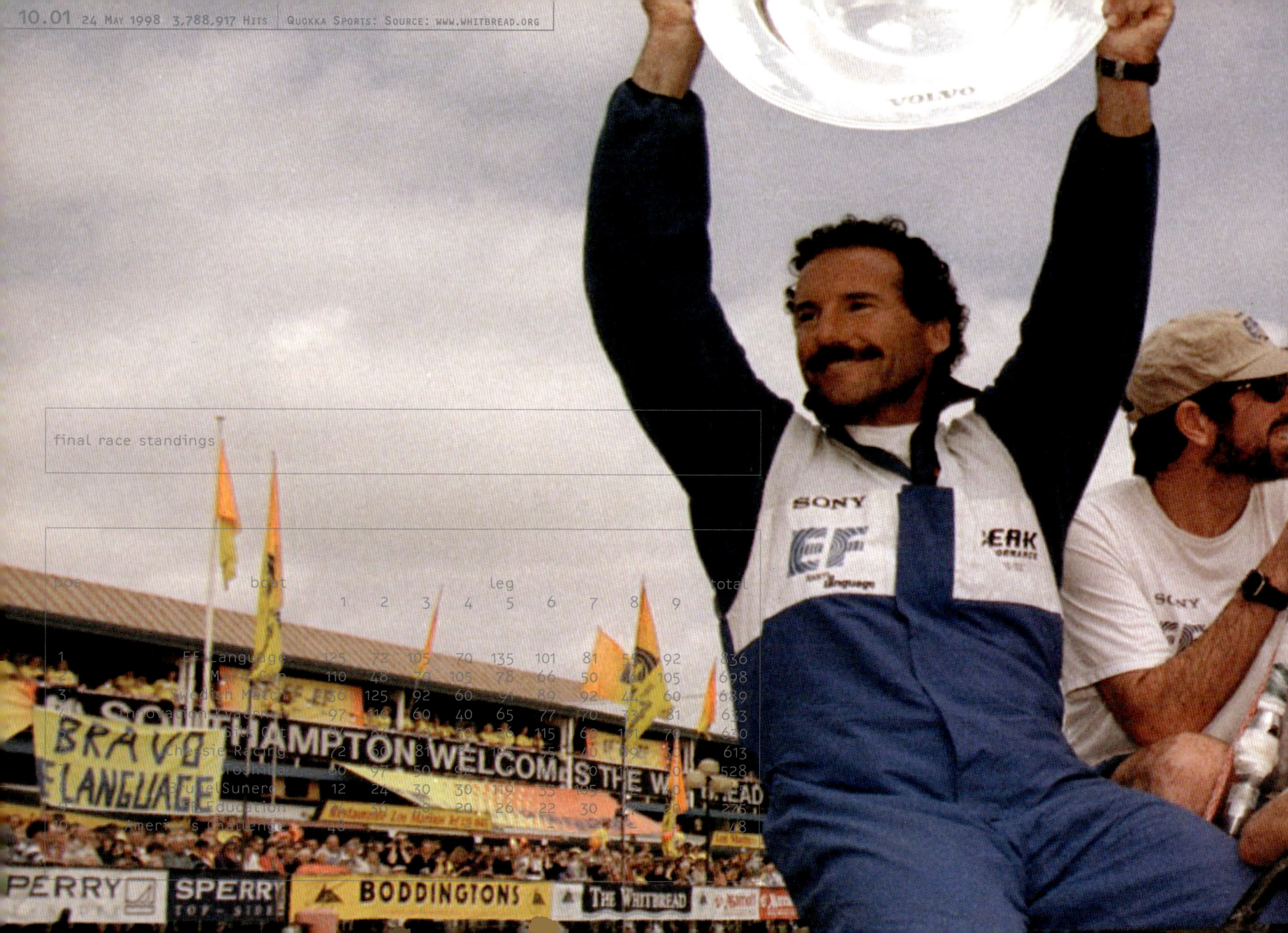

final race standings

pos	boat	leg 1	2	3	4	5	6	7	8	9	total
1	EF Language	125	72	105	70	135	101	81	55	92	836
2	Merit Cup	110	48	78	105	78	66	50	58	105	698
3	Swedish Match	130	125	92	60	91	89	92	42	60	689
4	Innovation Kvaerner	97	110	60	40	65	77	70	33	81	633
5	Silk Cut							115	63	71	630
6	Chessie Racing	72	60	81							613
7	Toshiba	60	97	50							528
8	BrunelSunergy	12	24	30	30	119	53				
9	EF Education				20	26	22	30			276
10	America's Challenge	48									48

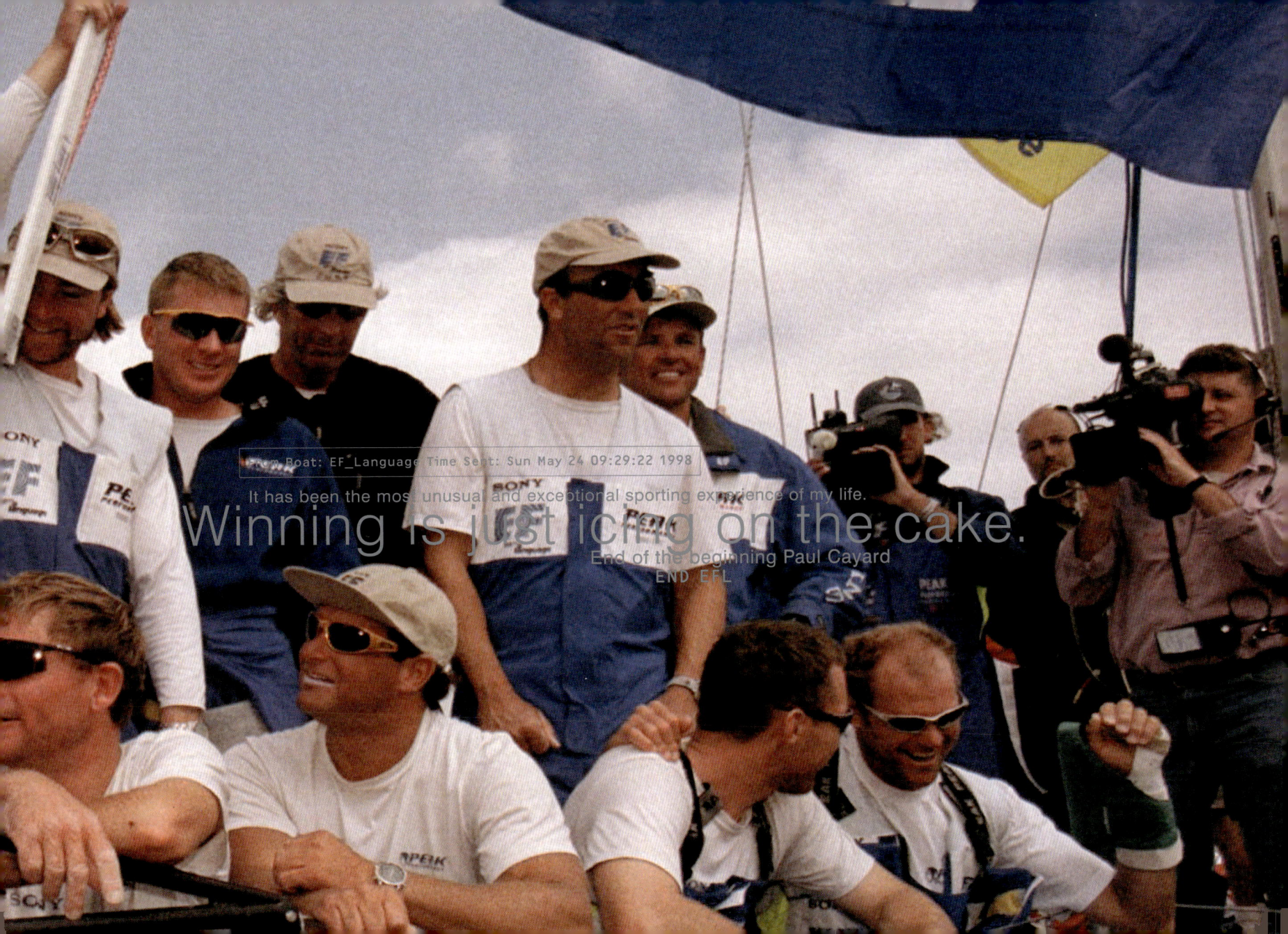

From Boat: EF_Language Time Sent: Sun May 24 09:29:22 1998

It has been the most unusual and exceptional sporting experience of my life. Winning is just icing on the cake.
End of the beginning Paul Cayard
END EFL

11.0.0 21 Sep 1997 – 24 May 1998   768,867,743 Hits   Quokka Sports: Source: www.whitbread.org

Conclusion

Distance:

The Wired Whitbread

31,600 nautical miles

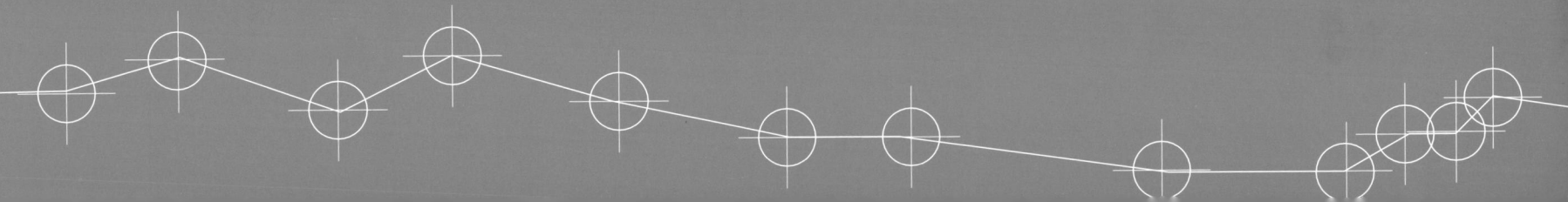

11.0.1 21 SEP 1997 – 24 MAY 1998   768,867,743 HITS   QUOKKA SPORTS: SOURCE: WWW.WHITBREAD.ORG

Welcome back. To your desk, your sofa, the bus you're riding.

Still feel the sting of the spray on your face? The intensity of falling off the face of a 40-foot wave? The heat of the tropics, the Antarctic cold? Are you exhausted after having experienced nine months of relentless competition condensed into an evening — or an hour?

You were there. For 32,000 nautical miles of the Whitbread Round The World Race, these pages, these images, these words transported you into the middle of the action. Perhaps they sparked your imagination, and in your mind you enacted your lifelong passion for the water. Or perhaps the scale — the vast, complete authority of sky and sea — left you longing for a battle with the wind and the waves, not the clock.

Maybe you came onboard in spite of yourself. Chronicles, scrapbooks — whatever you call travelogues — have a way of inviting us in. They titillate the voyeur in us. Perhaps we simply like the connection with the events and the people. We like vicarious experience. We like witnessing great events and rubbing against great people. To get in their shoes for a day, get in their heads, and yet be invisible.

We're no different at Quokka Sports. We're just in the business of engineering these vicarious experiences.

The Whitbread Round The World Race marked our debut, and, modesty aside, what we produced was a revolutionary way to view a sports event. What made it such a success? First, a commonsense understanding of how to immerse people into sports. Second, an unbridled thrill for new technology. Third, a vision — a crystal-clear construct of how to use that technology to immerse an audience in an event.

Let's take a look at the technology. Flip through the book again. A fleet of boats. Ten teams. Over 100 men and women in rigorous competition for nine months. Electronics everywhere to support the most technologically sophisticated racing machines on the planet. Quokka wired each boat from bow to stern. We mounted video cameras on deck. Placed sensors in the hull. Carefully installed a 'Sat-B' satellite dish just behind the mast step to transmit full-motion video and still pictures from boat to satellite to ground lines in England. Then powerful servers took over, processing a wealth of data, bouncing it to San Francisco, where we sifted it and instantly posted important race information, such as each boat's location and the current weather conditions.

However, the technology we used gave us more than data. It also gave us a set of eyes on the boats. We knew there were interesting stories onboard, and we wanted them to be true — true in the sense of 'from the source,' not filtered through a journalist or an editor. We wondered, would the participants be our camera operators, our storytellers, our guides? More importantly, would they have time, given the rigors of their odyssey?

They did. Paul Cayard, for one, took center stage in the digital world. To our delight, he sent us more digital video footage than we could manage! Paul's experience, and his visual interpretation, like that of many others, drove the technology and brought the race to us. The other competitors jostled for the limelight, flooding our studios with stories. Quokka took an editorial back seat. We let the athletes tell their stories and set the agenda.

It paid off. Our coverage sent shockwaves through the sports world. We broke new ground. We were pioneers. There had never been race coverage in the world like Quokka's Whitbread site.

It happened at a point in history where broadcast communications were redefining themselves, and they still are. We've jumped on the opportunity by fashioning a new genre of sports coverage. It's a hybrid of traditional television and classic documentary formats. This wide range of presentation and recording techniques will ultimately converge to create the next medium — a medium that will paint a broader, more detailed picture, getting all the way around the experience and inviting participation. Television just can't do as much.

Where television and Quokka's styles intersect is in storytelling. We, too, subscribe to storylines. However, our style diverges from television at two levels. First, at the level of content — the sheer quantity of experience we present. Second, at the level of audience choice. We believe that viewers like having control of what they watch. Give them multiple nonlinear streams of information, and yes, they'll build their own linear experiences. Our challenge is to create enough connections — and the right ones — so the experience is as direct as possible. It's a carefully balanced blend of data, news and emotional triggers, all within an interface that helps an audience stay oriented in time and space (geography).

Our presentations also differ from television in the way they reflect the rhythms of the real world. Think about where you are now. People may be talking around you. Halfway around the world the stock market just opened. It's a different season a hemisphere away. Delivering these multiple perspectives and multiple activities is the hallmark of Quokka's new class of presentation. We capture events in multiple dimensions. This makes the Quokka experience deeper, richer and more accurate than anything in conventional media.

This is Quokka's new conceptual and physical invention. We call it Quokka Sports Immersion, or QSI. We're engineering it as we go, but we're governed by a few simple 'muses' to keep us on track. First is affinity. Whatever we do must grab the audience's attention, and keep it for extended periods — up to months at a time. Next is location. Does the presentation leave us feeling like spectators at the venue? There's understanding. Does the information build interest in and feeling for the event? Next, empathy. Are we helping fans warm to the athlete, like they would to a friend or family member? Finally, participation. Involve the audience in the experience, not just with the content.

The Whitbread race was just a beginning in Quokka's experiment in sports entertainment. We know we're on to something that works, yet we've only scratched the surface of what we're capable of doing. We plan to use richer telemetry, for example, which will let us plot more than simple location. Soon, we'll be able to show the dynamic characteristics of moving objects and moving athletes, and biometric data like heart rate and respiration. We'll provide much more video as bandwidth increases and as bigger 'pipes' reach more and more people. We'll use all of this to show the multiple dimensions of any experience. There's no question — the more data, the more immersive the experience.

Whatever we look like in the future, we'll be ahead of the pack. Quokka is determined to change the way the world experiences sports. Count on this — it's going to be huge.

Glossary of Nautical Terms

Aft — Toward the stern; behind.
America's Cup — Historic yacht race held every three or four years since the 19th century.
Apparent Wind — The wind direction felt on the boat as it moves. A combination of the true wind angle and the change in wind angle created by the boat's movement.
Backstay — A mast support that runs aft to the deck or to another mast. Can be tightened to make the mast bend, or to tighten the forestay.
Ballast — Weight in the keel of a boat that adds stability (righting moment).
Batten — Thin strips of composite material inserted into a pocket in a sail, to support the curved leech of the sail.
Beam — A boat's greatest width.
Becalmed — Drifting with no wind.
Bilge — The lowest part of a boat's hull; area where water and diesel collects. Where you drop important bolts during repairs.
Blanketing — A tactical manoeuvre in which one boat slows a competitor by using her sails to obstruct the competitor's wind.
Boom — Spar to which a sail's lower edge or foot is attached. The boom is attached to the mast at the gooseneck.
Boom Vang or Kicking Strap — Tackle running between the boom and the deck that holds the boom down.
Bow — The front of the boat.
Broach — In a downwind situation, the boat turns uncontrollably and is pushed by the wind onto her side, lying with the mast parallel to the water.
Bulb — Torpedo-shaped weight on the bottom of the keel.
Chainplates — Metal plates on a boat's sides to which the shrouds are attached.
Chute — *See* Spinnaker.
Cleat — A fitting that holds a line against tension from the sails or rigging.
Clew — The corner of any sail where the leech intersects the foot.
Cockpit — A recessed area in the aft deck in which the crew work.
Companionway — Steps that lead from the deck to the cabin below.
Dead Reckoning (DR) — The calculation of a boat's position based on course and distance sailed.
Delamination — Failure of the bond between either of the hull's outer and inner skins, and the 'sandwich' spacing material in between — allowing either of the two outer layers to come off the centre layer.

Doldrums, the — Intertropical Convergence Zone (ITCZ): area near the equator with either squalls or no wind.
Downwind — The direction a balloon blows in the wind.
Ease — To let out a sail; take tension off a line.
Elapsed Time — A yacht's time, in days, hours and minutes, from the start of a leg or race to her finish of that leg/race.
Flyer — Choosing a course radically different than the majority of the fleet.
Foot — The bottom edge of a sail.
Foresail — Any sail used between the mast and the forestay.
Forestay — A mast support that runs from the top of the mast to the bow. It can be tightened to make the mast bend more, or to tighten the backstay.
Fractional Rig — The forestay is attached a 'fraction' below the top of the mast — usually seven-eighths or five-sixths of the height of the rig.
Furious Fifties — Area between 50 degrees south latitude and 60 S. Known for persistent gales and large seas.
Genniker (Gennaker) — Cross between a genoa and a spinnaker; a foresail used for reaching.
Genoa — A large foresail used for sailing upwind. It overlaps the mainsail.
Gradient Wind — Wind caused by the differential between high- and low-pressure systems.
GRIB (Gridded Binary) — File format used to send meteorological data.
Gybe — Turning the boat so that the stern passes through the wind, and the boat changes from port tack to starboard, or vice versa.
Halyard — Line that holds a sail up.
Head, the — The lavatory in a boat or ship.
Hounds — The point where the shrouds attach to the top of the mast.
Hull Speed — A boat's theoretical maximum speed, determined by multiplying the square root of her waterline length by 1.34.
Jacklines — The lines that run the length of the boat to which one attaches a safety harness.
Jib — Foresail used for upwind sailing.
Jury-rig — Emergency rigging using available gear. It typically involves a broken mast.
Keel — A ballasted appendage below the boat that keeps it from capsizing, and also supplies the hydrodynamic lateral force that enables the boat to sail upwind.
Kite — *See* Spinnaker.
Knot — One nautical mile per hour.
Lay — To sail a course that will clear an object or marker.
Leech — Trailing edge of a sail. Also, the curve of a sail.

Leeward, Lee — The downwind side of any object.
Lifelines — Cables that go around the deck to prevent the crew from falling overboard.
Lift — A wind shift allowing the helmsman to head up or alter course to windward, or the crew to ease sheets.
Luff — The forward edge of a mainsail or jib and the windward edge of a spinnaker.
Luff, to — Bubbling or flapping of a sail when it is not trimmed tightly enough, is being backwinded by another sail, or when the course sailed is too close to the wind.
Lines — A nautical term for ropes.
Mainsheet — The line used to adjust the mainsail's angle to the wind.
Mark — A buoy used in a race course.
Masthead Rig — The shrouds are attached to the 'masthead' — the top of the mast.
Nautical Mile — Unit of distance used on navigation charts. One nautical mile equals 6,076 feet, or 1.15 statute miles.
Off the Wind — Sailing away from the wind; also called downwind, reaching or running.
Peeling — Changing from one spinnaker to another.
Pitch — A boat pitches when the bow and stern move up and down about the transverse centre.
Plane — A boat planes when she sails over her own bow wave, so that only a small section of the hull is in the water. This allows the boat to go faster than the theoretical maximum hull speed.
Polars or Polar Table — The name for the database that holds all the information on the boat's projected speed at different angles to the wind. Crucial for maintaining performance when there are no other boats in sight.
Port — The left half of the boat when facing forward.
Port Tack — Sailing with the wind blowing onto the port side, and the mainsail on the starboard side.
Pulpit — Platform surrounded by a rail in the bow. It keeps crew and sails onboard during headsail changes.
Rail — Same as the gunwale, the edge between the hull and the deck.
Reaching — Sailing with the apparent wind between 45 and 135 degrees to the boat.
Reef, to — To decrease a sail's size.
Rhumb Line — The most direct course between two points.
Rigging — The gear used to adjust and support the sails.
Roaring Forties — The high-wind area between 40 degrees south latitude and 50 S.
Rod — Solid steel wire that replaces twisted cable in the rigging of large boats.
Roller Furling — A device to mechanically furl a sail, most often used on foresails.

Rolling — The hull's rotational oscillation, about the fore-and-aft axis.
Round-down — Ultimately wiping out to leeward into an uncontrolled gybe.
Running — Sailing with wind coming from behind the boat.
Running Backstay, Runner — Two adjustable stays that support the mast, one on the port side and one on the starboard. They run from the hounds to the stern. The stay has to be eased on the leeward side to let the mainsail out.
Running Rigging — All moving rods and lines that support and control the mast and sails.
Screaming Sixties — Area south of 60 S with high winds and rough seas. Here, winds and waves circle the Earth virtually unobstructed by any landmass.
Sheet — A line that controls a sail's angle to the wind.
Shroud — Cable or rod that supports the mast, from the chainplates at deck level on the port and starboard side, to the hounds just below the top of the mast.
Slatting — Becalmed with sails flapping uselessly.
Speed Made Good (SMG) — A boat's speed as measured by her progress relative to land, factoring in her speed through the water and current.
Spar — A basic term for a mast, boom or yard.
Spinnaker — Large, light triangular-shaped sails that are attached to spars at the sail's corners. They are used when running or reaching, sailing downwind.
Spreaders — Struts on the mast that spread the shrouds apart. They increase the 'working angle' of the shrouds.
Starboard — The right half of the boat when facing forward.
Starboard Tack — Sailing with the wind blowing onto the starboard side, and the mainsail on the port side.
Stanchions — Vertical supports that hold the lifelines in place around the boat.
Standing Rigging — The non-moving rods, stays or shrouds that support the mast and sails.
Step — (1) Support for the base of the mast. (2) Fixed or removable pegs used to climb the mast.
Stern — The rear of the boat.
Squall — A cell of violent rain and wind, normally in the area of thunderstorms. It begins abruptly, but typically lasts less than an hour.
Tacking — Turning the boat so that the bow passes through the wind while upwind of the stern, and the boat changes from port tack to starboard, or vice versa.
Transom — The flat rear end of a boat, the upper part of which tends to angle forward on modern racers.
Traveller — Track or bar on which the bottom part of the mainsheet runs across the boat.
Trim — To adjust the sail to make it the right shape and angle to the wind.

True Wind — The actual direction of the wind. Can only be directly measured on board when the boat is stationary.
24-Hour Run — The maximum distance in nautical miles a yacht achieves in a 24-hour period.
Upwind — Toward the direction from which the wind blows.
Velocity Made Good (VMG) — The average speed of a yacht since the start of a leg or race, if the yacht had sailed the shortest course.
Watch — The working teams into which the crew is divided. To be on watch means to be working. Free time is the free watch, or off-watch.
Watch Leader/Captain — The person in charge of a watch.
Way — Speed.
Winch Pedestal — Upright winch drive mechanism with two handles — increases purchasing power.
Yaw — To sail a wildly erratic course.

Glossary of Whitbread Slang
Big Kahuna — See Code 0.
Block to Block — Pull in a sheet or pulley system as far as it will go, i.e., block to block.
Bullet — A patch of wind.
Cheap Seats — Not doing well in a race; sailing at the back of the fleet.
Code 0 — A controversial 'upwind spinnaker' developed for the 1997-98 Whitbread. First used by EF Language on Leg 1.
Complete Dog, a — A very slow boat.
Death Roll — When sailing dead downwind, the sickening roll to windward and leeward that ends in a broach.
Down the Mine — Hurtling down a wave with no way out at the bottom.
Fantasyland — Everywhere that is not the bow.
Feeding the Fish — Vomiting.
Flossing — Checking the keel and rudder for kelp, garbage bags and other items hooked while sailing. Involves everything from dropping a looped line over the bow, to (in total frustration) diving over the side to clear it yourself.
Full Kit Up — Big genniker and full mainsail.
Full-on — Maximum; to the limit.
Fully Cocked — The best prepared; ready, great, excellent.
Going Over the Handlebars — When the boat hits something or stops suddenly.
Got a Bit On — When many things are happening on the boat at the same time.
Gunwale Bum — See Spotty Botty.
Haulin' the Mail, Haulin' the Chili — Sailing fast; when the boat is sailing at her optimum.
Heads On a Post — The so-called decision makers in the back of the boat.

Hour-glass — See Wrap In the Kite.
In the Pipe — In the groove, when the boat is sailing at her optimum.
Kip — Australian, British and New Zealand term for 'sleep.'
Marlboro Country — The bow, because you have to be very tough and a real cowboy to go there.
Mushrooms — What the crew forward of the companionway refer to themselves as, because they are kept in the dark until the absolute last minute.
Navi-guesser — The navigator.
Nipper — The youngest member of a crew; usually has to do the wet-sanding.
On Fire — Boat going fast compared to the competition.
On the Pace — Sailing well in relation to the rest of the fleet.
Pause for the Cause — That moment right before you chew something. A moment of divine worship because you are so happy to have something to eat.
Pitch-poling — Putting the bow into a wave and cartwheeling forward.
Pranging the Boat — Hitting a stationary object.
Pumped Up — When the boat is fully ballasted. Water in the ballast tanks.
Rack Her Down — To lean in an attempt to flatten the boat, using the weight of the crew.
Rag the Kite — Let the spinnaker flap, usually so the boat can sail to windward for a mark or to sail/manoeuvre against another boat.
Real Estate — Your area of ocean.
Riding Shotgun — On boats with two steering stations, when the breeze is very strong, two people need to helm, one on each wheel.
Sched/Sked — Each boat's scheduled position report. From schedule, when the boats would have to radio in to compile the daily schedule.
Sending It — To launch a boat down a wave.
Slot, the — Gap between the jib and the mainsail.
Smelling of Roses — A good tactical call.
Spotty Botty — Painful rash caused by sitting in salt water.
Strings — Lines / sheets / ropes.
Vision, the — Water tunnel created when you're haulin' a quarter-wake off both chainplates.
Wet-sanding — The worst job in boat preparation, smoothing the bottom of a boat to make it move faster through the water.
Wheels Came Off, the — Describing a series of problems.
Wrap In the Kite, a — When the spinnaker twists in the middle to form an hourglass shape, rendering it temporarily useless.

Thank you

We'd like to thank the support staff, crews, Whitbread staff, journalists, sponsors, Quokka Sports staff, port personnel, friends, family and dreamers that made the Whitbread Web site possible. Below is a list — admittedly incomplete — of the people who made www.whitbread.org happen every day. We began the race as individuals and finished it as one. Cheers!

All the volunteers and supporters in every host port • Charles Abrahams • David Abromowitz • Nathaniel Adkins • Yasmine Ahmed • Stuart Aitken • Kathy Alexander • Stuart Alexander • David Allen • Jim Allsopp • Enrique Alvarez • Michelle Amato • Fred Andersson • Alan Andrews • Peter Ansell • Rodney Ardern • Joylon Armstrong • Nysse Arruda • Sissel Tove Asberg • Isabelle Autissier • Ian Bailey-Willmot • Ed Baird • Mark Balicki • Beverley Ballinger • Stuart Bannatyne • Greg Barnhill • Neil Barth • Paolo Bassani • Michael Beasley • Lynnath Beckley • Chris Beeson • Rob Begg • Josh Belsky • Philippa Beresford • John Bergs • Rick Berman • Jean Yves Bernot • John Bertrand • Stuart Bettany • Nicola Binstead • David Blanchfield • Curtis Blewett • Stephen Bloom • Figge (Carl-Fredrik) Boksjö • Richard Bouzaid • Steve Bradley • Gavin Brady • David Branigan • Bravo Yacht Club and São Paulo Sailing Federation • Christine Briand • Phil Briars • Richard Brisius • Geoff Browning • Peg Buchan • Mark Bullingham • Ivan Bunner • Robert Buttress • Nicholas Campailla • Ken Campbell • Andrew Cape • John Capon • George Caras • Michael Carr • Jason Carrington • Paul Cayard • Al Chandler • Lisa Charles • Mark Chisnell • Mark Christensen • Sean Clarkson • Marleen Cleyndert • Jim Close • Julie Close • Justin Clougher • Kirk Clyne • Susan Colby • George Collins • Maureen Collins • Joe Collins • Dennis Conner • Marco Constant • Charles Cook • Chris Cooney • Lysiane Cotte • Steve Cotton • Cruising Yacht Club of Australia • Heather Dallas • Gene Dallosto • Grant Dalton • Susan Daly • Ramon Davies • Dirk de Ridder • Chris Deaton • Carlos Deihl • Dave Deiling • Jan Dekker • Rick Deppe • Dave Dilnott • Warren Douglas • Anna Drougge • David Duff • Laurence Duffy • Marina Dyfverman-Kock • Joe English • Paul Enriquez • Steve Erickson • Evan Evans • Jean-Louis Fabry • Tom Faire • Jez Fanstone • Bruce Farr • Campbell Field • Ross Field • Mark Fischer • Stephanie Fischer • Bryan Fishback • Kerry Fishback • Bob Fisher • Bob Fiske • Gail Fitzpatrick • Greg Flynn • Daniel Fong • Roch Fortin • Fremantle Sailing Club • Knut Frostad • Bob Gallagher • Brett Gardner • Shelley Garton • Vincent Geake • Greg Gendell • Howard Gibbons • John Gigichi • Marcus Giles • Emily Gist • Catarina Göthe • Michael Gough • Neil Graham • Lizzie Green • Alan Green • Jack Griffin • BJ Grimholt • Christine Guillou • Espen Guttormsen • Lisa Hackett • Kelvin Harrap • Sonia Harris • Cathy Harvey • Mick Harvey • Pat Healey • Kristi Hein • Roy Heiner • Richard Hellyer • Jared Henderson • Sarah Hewettson-Brown • Mark Hinkle • Marika Hejlm • Harald Hjort • Eric Hogan • Anders Holmquist • Henrik Holmquist • Jon Holstrum • Hans Horrevoets • Eileen Howard • Todd Howery •

Georgina Hyde • Will Ingham • David Ingham • Mubashar Iqbal • Brad Jackson • Rick Jarboe • Gary Jobson • Christen Horn Johanessen • Dennis Johnson • Janine Johnson • Linda Jones • Steve Jones • Pia Jonsson • Michael Joubert • Robin Judah • Judel/Vrolijk • Oscar Karlsson • Kaye Hopkins • Kellie Keating • Simon Keen • Simon Keijzer • Chris Kelly • Kyle Kendall • Daphne Kent • Marie-Claude Kieffer • Jerry Kirby • Rolf Kjeseth • Frits Koek • Sandry Koo • John Kostecki • Tim Kroger • Steve Kues • Richard Langdon • Christophe Lassegue • Lauderdale Yacht Club • Richard Lawson • Marcel Leeman • Esther Leune • Tom Levin • Cameron Lewis • Erik Lindkvist • Craig Lintott • Jack Lloyd • Kurt Loman • Jeremy Lomas • Matthew Lovett • Mikael Lundh • Brion Lutz • Gordon Maguire • Guido Maisto • Paddy Mant • Andy Marks • Ralph Marrinson • Thierry Martinez • Clive Mason • Anne Massot • Kate Maudslay • Jack Mauger • Sonia Mayes • Scott McAllister • Andrew McCall • Neal McDonald • Murray McDonnell • Keryn McMaster • Bob Meagher • Henry Menin • Brett Miller • George Miller • Gerry Mitchell • Nick Moloney • Tony Mooney • Roxanne Moore • Alison Moore • Brian Morris • Steve Munday • Sam Murch • Paul Murray • Tony Mutter • Geoffrey Myburgh • Rob Myers • Steve Nelson • Leah Newbold • Tom Newell • Janine Newman • Sasha Nice • James Nicholls • Pieter van Nieuwenhuyzen • Roger Nilson • Donna North • Craig Nutter • Anna Nycander • Klas Nylof • Fredrik Nylöf • Mark O'Brien • Curt Oetking • Kaoru Ogimi • Magnus Olsson • Andreas Olsson • Graeme Owens • Louise Palmstierna • Kiny Parade • Bruce Parker-Forsyth • Jonathan Patton • Rita Pearce • Josh Peerless • Mary Pera • Kim Pervan • Klaus Peters • Goran Peterssen • Katherine Pettibone • Russel Pickthall • Barry Pickthall • Phil Pierotti • Jim Pimentel • Alex Pineda • Antonio Piris • Steve Pizzo • Carol Pogash • Tatjana Pokorny • Dalia Pons • Tim Powell • Veronique Powell • Andrew Preece • Anne Prees • Mel Pyatt • Stuart Quarrie • Mike Quilter • Paul Quinn • Jasinta Rajan • Alan Ramadan • Magnus Rastrom • Bud Reiss • Tony Rey • Pam Rickman • Paul Reid • John Ripard • John Roberson • Staveley Roberts • Neil Robertshaw • Emily Robertson • Rene Rochat • Parker Rockefeller • Phil Rose • Eric Rodenbeck • Rudi Rodriguez • David Rolfe • Murray Ross • The Royal Cape Yacht Club • Royal New Zealand Yacht Squadron • The Royal Southampton Yacht Club • Mark Rudiger • Todd Russell • Johan Salen • Mike Sanderson • Anne Sandison • Craig Satterthwaite • Ted Schachter • Bill Schaefer • Les Schmidt • Elissa Schreck • Dave Scott • Sally Scott • Gaither Scott • Jenny Sharman • Kevin Shoebridge • Steve Shugh • Dee Siebert • Peter Siemens • Dave Sinclair • Priscila Siqueira • Rob Slade • Dee Smith • Lawrence Smith • Lawrie Smith • Alan Smith • Eileen Quinn Smith • Franz Smolkovic • Societe des Regates Rochelaises • Marit Söderström • Rod Solomons • Soraya Hearn • Tim Spalding • Grant Spanhake • Laura Spanhake • Bertie de Speville • Joanne Stallard • Paul Standbridge • Barbara Stange • Adrian Stead • Todd Steele • Ian Stewart • Mick Stickney • Allison Stoneham • Sally Stump • Bridget Suckling • Jeff Sussna • Jonathan Swain • Cary Swain • Les Symes • Peter Tans • Lee Tawney • Murray Taylor • Fred Teale • Michael Tette • John Thackwray • David Thomas • Rick Thomas • Tucker Thompson • Sveinung Togersen • Rick Tomlinson • Mike Toppa • Juan Torruella • Steven Travers • Laurie Tucker • Vince Tyson • Arend van Bergeijk • Paul van Dyke • Arjen Van Gent • Peter van Niekerk • Marcel van Triest • Stef van't Zant • Ann Veibig • Christophe Vieux • Juan Vila • Jacque Vincent • Howard Voght • Hal Wagstaff • Ian Walker • Chris Walter • Mark Ward • Phil Wardrop • Beth Weatherston • David White • Nicholas White • Stuart Whittle • Frieda Wildey • Erle Williams • Dick Williams • Bryan Willis • Stuart Wilson • David Wise • Neville Wittey • Michael Woods • Dennis Woodward • Kimo Worthington • Magnus Woxen • Julian Yeomans •

The following companies were instrumental in creating and supporting www.whitbread.org. Whether as a sponsor, partner or content partner, these companies took the site to a new level. Quokka Sports would like to thank each individually and as a group. We couldn't have done it without you.

Sponsors

COMPAQ

When a crew's only link to the outside world is through a computer, the systems in place had better be reliable. Compaq proved that its systems have the speed, endurance and reliability to survive the toughest challenges in the world.

The Whitbread Web site was powered by a 'best of both worlds' combination of technology. Highly reliable NonStop® Himalaya® servers, using a total of 16 processors, worked to manage the phenomenal electronic traffic. The Himalaya servers were clustered with 18 Compaq ProLiant servers running Microsoft® Windows NT® Server. This 'supercluster' allowed fans to experience — through video, voice, and email — the feverish excitement of the Whitbread race first-hand.

A NonStop Integrity® server located at Whitbread headquarters in England acted as the hub of the race management network, receiving satellite transmissions of voice and video clips, crew reports, telemetric data and email from the yachts, then sending them to the Web. On board, Whitbread navigators received live weather data and other communications four times a day. This global network provided 24-hour availability for every boat, every minute of the race's nine grueling months.

Almost two million people visited the site in order to be immersed in the world's premier ocean race. With the help of Compaq's Tandem Division, the Web site turned the Whitbread race into a major international sporting event.

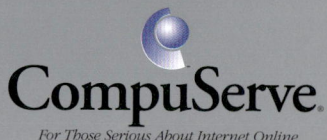

CompuServe was proud to be the Official Supplier of Internet and Online Services to the Whitbread race and official Web site. Online coverage of international yacht racing was pioneered on CompuServe in its legendary sailing forums, and has continued with its sponsorship of The Whitbread.

Throughout The Whitbread, the CompuServe Sail Racing Forum® served as the official Chat and Messaging area for the race, and showcased CompuServe's new Web-based Forums. More than just a chat room, CompuServe Forums include chat and moderated conferencing, 'threaded' message boards and extensive libraries of information. The Forum was available to both CompuServe members and guests from the entire Web during the race. In addition, CompuServe provided the Web site with state-of-the-art Web public conferencing facilities and conference moderators. These facilities included photo presentations and moderated audience Q&A, with the added fun of in-row person-to-person chat during conferences. Conference participants included John Bertrand and Paul Cayard, as well as live coverage of the race restarts.

CompuServe provided high-speed Internet connections at each port of call in the Media Centres and at a 'Cybercafe' in most ports. The Cybercafes, which CompuServe co-hosted with Tandem, a Compaq division, introduced port visitors to the official Web site and the Sail Racing Forum. Visitors could participate in the Forum, get the latest news, photos and emails from the boats, surf the Web, participate in the Virtual Race and send postcards to friends. CompuServe provided over 100 free CompuServe accounts to race syndicates, the press and race personnel, to enable them to reliably stay in touch by email from almost anywhere in the world.

Kodak

As a technology partner to the Whitbread Round The World Race for the Volvo Trophy, Eastman Kodak Company was proud to provide the equipment that brought exciting images of The Whitbread to race enthusiasts' desktops — and beyond. Through film, on-board digital cameras, image scanning, storage and printers, Kodak technology was put through the rugged paces of sailboat racing. Kodak was there to visually document the event — helping the Whitbread teams Take Pictures. Further.

NERA TELECOMMUNICATIONS

If not for the satellites provided by NERA, the information exchange between the Whitbread yachts, race headquarters and millions of fans would not have been possible.

Before the 1997-98 Whitbread, sailors would face the dangerous waters alone without any contact with the outside world. Last year, during the Vendee Globe 'round-the-world race, world-renowned yachtsman Tony Bullimore survived five days in his upturned yacht, Exide Challenger, in the Southern Ocean. Bullimore commented, "If I'd had NERA WorldPhone Marine Equipment on board, I could have made a couple of telephone calls and the rescue services would have known I was alive and where I was. As far as safety is concerned, the NERA solution is an Olympian technological leap forward."

marimba

Since its introduction in early 1997, Marimba's Castanet software has rapidly emerged as the technology-of-choice for businesses that wish to reduce the cost and simplify the complexity of deploying, managing and updating applications and information services over corporate networks and the Internet. Castanet allows existing or new applications written in all of the popular languages to be published to a Castanet Transmitter server. The Transmitter then provides personalised deployment, management and updating of the application and data to appropriate end-user clients on an iterative basis.

Castanet uses network bandwidth efficiently, in that only the actual bytes that change from one update to the next are transmitted over the network. This allows the applications to be fully functional for the end-user — both on- and off-line. Castanet provides the flexibility of distributed or centralised control of update activity, scalability and version control. It is the only product in the industry to provide all of this functionality with the highest level of security possible, including access control, encryption, authentication and digital code signing.

Partners

RODES PROFESSIONAL APPAREL
A Rodes Company

Whitbread enthusiasts from every continent visited the official www.whitbread.org Shop, hosted by Whitbread Sportswear, Inc., a division of Rodes Apparel. Quokka Sports chose Rodes as a fulfilment partner because of its commitment to offer licensed sport event merchandise worldwide. Rodes was one of the first companies to set up an e-commerce solution that could offer global shipping of exclusive merchandise. Being able to purchase merchandise internationally is an important part of any sports experience — this is especially true with online sports events. Rodes provided an end-to-end solution for the production of the Whitbread Web site, while offering unique, quality merchandise and total customer interaction.

amazon.com
BOOKS, MUSIC & MORE

Amazon.com offers more than 3.5 million titles — books, CDs, DVDs and more! Search our catalogues to find a particular title, or browse for books and CDs that suit your tastes. We're open 24 hours a day, 365 days a year, so you can get what you want, any time. Amazon.com — books, music & more.

Content Partners

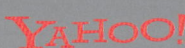 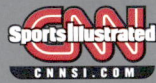

Image Credits

1.01:	John Gichigi – Allsport
1.02:	Innovation Kvaerner video
1.03:	Swedish Match
1.04:	Merit Cup video
1.05:	Innovation Kvaerner video
1.06:	Rick Tomlinson – EF Education
1.07:	(background) Rick Tomlinson – EF Education
	(video grab series) Merit Cup
1.08:	Innovation Kvaerner video
1.09:	(background) Swedish Match
	(video grab far left) EF Education
	(video grab left) Swedish Match
	(video grab right) EF Language
1.10:	Rick Tomlinson – EF Education
1.11:	(background) Rick Tomlinson – EF Education
	(video grab series) BrunelSunergy
1.12:	EF Language video
1.13:	(background) Rick Tomlinson – EF Education
	(video grab series) EF Language
1.14:	(background) Merit Cup video
	(video grab series) Merit Cup
1.15:	America's Challenge
1.16:	Stephen Munday – Allsport
2.01:	(background) Kos Picture Source
	(video grab series) Swedish Match
2.02:	(background) Toshiba video
	(video grab series) Chessie Racing
2.03:	(background) Innovation Kvaerner
	(video grab series) EF Education
2.04:	(background) Merit Cup
	(video grab right) Swedish Match
	(video grab left) Silk Cut
2.05:	(background) BrunelSunergy video
	(video grab series) Innovation Kvaerner
2.06:	(background) Rick Tomlinson – EF Language
	(video grab series) BrunelSunergy
2.07:	(background) Rick Tomlinson – EF Language
2.08:	Innovation Kvaerner
3.01:	Innovation Kvaerner
3.02:	(background) Innovation Kvaerner
	(video grab top) Innovation Kvaerner
	(video grab bottom) Swedish Match
3.03:	EF Education
3.04:	(background) Swedish Match
	(small photo) Swedish Match
3.05:	Clive Mason – Allsport
4.01:	Clive Mason – Allsport
4.02:	(background) EF Education
	(video grab series) EF Education
4.03:	Stephen Munday – Allsport
5.01:	(background) Stephen Munday – Allsport
	(left image) Stephen Munday – Allsport
5.02:	(background) EF Education
	(small image top) Swedish Match
	(small image middle) BrunelSunergy
	(bottom two images) EF Education
5.03:	Swedish Match
5.04:	(background) EF Education
	(small image) Swedish Match video
5.05:	(background) Rick Tomlinson – EF Language
	(video grab series) EF Education
5.06:	Toshiba video
5.07:	(background) Chessie Racing video
	(small image) Chessie Racing video
5.08:	(background) Allsport
	(video grab series) EF Education
5.09:	(background) Allsport
	(small upper left) Sea & See / Merit Cup
	(middle left) Swedish Match
	(middle right) BrunelSunergy
	(right) Toshiba video
5.10:	(background) BrunelSunergy video
	(small image) Merit Cup video
5.11:	Merit Cup video
5.12:	BrunelSunergy video
5.13:	Chessie Racing video
5.14:	Mike Hewitt – Allsport
6.01:	(background) John Gichigi – Allsport
	(video grab series) BrunelSunergy
6.02:	(background) BrunelSunergy
	(video grab far left) Innovation Kvaerner
	(video grab middle) Merit Cup
	(video grab right) BrunelSunergy
6.03:	(background) EF Language
	(video grab) Toshiba
6.04:	(background) EF Language
	(video grab series) EF Language
6.05:	Toshiba – Kos Picture Source
6.06:	(background) Swedish Match video
	(video grab series) Swedish Match
	(small photo far left) Chessie Racing
6.07:	Toshiba – Kos Picture Source
6.08:	(background) Merit Cup
	(video grab series) Chessie Racing
7.01:	Stephen Munday – Allsport
7.02:	Merit Cup video
8.01:	(background) Toshiba video
	(video grab series) Toshiba
	(small photo) Stephen Munday – Allsport
8.02:	Innovation Kvaerner
8.03:	(background) Swedish Match
	(video grab series) Chessie Racing
8.04:	Merit Cup video
8.05:	(background) Toshiba
	(video grab series) Innovation Kvaerner
8.06:	EF Language video
8.07	Kos – Kos Picture Source
9.01:	EF Language video
9.02:	Carlo Borlenghi – Sea & See
10.01:	Stephen Munday – Allsport
Cover:	EF Language video

Colophon

Hardware: Macintosh G3 workstations: 288 mb / 8 gb, 300 mHz. Stored on a 48 gb RAID array. Proofed on an EFI Fiery 200i with a Canon 700 color laser printer.

Software: QuarkXPress 3.32, Adobe Photoshop 5.0, Adobe Illustrator 7.0, Adobe Premiere 5.0, QuickTime 3.0.

Tracks: 44 EURONAV LiveChart vector-format nautical charts. Drawn with a custom Java app and RDBMS back-end on a 400 mHz PII PC.

Production: Set in BitStream Swiss 721 and FontFont OCR-F. 175 line-screen process; PANTONE Metal 8400.

Materials: Pedigree Velvet 150 gsm gloss text.